Demos Surgical Pathology Guides

Lymph Nodes

Demos Surgical Pathology Guides

SERIES EDITOR

Saul Suster, MD
Professor and Chairman
Department of Pathology
Medical College of Wisconsin
Milwaukee, Wisconsin

TITLES

- ***Head and Neck Pathology***
  Paul E. Wakely

- ***Breast Pathology***
  Giovanni Falconieri, Janez Lamovec, and Abiy B. Ambaye

- ***Inflammatory Skin Disorders***
  Jose A. Plaza and Victor G. Prieto

- ***Lymph Nodes***
  Horatiu Olteanu, Alexandra M. Harrington, and Steven H. Kroft

FORTHCOMING TITLES

- ***Skin Tumors***
  Jose A. Plaza and Victor G. Prieto

- ***Pulmonary Pathology***
  R. Nagarjun Rao and Cesar A. Moran

- ***Soft Tissues***
  Eduardo V. Zambrano

- ***Gastrointestinal Pathology***
  Richard A. Komorowski

Demos Surgical Pathology Guides

Lymph Nodes

HORATIU OLTEANU, MD, PhD
Department of Pathology
Medical College of Wisconsin
Milwaukee, Wisconsin

ALEXANDRA M. HARRINGTON, MD
Department of Pathology
Medical College of Wisconsin
Milwaukee, Wisconsin

STEVEN H. KROFT, MD
Department of Pathology
Medical College of Wisconsin
Milwaukee, Wisconsin

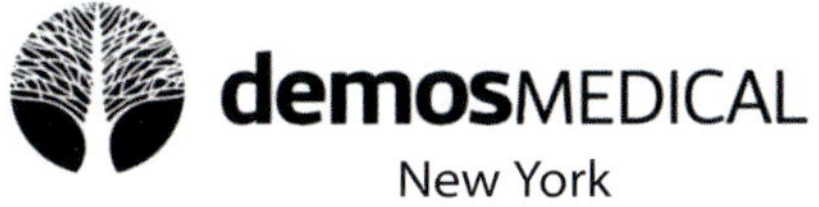

New York

ISBN: 9781936287086
e-book ISBN: 9781617050206

Acquisitions Editor: Rich Winters
Compositor: diacriTech

Visit our website at www.demosmedpub.com

Medicine is an ever-changing science. Research and clinical experience are continually expanding our knowledge, in particular our understanding of proper treatment and drug therapy. The authors, editors, and publisher have made every effort to ensure that all information in this book is in accordance with the state of knowledge at the time of production of the book. Nevertheless, the authors, editors, and publisher are not responsible for errors or omissions or for any consequences from application of the information in this book and make no warranty, express or implied, with respect to the contents of the publication. Every reader should examine carefully the package inserts accompanying each drug and should carefully check whether the dosage schedules mentioned therein or the contraindications stated by the manufacturer differ from the statements made in this book. Such examination is particularly important with drugs that are either rarely used or have been newly released on the market.

Library of Congress Cataloging-in-Publication Data
Olteanu, Horatiu.
Lymph nodes / Horatiu Olteanu, Alexandra Harrington, Steven H. Kroft.
p. cm. — (Demos surgical pathology guides)
ISBN 978-1-936287-08-6
1. Lymph nodes—Diseases. 2. Histology, Pathological. I. Harrington, Alexandra, MD. II. Kroft, Steven H. III. Title.
RC646.O48 2013
616.99'442—dc23

2012031280

Printed in the United States of America by Bradford & Bigelow.
12 13 14 15 / 5 4 3 2 1

Contents

Series Foreword *ix*
Preface *xi*

The Normal Lymph Node xiv

1. Infectious Lymphadenopathies ***1***

Infectious Mononucleosis Lymphadenitis ***2***

Cytomegalovirus Lymphadenitis ***4***

Herpes Simplex Virus Lymphadenitis ***6***

Human Immunodeficiency Virus Lymphadenitis ***8***

Nonspecific Bacterial Lymphadenitis ***10***

Cat Scratch Lymphadenitis ***12***

Bacillary Angiomatosis ***14***

Syphilis (Luetic) Lymphadenitis ***18***

Mycobacterium Tuberculosis Lymphadenitis ***22***

Mycobacterium Avium-Intracellulare Lymphadenitis ***24***

Histoplasma Lymphadenitis ***26***

Coccidioides Lymphadenitis ***28***

Filariasis ***30***

2. Reactive Lymphadenopathies ***33***

Follicular Hyperplasia ***34***

Paracortical Hyperplasia ***36***

Sinus Histiocytosis ***38***

Progressive Transformation of Germinal Centers (PTGC) ***40***

Dermatopathic Lymphadenopathy ***42***

3. Lymphadenopathies Associated With Systemic Disorders ***45***

Kimura Lymphadenopathy ***46***

Sinus Histiocytosis with Massive Lymphadenopathy (Rosai-Dorfman Disease) ***48***

Kikuchi-Fujimoto Lymphadenopathy *50*

Sarcoidosis *52*

Systemic Lupus Erythematosus Lymphadenopathy *54*

Rheumatoid Lymphadenopathy *56*

Castleman Disease *58*

Hyaline Vascular Castleman Disease *58*
Unicentric Castleman Disease, Plasma Cell Variant *60*
Multicentric Castleman Disease *62*

Still's Disease *64*

IgG4-Related Sclerosing Disease *66*

Autoimmune Lymphoproliferative Syndrome *68*

4. Lymph Node Inclusions *71*

Epithelial Cell Inclusions in Lymph Nodes *72*

Nevus Cell Inclusions in Lymph Nodes *74*

5. Spindle Cell Neoplasms of Lymph Nodes *77*

Palisaded Myofibroblastoma *78*

Inflammatory Pseudotumor of Lymph Node *80*

6. Vascular Lymphadenopathies and Neoplasms of Lymph Nodes *83*

Vascular Transformation of Lymph Node Sinuses *84*

Angiomymatous Hamartoma *86*

Hemangiomas and Hemangioendotheliomas *88*

Kaposi Sarcoma *90*

7. Foreign Body Lymphadenopathies *93*

Metal Debris-Associated Lymphadenopathy *94*

Lymphangiography-Associated Lymphadenopathy *96*

8. Mature B-Cell Neoplasms *99*

Nomenclature and Classification *100*

Chronic Lymphocytic Leukemia/Small Lymphocytic Lymphoma (CLL/SLL) *102*

Splenic B-Cell Marginal Zone Lymphoma (SMZL) *106*

Hairy Cell Leukemia (HCL) *108*

Lymphoplasmacytic Lymphoma (LPL) *110*

Heavy Chain Diseases (HCDs) *112*

Extraosseous Plasmacytoma *114*

Nodal Marginal Zone Lymphoma (MZL) *116*

Follicular Lymphoma (FL) *118*

Mantle Cell Lymphoma (MCL) *122*

Diffuse Large B-Cell Lymphoma, Not Otherwise Specified (DLBCL, NOS) *124*

DLBCL Subtypes *126*

Primary Mediastinal Large B-Cell Lymphoma (PMLBCL) *128*

ALK Positive Large B-Cell Lymphoma *130*

Plasmablastic Lymphoma (PBL) *132*

Large B-Cell Lymphoma Arising in HHV8-Associated Multicentric Castleman Disease *134*

Burkitt Lymphoma (BL) *136*

B-Cell Lymphoma, Unclassifiable, with Features Intermediate Between Diffuse Large B-Cell Lymphoma and Burkitt Lymphoma *138*

B-Cell Lymphoma, Unclassifiable, with Features Intermediate Between Diffuse Large B-Cell Lymphoma and Classical Hodgkin Lymphoma *140*

9. Mature T- and NK-Cell Neoplasms *143*

T-Cell Prolymphocytic Leukemia *144*

Aggressive NK-Cell Leukemia/Lymphoma *146*

Adult T-Cell Leukemia/Lymphoma *148*

Sezary Syndrome/Mycosis Fungoides *150*

Peripheral T-Cell Lymphoma, Not Otherwise Specified *152*

Angioimmunoblastic T-Cell Lymphoma *156*

Anaplastic Large Cell Lymphoma, ALK Positive *160*

Anaplastic Large Cell Lymphoma, ALK Negative *166*

10. Hodgkin Lymphoma *169*

Nodular Lymphocyte Predominant Hodgkin Lymphoma *170*

Nodular Sclerosis Classical Hodgkin Lymphoma *172*

Mixed Cellularity Classical Hodgkin *176*

Lymphocyte Rich Classical Hodgkin Lymphoma *178*

Lymphocyte-Depleted Classical Hodgkin Lymphoma *180*

11. Immunodeficiency-Associated Lymphoproliferative Disorderss ***183***

Lymphomas Associated with HIV Infection ***184***

Post-Transplant Lymphoproliferative Disorders (PTLD) ***186***

Early Lesions: Plasmacytic Hyperplasia and Infectious Mononucleosis (IM)-Like PTLD ***188***
Polymorphic PTLD ***190***
Monomorphic PTLD ***192***
Classical Hodgkin Lymphoma Type PTLD ***196***

Other Iatrogenic Immunodeficiency-Associated Lymphoproliferative Disorders ***198***

12. Histiocytic and Dendritic Cell Neoplasms ***201***

Histiocytic Sarcoma ***202***

Langerhans Cells Histiocytosis ***204***

Langerhans Cell Sarcoma ***206***

Interdigitating Dendritic Cell Sarcoma ***208***

Follicular Dendritic Cell Sarcoma ***210***

13. Precursor Lymphoid Neoplasms ***213***

Lymphoblastic Leukemia/Lymphoma ***214***

14. Acute Myeloid Leukemia and Related Precursor Neoplasms ***217***

Myeloid Sarcoma ***218***

Blastic Plasmacytoid Dendritic Cell Neoplasm ***220***

15. Metastatic Tumors in Lymph Nodes ***223***

References *227*

Index *241*

Series Foreword

The field of surgical pathology has gained increasing relevance and importance over the years as pathologists have become more and more integrated into the health care team. To the need for precise histopathologic diagnoses has now been added the burden of providing our clinical colleagues with information that will allow them to assess the prognosis of the disease and predict the response to therapy. Pathologists now serve as key consultants in the patient management team and are responsible for providing critical information that will guide their therapy. With the progress gained due to the insights obtained from the application of newer diagnostic techniques, surgical pathology has become progressively more complex. As a result, diagnoses need to be more detailed and specific and the number of data elements required in the generation of a surgical pathology report have increased exponentially, making management of the information required for diagnosis cumbersome and sometimes difficult.

The past 15 years have witnessed an explosion of information in the field of pathology with a massive proliferation of specialized textbooks appearing in print. For the most part, such texts provide in-depth and detailed coverage of the various areas in surgical pathology. The purpose of this series is to bridge the gap between the major subspecialty texts and the large, double-volume general surgical pathology textbooks, by providing compact, single-volume monographs that will succinctly address the most salient and important points required for the diagnosis of the most common conditions. The series is organized following an organ-system format, with single volumes dedicated to individual organs. The volumes are divided on the basis of disease groups, including benign reactive, inflammatory, infectious or systemic conditions, benign neoplastic conditions, and malignant neoplasms. Each chapter consists of a bulleted list of the most pertinent clinical data related to the condition, followed by the most important histopathologic criteria for diagnosis, pertinent use of immunohistochemical stains and other ancillary techniques, and relevant molecular tests when available. This is followed by a section on differential diagnosis. References appear at the back of the volume. Each entity is illustrated with key, high-quality histological images that highlight the most salient and distinctive features that need to be recognized for the correct diagnosis.

These books are intended for the busy practicing pathologist, and for pathology residents and fellows in training who require an easy and simple overview of major diagnostic criteria and key points during the course of routine daily practice. The authors have been carefully chosen for their experience in the field and clarity of exposition in the various topics. It is hoped that this series will fulfill its purpose of providing quick and easy access to critical information for the busy practitioner or trainee, and that it will assist pathologists in their routine practice of the specialty.

Saul Suster, MD
Professor and Chairman
Department of Pathology
Medical College of Wisconsin
Milwaukee, Wisconsin

Preface

Lymph node pathology, like many other subspecialty areas of diagnostic pathology, has evolved to a level of complexity that sometimes makes it seem unapproachable to students, residents, and even general pathologists. This complexity derives in part from the ever-changing and ever-growing classification schemes for hematolymphoid neoplasia. It also stems in part from the critical and expanding role of immunophenotyping and molecular genetics in the diagnosis of lymph node disorders; every day, it would seem, there are new CD markers to stain for or new gene mutations to assay. However, despite this overlay of modern diagnostic tools, lymph node pathology remains at its core a morphologic discipline, and there is no doubt that lymph nodes are complex organs, both anatomically and functionally. Consequently, this volume focuses on histopathologic features of lymph node diseases, although important ancillary studies useful for diagnosis are discussed, where appropriate.

As highlighted in the "Normal Lymph Node" section at the start of this book, lymph nodes can be broken down into several anatomic and functional compartments. Each of these compartments can be independently affected by various non-neoplastic and neoplastic processes. Consequently, a low-power assessment of the architecture of a lymph node is an important and highly informative part of the pathologic evaluation of this organ, and this explains why many of the sections in this book contain a low-power image illustrating the architectural features of pathologic nodal processes. However, high-power analysis of the cytologic features of constituent cells is just as important as understanding the architecture of a lymph node. Even normal lymph nodes contain a daunting array of various types of cells, mixed together in what may seem a haphazard and bewildering fashion. Thus, the ability to make fine cytologic discrimination of various cells types is an essential skill for lymph node interpretation. This complex admixture of different cell types also creates challenges for the assessment of immunohistochemical stains; a low-power assessment of "brown or not brown" often does not suffice when assessing lymph node immunohistochemistry. It is important to look closely at which cells are brown, and which are not brown. Finally, clinical features often impart critical clues to diagnosis; important clinical characteristics of lymph node disorders are therefore highlighted in this text, where appropriate.

This book is not, of course, intended as a comprehensive reference for the myriad diseases within its pages. Instead, we hope that it provides concise descriptions of the most important diagnostic features of a wide array of disorders affecting lymph nodes, hopefully to serve as a convenient, concise source of information for those interested in learning about or diagnosing disorders of this very interesting organ.

Demos Surgical Pathology Guides

Lymph Nodes

The Normal Lymph Node

DEFINITION

The normal lymph node has intact follicular, paracortical, and sinusoidal architecture and is populated mostly by lymphocytes in various states of activation and dendritic cells. Normal lymph nodes are usually <1 cm in size.

HISTOLOGIC FINDINGS

- Lymph nodes have a thin fibrous capsule, which allows entry of afferent lymphatics and the hilar structures: artery, vein, and efferent lymphatic (Figure 1).
- Multiple afferent lymphatic vessels deliver relatively acellular lymph into the subcapsular sinuses, which further divide into cortical and medullary sinuses (Figure 2). Sinuses are lined by bland, flattened endothelial cells, and are normally patent structures, containing few histiocytes. Lymph containing activated lymphocytes and macrophages exits through the efferent lymphatic at the hilum.
- Broadly, the lymph node can be divided into the cortex, paracortex, and medulla. The cortex contains B cell-rich follicles, and the paracortex is predominantly composed of T cells. The medulla is composed of sinuses surrounded by plasma cells.
- Follicles are peripherally distributed, evenly spaced, variable in size and show varying states of activation in the normal lymph node, ranging from the quiescent primary follicles to secondary follicles with germinal centers. Primary follicles are composed of monotonous, small B cells with round to mildly irregular nuclei, mature chromatin, and indistinct cytoplasmic borders. Secondary follicles contain a central germinal center, rimmed by a mantle zone, and are composed of small and medium-sized, irregular centrocytes, and variable numbers of transformed centroblasts and follicular dendritic cells (Figure 3). Reactive follicles have polarized germinal centers, showing both light (centrocyte-rich) and dark (centroblast-rich) zones.
- The paracortex (Figure 4) is composed of small, mature lymphocytes lacking atypia and variable numbers of dendritic cells and rare immunoblasts. High endothelial, post-capillary venules are also found in the paracortex. They are lined by plump endothelial cells with ovoid nuclei, small nucleoli, and indistinct cell borders; activated lymphocytes and macrophages can cross these endothelial cells and enter the systemic circulation.

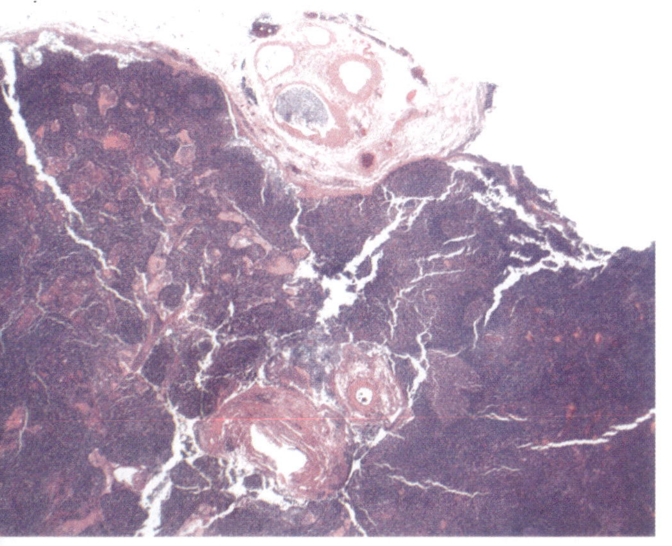

FIGURE 1

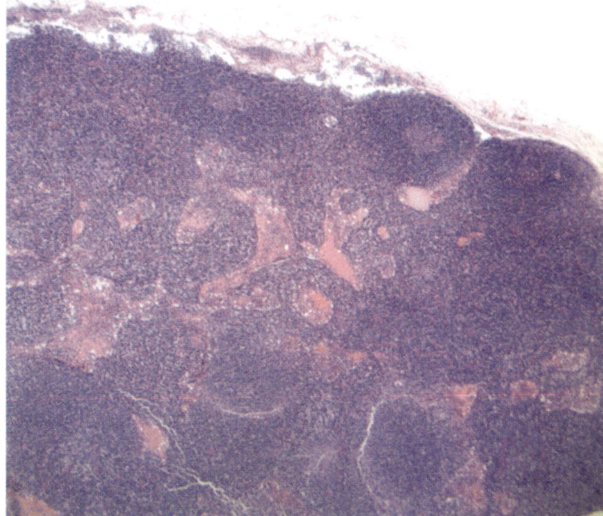

FIGURE 2

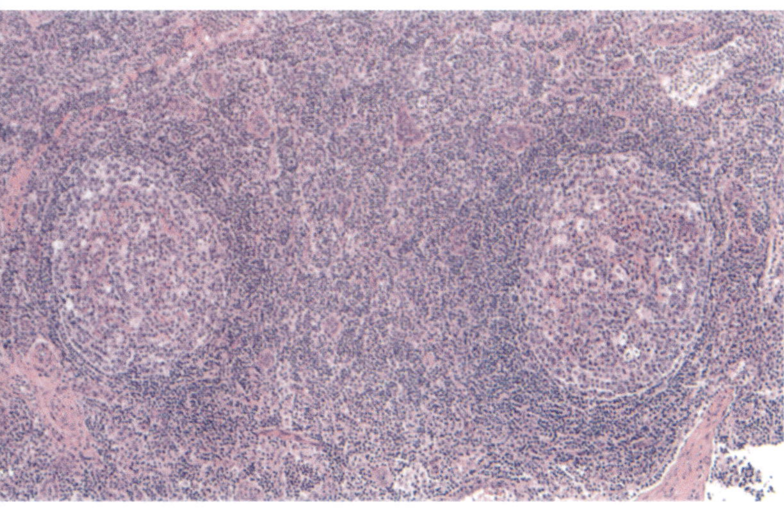

FIGURE 3

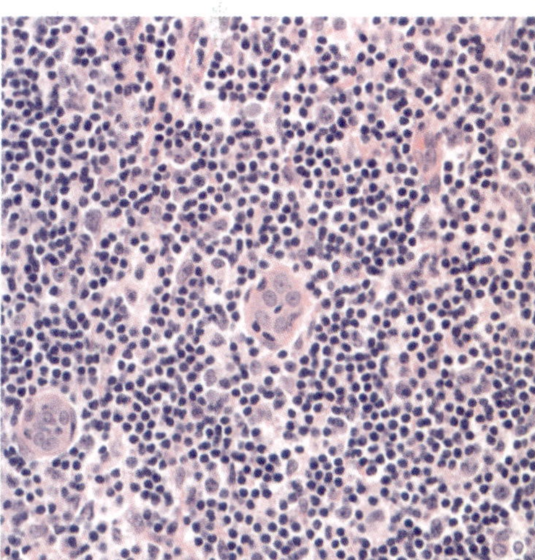

FIGURE 4

FIGURE 1 The lymph node hilum contains an artery, vein, and efferent lymphatic.

FIGURE 2 The normal lymph node shows intact follicular and paracortical architecture with patent cortical sinuses.

FIGURE 3 Two secondary follicles are present, showing reactive germinal centers and well-defined mantle zones.

FIGURE 4 High power magnification of the paracortex reveals high endothelial venules surrounded by small, mature lymphocytes, dendritic cells, and rare immunoblasts.

1

Infectious Lymphadenopathies

INFECTIOUS MONONUCLEOSIS LYMPHADENITIS

CYTOMEGALOVIRUS LYMPHADENITIS

HERPES SIMPLEX VIRUS LYMPHADENITIS

HUMAN IMMUNODEFICIENCY VIRUS LYMPHADENITIS

NONSPECIFIC BACTERIAL LYMPHADENITIS

CAT SCRATCH LYMPHADENITIS

BACILLARY ANGIOMATOSIS

SYPHILIS (LUETIC) LYMPHADENITIS

MYCOBACTERIUM TUBERCULOSIS LYMPHADENITIS

MYCOBACTERIUM AVIUM-INTRACELLULARE LYMPHADENITIS

HISTOPLASMA LYMPHADENITIS

COCCIDIOIDES LYMPHADENITIS

FILARIASIS

Infectious Mononucleosis Lymphadenitis

DEFINITION

Infectious mononucleosis (IM) is caused by Epstein-Barr virus (EBV), and refers to the acute clinical syndrome of pharyngitis, lymphadenopathy, and fever.

CLINICAL FEATURES

- IM occurs in 35–50% of adolescents first exposed to EBV during their teenage years. Most are exposed to EBV during childhood and have asymptomatic infections.
- IM presents classically with fever, pharyngitis, and cervical adenopathy. Lymph nodes may show generalized enlargement. Abdominal pain may also occur from hepatosplenomegaly. Rare cases can present with splenic rupture.
- Symptoms dissipate in 1–2 months.
- Laboratory tests reveal a positive heterophil antibody test and an elevated white blood cell count with the characteristic triad of >50% mononuclear cells, heterogeneous lymphocyte morphology, and >10% reactive lymphocytes (of total leukocytes).

HISTOLOGIC FINDINGS

- The lymph node shows variable architectural distortion by follicular and paracortical hyperplasia and sinus histiocytosis (Figure 1-1). The paracortex preferentially becomes expanded, occasionally organizing into nodular expansions. There is increased vascularity.
- The paracortex is expanded by a heterogeneous population of small, mature lymphocytes, histiocytes, and variable numbers of T and B-immunoblasts (Figures 1-2 and 1-3). Large numbers of paracortical immunoblasts may be observed in some cases, though sheets of these cells should raise suspicion for a large cell lymphoma.
- Immunoblasts (Figure 1-3) are large in size and have generally oval nuclei with single to multiple distinct, often irregular nucleoli and small amounts of dense, amphophilic, variably vacuolated cytoplasm; occasionally, these cells may resemble Reed-Sternberg cells. The immunoblasts stain positively for CD30 and CD45.
- Several reports describe monocytoid B-cell aggregates in IM.
- Foci of necrosis may be observed.
- EBV small encoded RNA (EBER) in situ hybridization studies are positive in subsets of paracortical lymphocytes and B-immunoblasts and occasionally in the germinal center cells. EBER positive cells are numerous in IM, in contrast to the rare EBER staining observed in small lymphocytes in the context of latent infection.
- EBV latent membrane protein type 1 (LMP) is not as sensitive for EBV infection as EBER in situ hybridization studies.

DIFFERENTIAL DIAGNOSIS

- Non-specific reactive lymphadenopathy
- Cytomegalovirus lymphadenitis
- *Toxoplasma* lymphadenitis
- Large B-cell lymphoma
- Peripheral T-cell lymphoma, not otherwise specified
- Angioimmunoblastic T-cell lymphoma
- Anaplastic large cell lymphoma
- Classical Hodgkin lymphoma

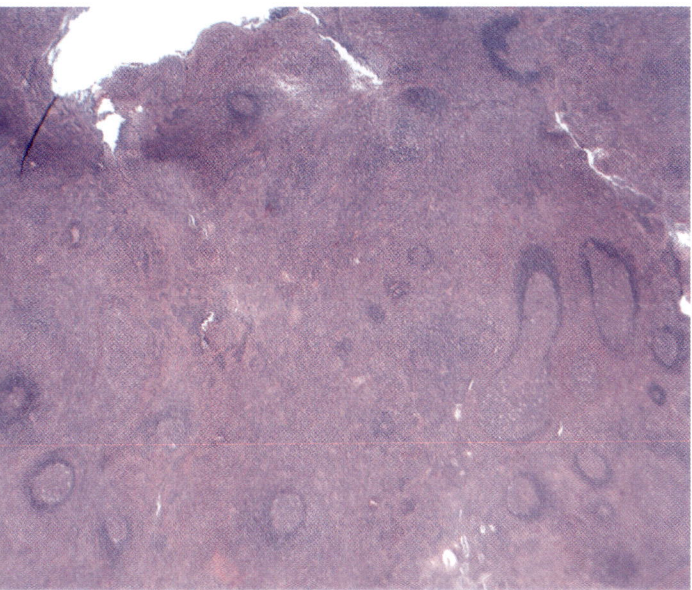

FIGURE 1-1

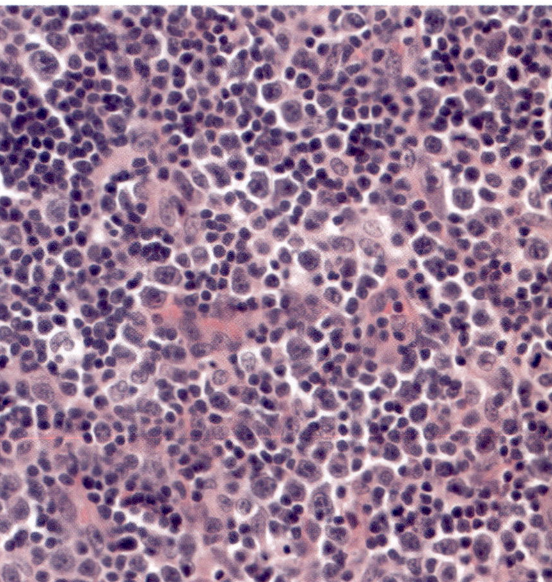

FIGURE 1-2

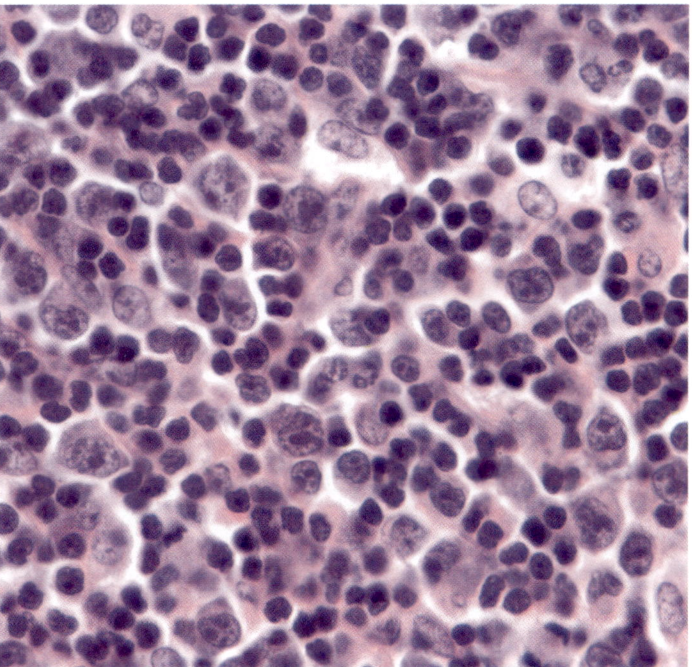

FIGURE 1-3

FIGURE 1-1 This lymph node shows prominent paracortical hyperplasia with several reactive secondary follicles.

FIGURE 1-2 Intermediate power reveals increased vascularity and a heterogeneous infiltrate with many immunoblasts.

FIGURE 1-3 Numerous immunoblasts are observed within the paracortex of this EBV-infected lymph node.

Cytomegalovirus Lymphadenitis

DEFINITION

Cytomegalovirus is a herpesvirus, which can cause an infectious mononucleosis-like (IM-like) syndrome, including lymphadenitis in the immunocompetent host, and widespread organ involvement in immunosuppressed patients.

CLINICAL FEATURES

- Lymphadenopathy can occur in perinatal infections, IM-like syndrome, and infections in immunosuppressed patients.
- An IM-like syndrome occurs most commonly in young, sexually active adults, and is characterized by fever, fatigue, lymphadenopathy, splenomegaly, hepatitis, and malaise, but not pharyngitis. The heterophil antibody test is negative. Patients have a lymphocytosis with reactive morphology.
- Infections in immunocompromised patients can cause severe organ impairment, most notably pneumonitis, hepatitis, and gastroenteritis.

HISTOLOGIC FINDINGS

- Lymph nodes show distorted architecture with follicular and paracortical hyperplasia (Figure 1-4), mimicking IM (see Chapter 2).
- The paracortex is expanded by a heterogeneous infiltrate consisting of small, mature lymphocytes, histiocytes, plasma cells, and variable numbers of immunoblasts, similar to IM (see Chapter 2).
- Collections of monocytoid B-cells may be observed at the periphery of the follicle (in the marginal zone) or within the paracortex in a perivascular distribution (Figure 1-5).
- Intracytoplasmic inclusions may be observed in the T-immunoblasts or sinusoidal endothelial cells (Figure 1-6). CMV immunohistochemistry is positive in these cells.

DIFFERENTIAL DIAGNOSIS

- Non-specific reactive lymphadenopathy
- Infectious mononucleosis
- *Toxoplasma* lymphadenitis
- HIV lymphadenopathy
- Large B-cell lymphoma
- Peripheral T-cell lymphoma, not otherwise specified
- Anaplastic large cell lymphoma

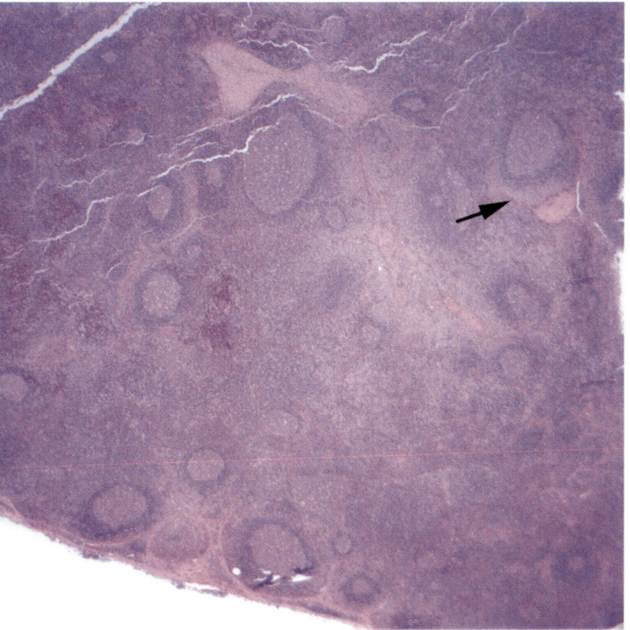

FIGURE 1-4

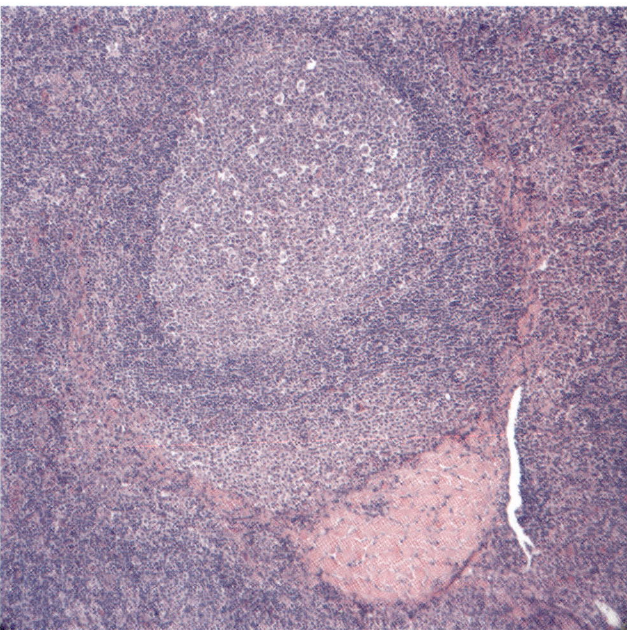

FIGURE 1-5

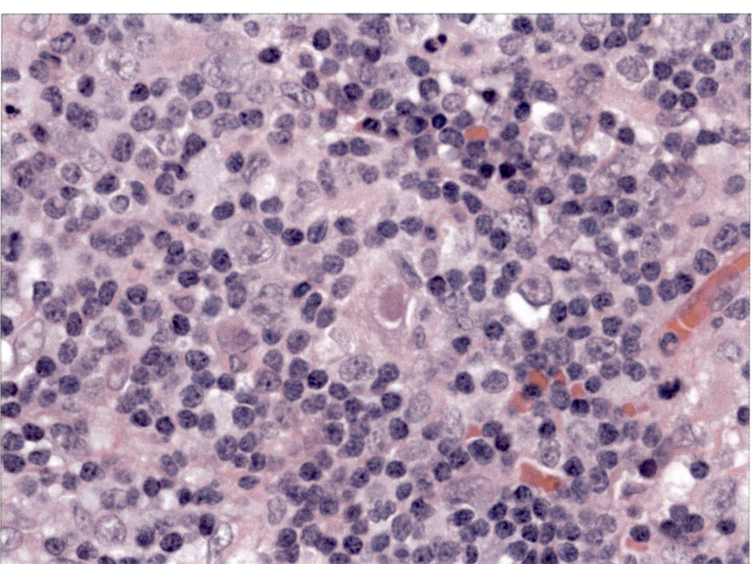

FIGURE 1-6

FIGURE 1-4 The lymph node reveals both follicular and paracortical hyperplasia with monocytoid B-cell collections (arrowed).

FIGURE 1-5 A higher power magnification of the case illustrated in Figure 1-4 reveals a collection of monocytoid B-cells adjacent to the mantle zone.

FIGURE 1-6 This high-power image demonstrates a large cell in the center of the field with an eosinophilic viral inclusion occupying most of the nucleus. Granular eosinophilic material may also be seen in the cytoplasm, corresponding to cytoplasmic viral inclusions.

Herpes Simplex Virus Lymphadenitis

DEFINITION

Herpes simplex virus (HSV) lymphadenitis is a rare clinical entity and is most commonly reported in patients with hematologic malignancies.

CLINICAL FEATURES

- HSV lymphadenitis presents with fever, generalized lymphadenopathy, and skin erythema. Involved lymph nodes are often tender. Patients may have oral or genital herpetic lesions.
- HSV lymphadenitis has been described mostly in patients with hematologic malignancies, notably chronic lymphocytic leukemia/small lymphocytic lymphoma (CLL/SLL).
- HSV lymphadenitis may follow a self-limited course, though other cases require anti-viral therapy.

HISTOLOGIC FINDINGS

- Lymph nodes show variably distorted architecture. The paracortex is expanded in either a diffuse or nodular pattern. Sinus histiocytosis is described in some cases. Follicular hyperplasia is not a characteristic finding.
- The paracortex is expanded by a heterogeneous infiltrate composed of small lymphocytes, histiocytes, eosinophils, and variable numbers of immunoblasts, thus mimicking infectious mononucleosis and cytomegalovirus lymphadenitis (see earlier sections in this chapter).
- Immunoblast proliferations can be florid, though sheets of immunoblasts are worrisome for a large cell lymphoma.
- Necrosis can range from individual cells to focal areas to suppurative, geographic necrosis (Figures 1-7 and 1-8). Viral inclusions are found most commonly in or at the edge of these necrotic areas.
- Intranuclear HSV inclusions are observed in the T-immunoblasts or stromal cells. The inclusions are eosinophilic and associated with marginated chromatin (Figure 1-9). HSV immunohistochemistry is positive in these cells (Figure 1-10).

DIFFERENTIAL DIAGNOSIS

- Non-specific reactive lymphadenopathy
- Infectious mononucleosis
- Cytomegalovirus lymphadenitis
- Large B-cell lymphoma/Richter's transformation in CLL/SLL
- Angioimmunoblastic T-cell lymphoma

FIGURE 1-7 This low-power image of a lymph node involved by chronic lymphocytic leukemia/small lymphocytic lymphoma demonstrates large areas of geographic necrosis.

FIGURE 1-8 High-power image of a necrotic area demonstrates eosinophilic necrotic material, apoptotic debris, histiocytes, and scattered neutrophils.

FIGURE 1-9 At the edge of the necrotic areas there are frequent nuclei with marginated chromatin containing eosinophilic, "ground glass" inclusions.

FIGURE 1-10 HSV immunohistochemistry demonstrates numerous positive cells at the edge of a necrotic focus.

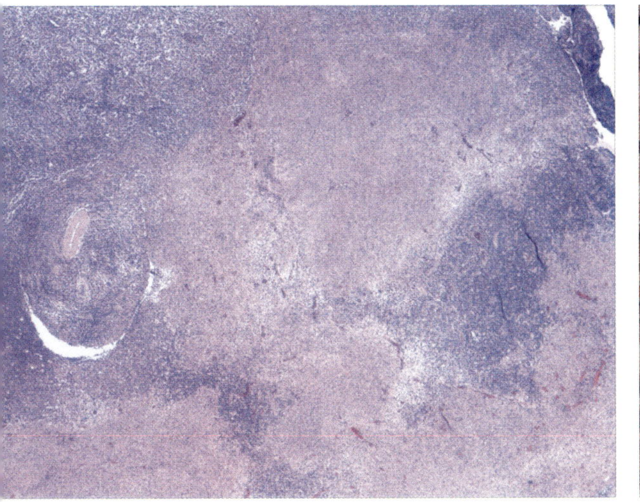
FIGURE 1-7

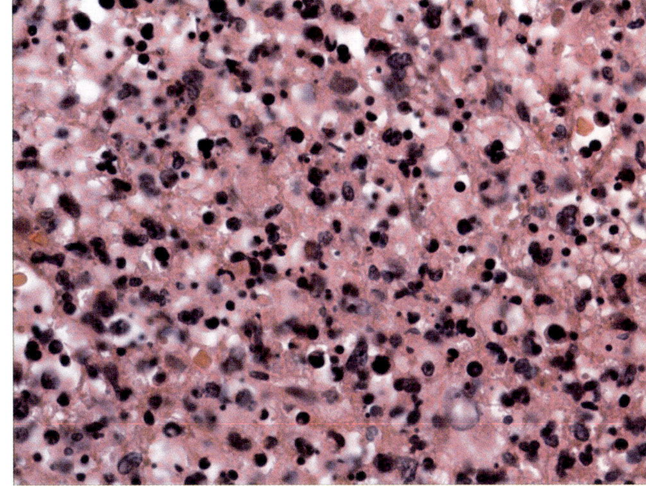
FIGURE 1-8

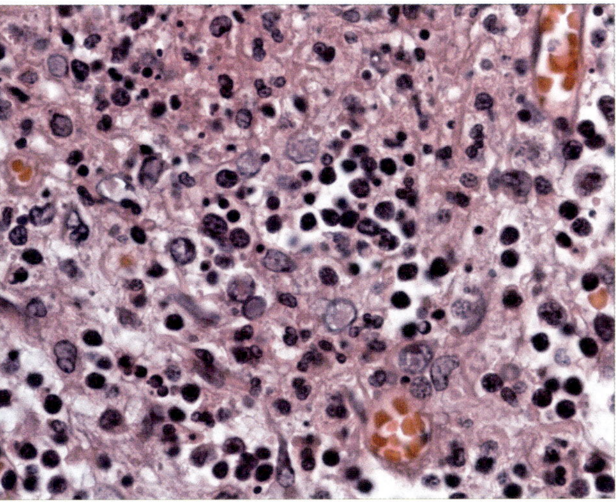
FIGURE 1-9

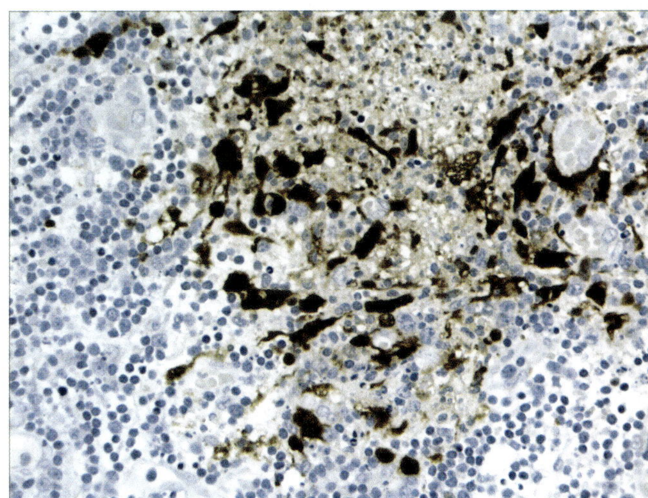
FIGURE 1-10

Human Immunodeficiency Virus Lymphadenitis

DEFINITION

Human immunodeficiency virus (HIV) lymphadenitis is a lymphadenopathy associated with HIV infection and not caused by a secondary infectious agent.

CLINICAL FEATURES

- Lymphadenopathy is a characteristic finding in acute HIV infection. It is often accompanied by nonspecific features such as fever and malaise. Some acute HIV infections are asymptomatic, however.
- HIV infection can be acquired through sexual activity, intravenous drug use, transfusion, occupational exposures, and congenitally.
- Depressed CD4(+) T cells are observed as the HIV infection progresses.

HISTOLOGIC FINDINGS

- Three histologic patterns have been described in HIV lymphadenitis: pattern A (acute infection), pattern B (chronic infection), and pattern C (burnout).
- Pattern A (Figure 1-11) is characterized by florid follicular hyperplasia with enlarged and often irregular secondary follicles showing exuberant germinal centers. Some follicles may show lysis. Mantle zone may be attenuated, and germinal centers may be confluent. Monocytoid B-cell hyperplasia is common.
- Pattern B is characterized by progressive involution of follicles, resulting in variably sclerotic, lymphocyte-depleted germinal centers. The paracortex shows hyperplastic vasculature and polytypic plasmacytosis.
- Pattern C is characterized by depleted follicles and paracortex with increased nodal fibrosis (Figures 1-12 and 1-13). Germinal centers show "Castleman-like" changes with hyalinization, lymphocyte depletion, and penetrating vessels. The paracortex is depleted of lymphocytes as well, and shows increased polytypic plasma cells, histiocytes, and vasculature- a pattern which is sometimes referred to as "angioimmunoblastic-like."

DIFFERENTIAL DIAGNOSIS

- CMV lymphadenitis
- Infectious mononucleosis
- *Toxoplasma* lymphadenitis
- Syphilis (luetic) lymphadenitis
- Lupus lymphadenitis
- Non-specific reactive lymphadenopathy
- Progressive transformation of germinal centers
- Castleman lymphadenopathy
- Kaposi's sarcoma
- Angioimmunoblastic T-cell lymphoma

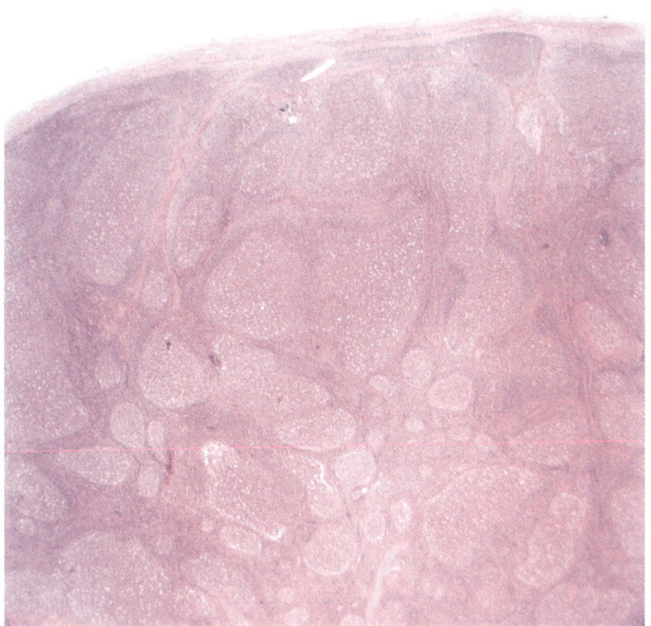

FIGURE 1-11

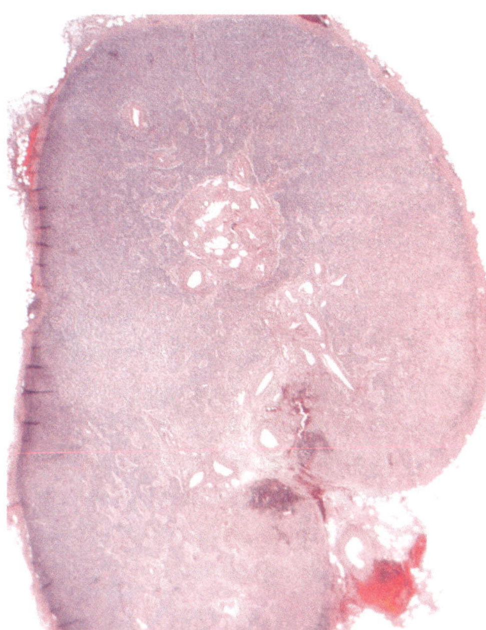

FIGURE 1-12

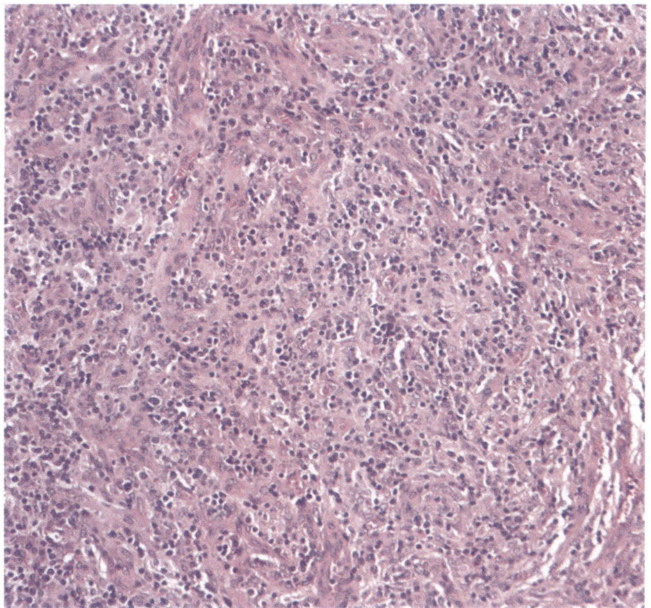

FIGURE 1-13

FIGURE 1-11 Pattern A. This lymph node from an HIV patient represents pattern A (acute infection) showing florid follicular hyperplasia.

FIGURE 1-12 Pattern C. This small atrophic lymph node shows loss of the normal follicular architecture with prominent vasculature.

FIGURE 1-13 Pattern C. Higher magnification reveals increased vasculature and fibrosis with lymphocytic depletion during the burnout stage.

Nonspecific Bacterial Lymphadenitis

DEFINITION

Bacterial lymphadenitis is most commonly caused by *Staphylococcus aureus* and *Streptococcus pyogenes* and is characterized by suppurative inflammation. Other etiologic agents include: *Yersinia sp, Francisella tularensis,* and *Neisseria sp.* Bacterial infections with more specific histologic findings are excluded from this category.

CLINICAL FEATURES

- Cervical, axillary, and inguinal lymph nodes are most frequently involved.
- Lymph nodes are tender, soft, and mobile.
- Clinical features are dependent on the underlying infected site.

HISTOLOGIC FINDINGS

- Lymph nodes show variable infiltration by neutrophils, ranging from sinusoidal infiltrates to microabscess formation and geographic necrosis (Figure 1-14). Areas of edema may be observed in association with these infiltrates (Figure 1-15). The inflammation and edema may extend into the perinodal tissue.
- Non-suppurative areas show follicular and/or paracortical hyperplasia. Immunoblast proliferation can mimic a viral lymphadenitis (Figure 1-15).
- Organisms can be identified by fresh or fixed tissue gram stain. Confirmatory identification requires microbiological culture of fresh tissue.

DIFFERENTIAL DIAGNOSIS

- Cat scratch lymphadenitis
- Lymphogranuloma venereum
- *Histoplasma* lymphadenitis
- Viral lymphadenitis: EBV, HSV

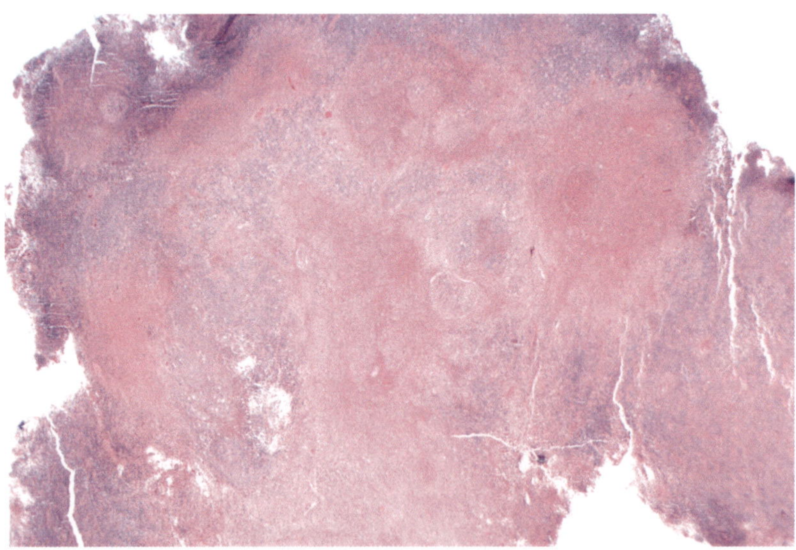

FIGURE 1-14 This inguinal lymph node shows geographic necrosis.

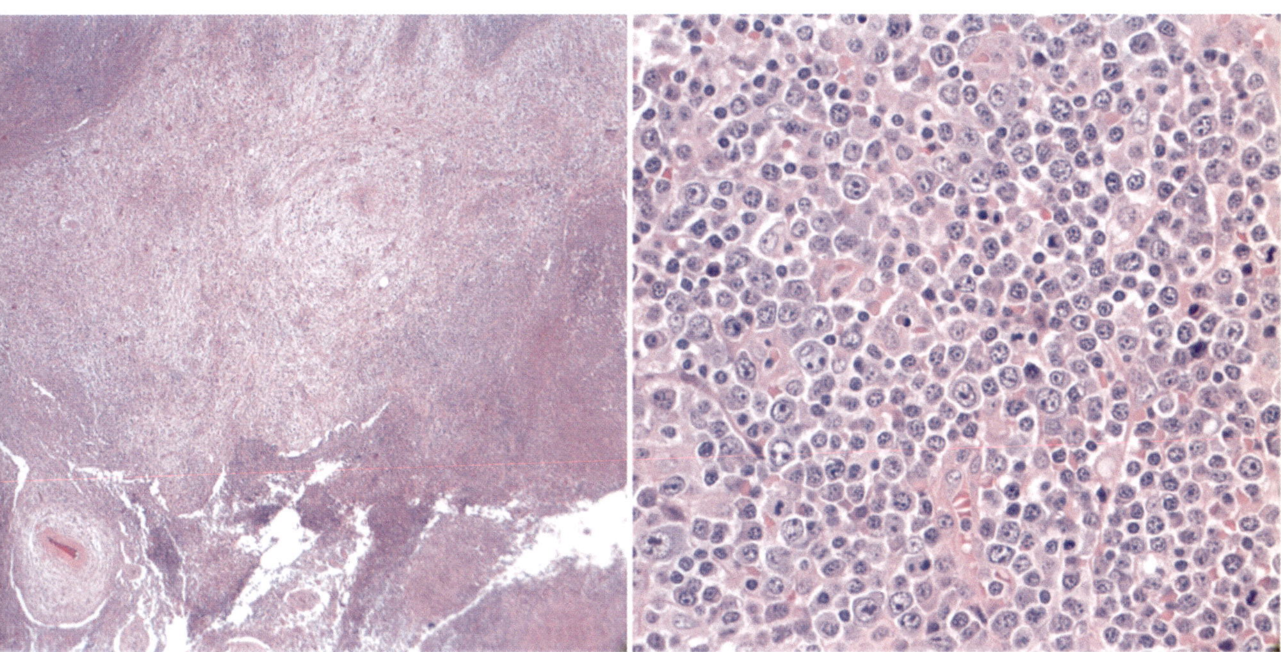

FIGURE 1-15

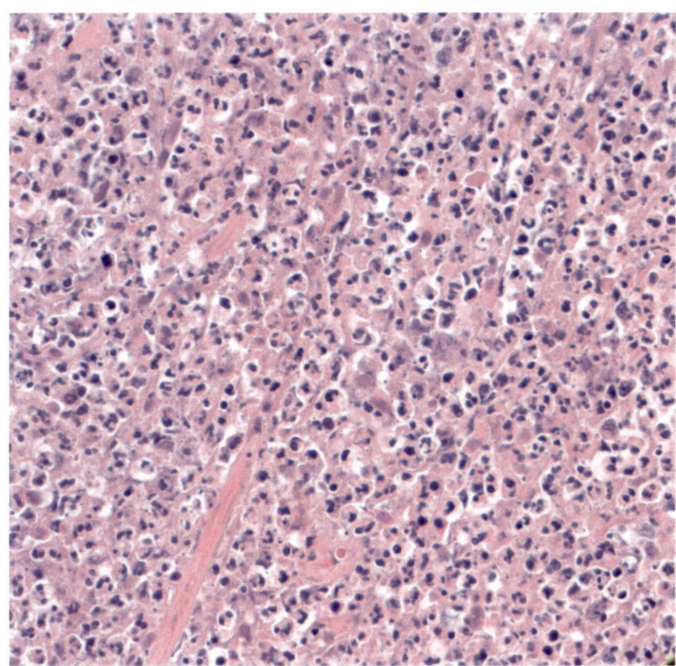

FIGURE 1-16

FIGURE 1-15 Necrotic areas alternate with areas showing severe edema (left) and paracortical immunoblast proliferation (right).

FIGURE 1-16 High-power magnification of a necrotic area within the lymph node illustrated in Figures 1-14 and 1-15 shows numerous neutrophils and histiocytes.

Cat Scratch Lymphadenitis

DEFINITION

Cat scratch lymphadenitis is caused by the bacterium *Bartonella henselae* and is one of the most common causes of lymphadenopathy in children and young adults.

CLINICAL FEATURES

- The majority of cases present in children, adolescents, and young adults, with males more commonly affected than females.
- Patients present with regional, tender enlargement of lymph nodes draining sites of cat bites or scratches. The most common affected lymph nodes include those of the head, neck, axilla, and inguinal area. Adenopathy may be accompanied by fever and fatigue.
- Complications of *Bartonella* infection include localized processes related to inoculation sites, such as conjunctivitis and bacillary angiomatosis of the skin; and disseminated disease in immunosuppressed patients such as retinitis, atypical pneumonia, hepatitis, encephalitis, and bacillary angiomatosis.
- Elevated IgG or IgM antibodies (elevated titers or 4-fold increases in titers) are detected in the majority of cases. Polymerase chain reaction (PCR) methods are also available for fresh and formalin-fixed paraffin tissue. *Bartonella* organisms are difficult to culture.
- Regional cat scratch disease is a self-limited infection.

HISTOLOGIC FINDINGS

- Lymph nodes show effaced architecture with necrotizing granulomatous inflammation and multiple stellate microabscesses (Figures 1-17 and 1-18). Follicular hyperplasia and monocytoid B-cell hyperplasia may be observed early in the infection.
- Microabscesses and granulomas contain central necrotic debris and numerous neutrophils and histiocytes (Figure 1-19), in contrast to the acellular caseation of tuberculous granulomas.
- Organisms may be observed with Warthin-Starry (Figure 1-20) and/or *Bartonella henselae*-specific immunohistochemical stains. Approximately 50% of PCR-positive cases are positive with these stains. The organisms are pleomorphic bacilli and may be present in few numbers.

DIFFERENTIAL DIAGNOSIS

- Mycobacterial lymphadenitis
- *Histoplasma* lymphadenitis
- *Coccidioides* lymphadenitis
- Non-specific bacterial lymphadenitis
- Lymphogranuloma venereum lymphadenitis
- *Tularemia* lymphadenitis

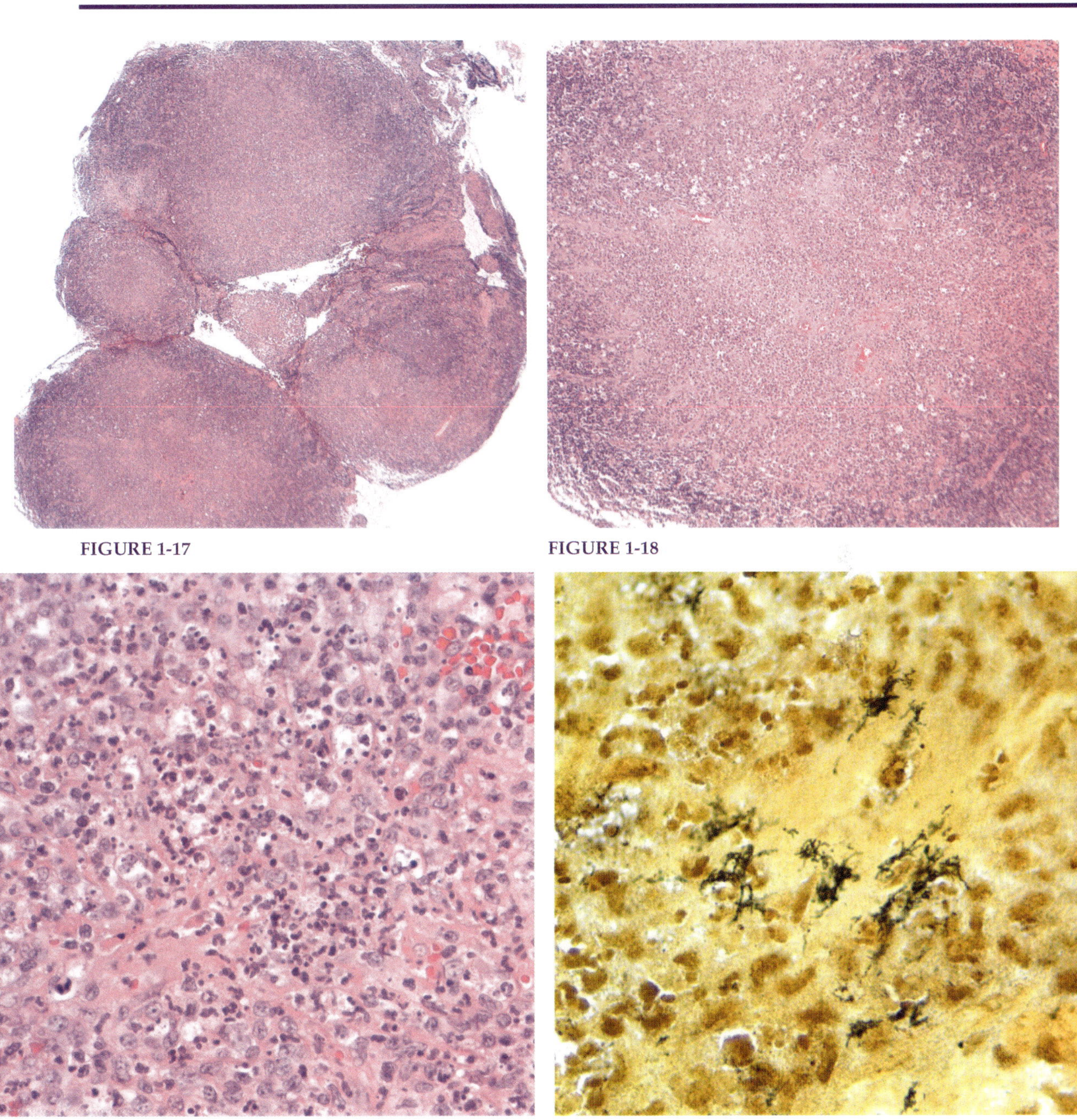

FIGURE 1-17

FIGURE 1-18

FIGURE 1-19

FIGURE 1-20

FIGURE 1-17 This axillary lymph node shows effaced architecture with multiple stellate microabscesses.

FIGURE 1-18 An intermediate view of an irregularly-shaped microabscess containing central neutrophils rimmed by histiocytes and residual lymphoid tissue.

FIGURE 1-19 High-power magnification of the central portion of a microabscess containing numerous neutrophils.

FIGURE 1-20 A Warthin-Starry stain reveals numerous bacilli within a microabscess.

Bacillary Angiomatosis

DEFINITION

Bacillary angiomatosis is a benign vascular proliferative lesion caused by the bacterium *Bartonella henselae* that most commonly presents in the skin and lymph nodes of immunosuppressed patients.

CLINICAL FEATURES

- All affected patients have recent exposure to a cat scratch or bite, with rare exceptions.
- Bacillary angiomatosis presents almost uniformly in immunosuppressed patients, including HIV/AIDS and transplant patients, though occasionally it may be diagnosed as a localized skin process at the inoculum site in immunocompetent hosts.
- Sites of involvement include: skin, lymph nodes, liver, and spleen.
- Involved lymph nodes are tender and mobile and associated with persistent fever, chills, night sweats, fatigue, and myalgias. Skin manifestations are described as nontender, erythematous or hyperkeratotic nodular lesions.
- Positive *Bartonella* serology (see Chapter 7) and/or PCR studies on fresh or formalin-fixed tissue are confirmatory. *Bartonella* organisms are difficult to culture.
- Patients are treated with antibiotic therapy.

HISTOLOGIC FINDINGS

- Lymph nodes show effaced, nodular architecture. Nodules are variably sized, pale pink, and composed of numerous vascular structures (Figures 1-21–1-23).
- The vascular structures are lined by plump endothelial cells with oval, uniform nuclei, single to multiple small nucleoli, vesicular chromatin, and moderate amounts of pale, finely vacuolated cytoplasm. Mild nuclear atypia may be observed in some cases.
- Vascular structures may be widely separated or closely packed, forming solid areas and have variably patent lumina, ranging from poorly formed to dilated.

(*continued*)

FIGURE 1-21 This axillary lymph node from an HIV(+) patient shows obliteration of the normal architecture by pale pink-staining, vascular lobules.

FIGURE 1-22 Numerous, variable caliber vascular structures are observed on intermediate power of the case illustrated in Figure 1-21 (left). High-power magnification reveals plump endothelial cells with bland nuclear features embedded within an eosinophilic, fibrillary stroma (right).

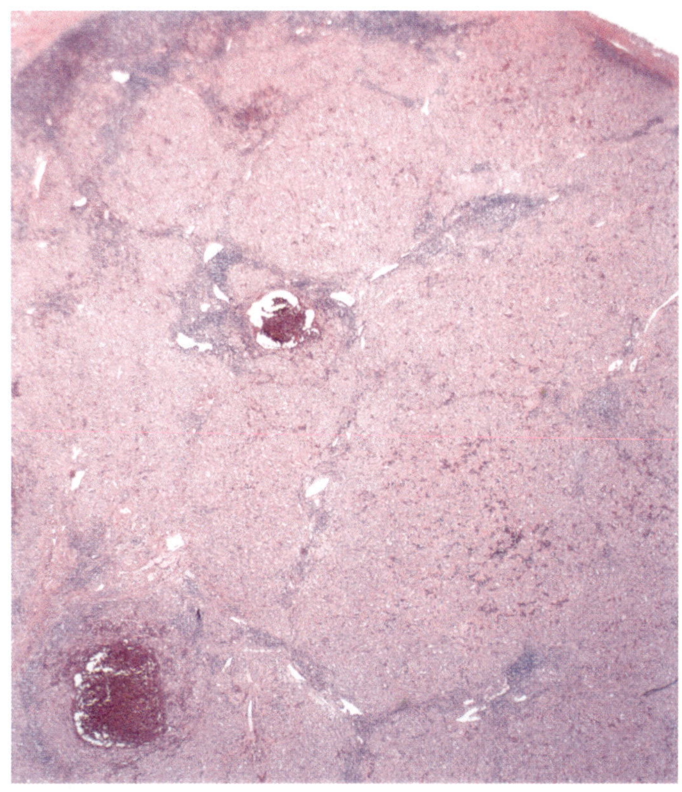

FIGURE 1-21

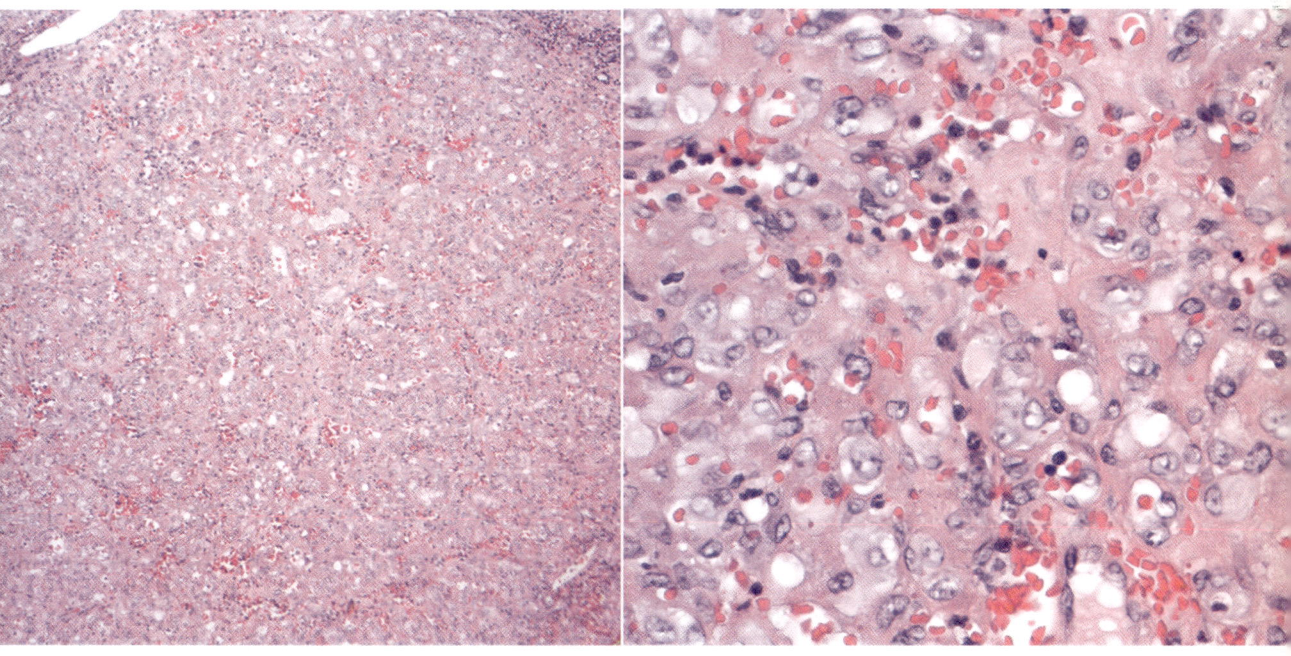

FIGURE 1-22

Bacillary Angiomatosis *(continued)*

- The proliferative blood vessels are embedded in a distinct stroma, which consists of eosinophilic, fibrillary and/or granular material, representing bacteria. Some cases show condensation of bacilli in basophilic, granular clumps (Figure 1-24). Variable numbers of neutrophils are present within the stroma.
- The *Bartonella* organisms stain positive with the Warthin-Starry stain but stain poorly with a gram stain.

DIFFERENTIAL DIAGNOSIS

- Kaposi's sarcoma
- Epithelioid hemangioma/hemangioendothelioma
- Angiosarcoma
- Nodal hemangioma
- Vascular transformation of lymph node sinuses

FIGURE 1-23 Intermediate magnification of this axillary lymph node from an HIV(+) patient reveals numerous vessels lined by flattened to plump endothelial cells and eosinophilic stroma with acute inflammatory cells.

FIGURE 1-24 Higher power of the lymph node illustrated in Figure 1-23 reveals basophilic clumps of bacteria (arrowed) and acute and chronic inflammatory cells within the stroma.

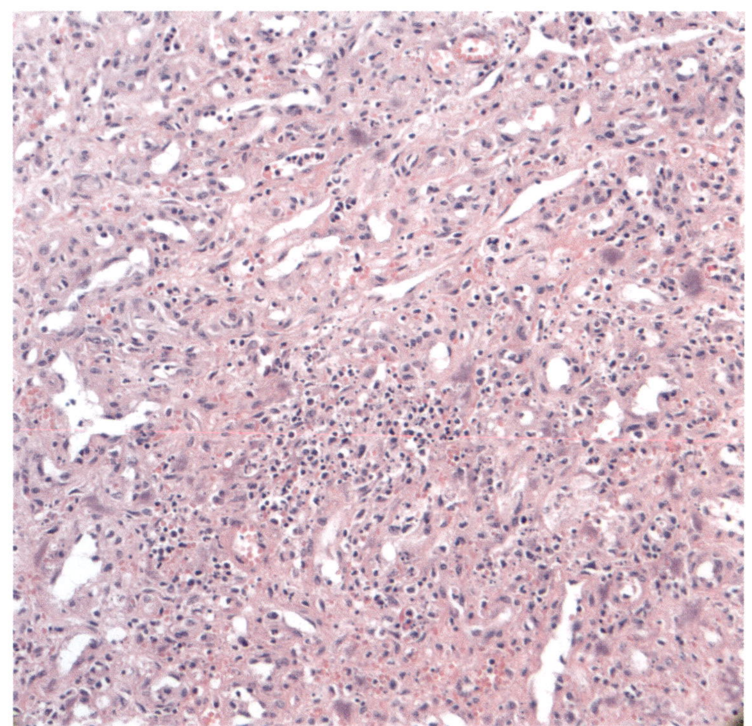

FIGURE 1-23

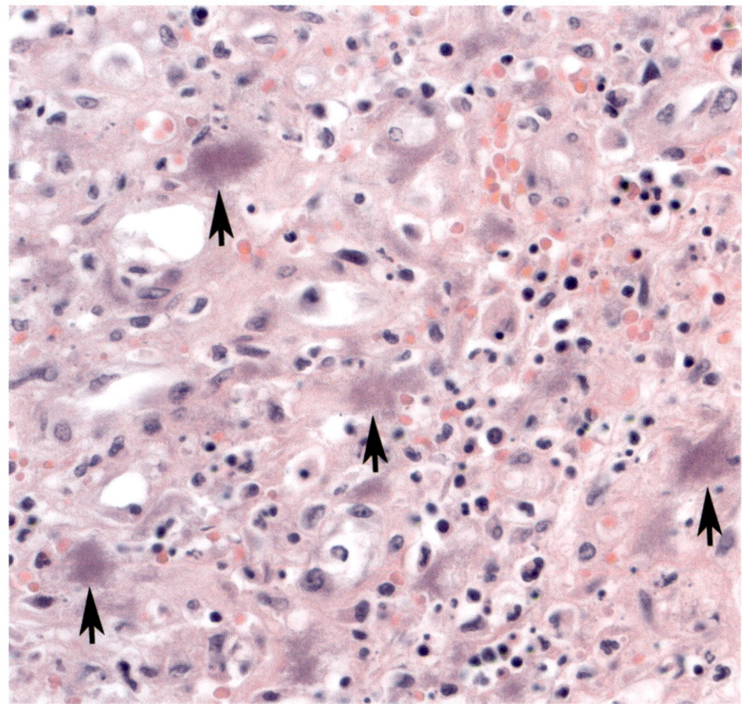

FIGURE 1-24

Syphilis (Luetic) Lymphadenitis

DEFINITION

Luetic lymphadenitis is caused by the spirochete, *Treponema pallidum*, and is observed during the primary and secondary stages of the infection.

CLINICAL FEATURES

- Inguinal lymph nodes are most frequently involved, though cervical, axillary and occipital lymph node involvement has been reported. Most cases are in males.
- Regional non-tender lymphadenopathy is common during primary syphilis and is associated with a painless genital or oral ulcer.
- Generalized lymphadenopathy can also be observed during the maculopapular rash characteristic of secondary syphilis.
- Non-treponemal antibody tests, such as the VDRL (venereal disease research laboratory), and specific treponemal antibody tests are positive.

HISTOLOGIC FINDINGS

- Involved lymph nodes show retained architecture, frequently with follicular hyperplasia (Figure 1-25), which may mimic follicular lymphoma. Follicular hyperplasia may be the only histologic finding in lymph nodes of the head, neck, and axilla.
- There is capsular thickening by fibrosis and chronic inflammation, consisting of lymphocytes and plasma cells. Vessels within the capsule show endothelitis and are cuffed by lymphocytes and plasma cells (Figure 1-26).

(*continued*)

FIGURE 1-25 This inguinal lymph node shows florid follicular hyperplasia.

FIGURE 1-26 High-power magnification reveals endothelitis and perivascular cuffing by plasma cells and lymphocytes.

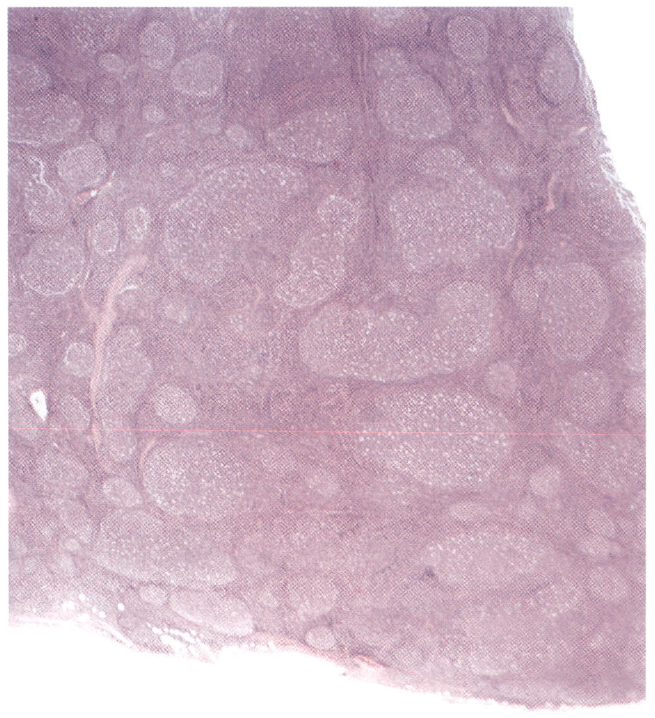

FIGURE 1-25

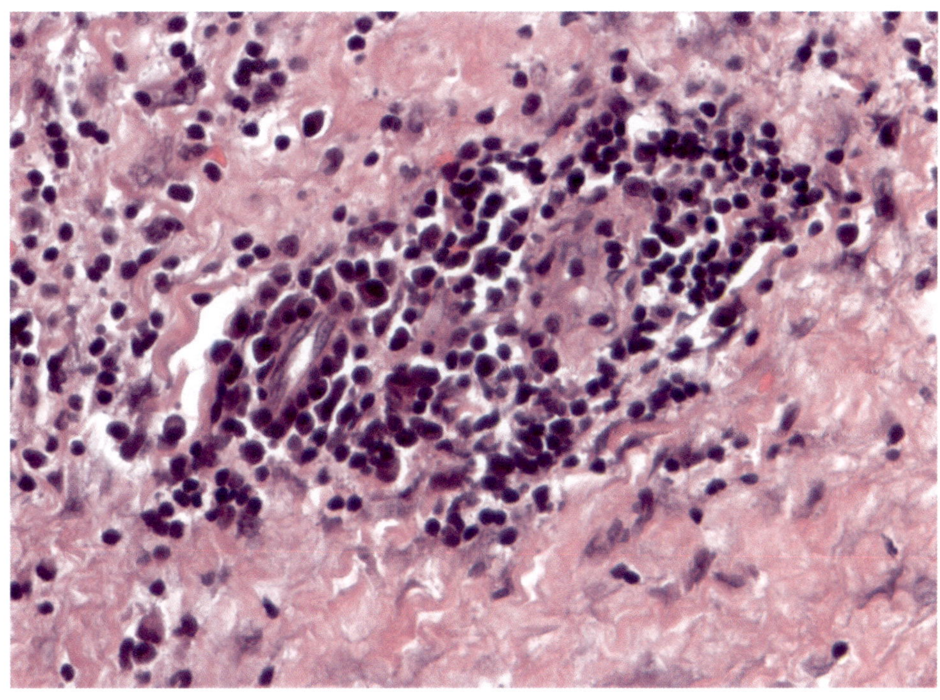

FIGURE 1-26

Syphilis (Luetic) Lymphadenitis *(continued)*

- Sheets of plasma cells may be observed in the interfollicular and medullary zones (Figure 1-27). The plasma cells are morphologically unremarkable and polytypic by immunohistochemistry.
- Foci of acute inflammation, including microabscess formation, are observed in some cases.
- Noncaseating granulomas associated with the hyperplastic follicles may be present in a subset of cases (Figure 1-28).
- Spirochetes can be observed with Warthin-Starry or immunohistochemical stains. The organisms are located in the microabscesses, granulomas, germinal centers, and/or walls of vessels.

DIFFERENTIAL DIAGNOSIS

- Lupus lymphadenitis
- Rheumatoid lymphadenitis
- Follicular lymphoma
- Nodal marginal zone lymphoma
- Nonspecific bacterial lymphadenitis
- Mycobacterial lymphadenitis
- Fungal lymphadenitis
- *Toxoplasma* lymphadenitis
- Inflammatory pseudotumor of lymph node
- Kaposi's sarcoma

FIGURE 1-27 The interfollicular and medullary areas are expanded by a prominent plasma cell infiltrate.

FIGURE 1-28 Scattered granulomas and microabscesses were observed in this inguinal lymph node.

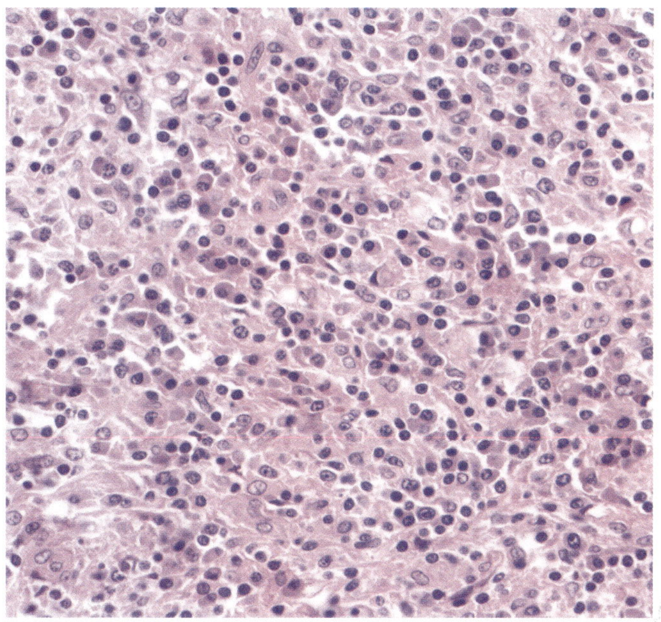

FIGURE 1-27

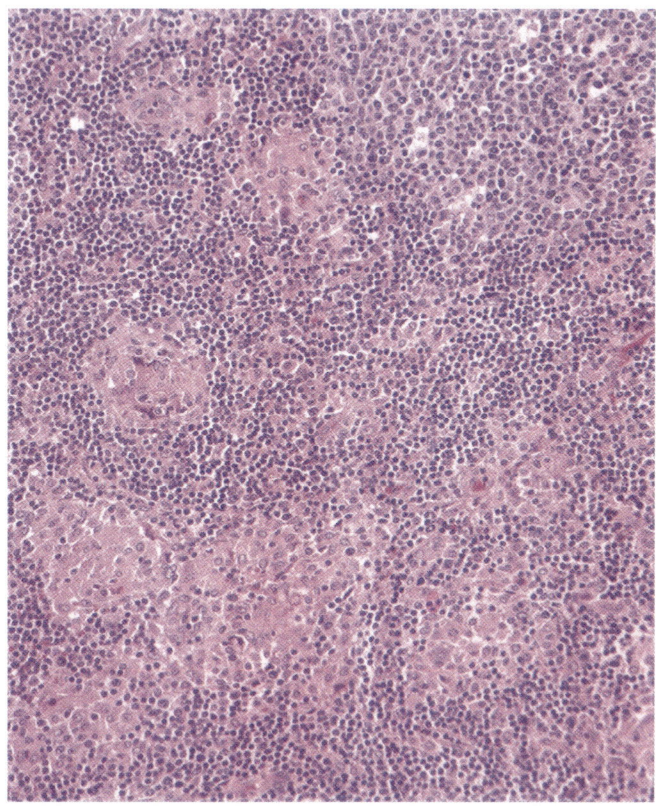

FIGURE 1-28

Mycobacterium Tuberculosis Lymphadenitis

DEFINITION

This entity represents granulomatous lymphadenitis due to infection with *Mycobacterium tuberculosis* (Mtb).

CLINICAL FEATURES

- Tuberculous lymphadenitis is relatively common in Western countries, especially in HIV-infected individuals.
- Cervical and mediastinal lymph nodes are frequently involved.

HISTOLOGIC FINDINGS

- Involved lymph nodes show granulomatous inflammation, with typical granulomas consisting of a caseating necrotic center, surrounded by concentric epithelioid cells, multinucleated giant cells, and small lymphocytes (Figure 1-29).
- Special stains (Fite, Ziehl-Neelsen, or Kinyoun) demonstrate the presence of rod shaped acid-fast bacilli, with a beaded staining pattern.
- Fibrosis and calcification are present in variable amounts, depending on the time course of the infection.

DIFFERENTIAL DIAGNOSIS

- Non-tuberculous lymphadenitis
- *Histoplasma capsulatum* lymphadenitis
- Cat-scratch lymphadenitis
- Sarcoidosis

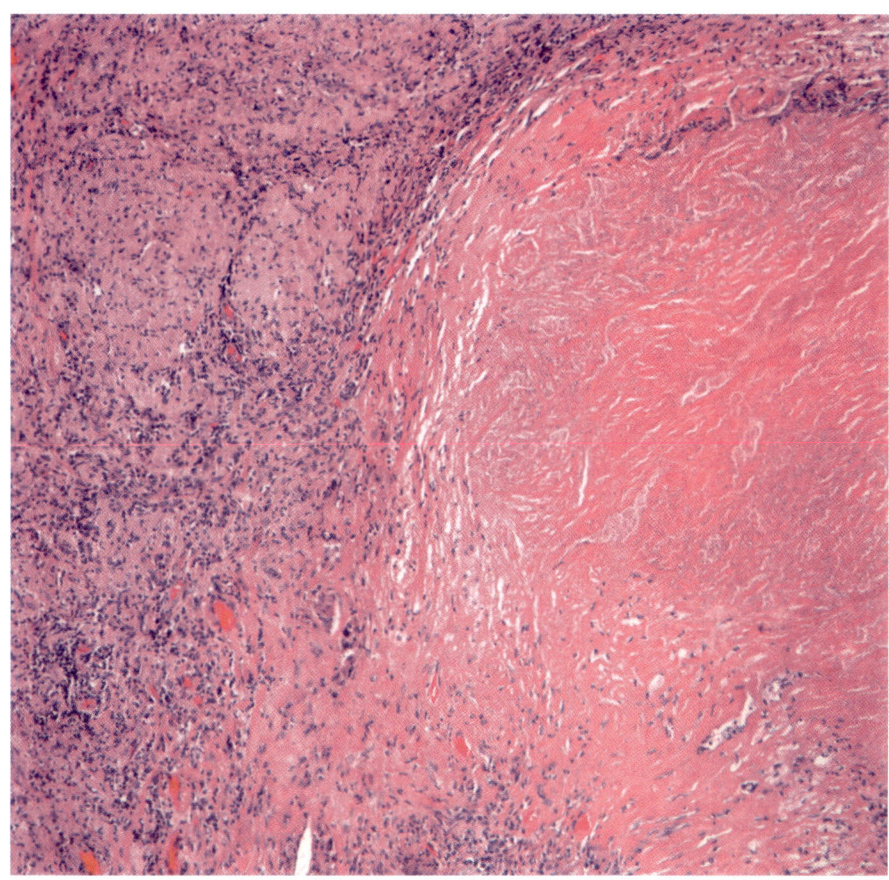

FIGURE 1-29

FIGURE 1-29 Large area of caseous necrosis, surrounded by epithelioid histiocytes and lymphocytes.

Mycobacterium Avium-Intracellulare Lymphadenitis

DEFINITION

Lymphadenitis due to *Mycobacterium avium-intracellulare* usually represents massive lymph node infiltration by histiocytes containing abundant microorganisms in the setting of severe immune suppression.

CLINICAL FEATURES

- This infection is commonly seen in patients with AIDS, usually in patients with severe depression of CD4 counts.

HISTOLOGIC FINDINGS

- Lymph nodes architecture is effaced by an infiltrate of large histiocytes, either diffusely or in the form of ill-formed granulomas. The histiocytes have abundant pink/grey cytoplasm with a foamy or striated appearance. (Figures 1-30 and 1-31). Some cases have prominent admixed neutrophils.
- Special stains (Fite, Ziehl-Neelsen, or Kinyoun) demonstrate the presence of numerous acid-fast bacilli in the histiocytes (Figure 1-32).

DIFFERENTIAL DIAGNOSIS

- Tuberculous lymphadenitis
- *Histoplasma capsulatum* lymphadenitis
- Cat-scratch lymphadenitis
- Sarcoidosis

FIGURE 1-30 Lymph node with sheets of foamy histiocytes and frequent neutrophils.
FIGURE 1-31 Histiocytes with abundant foamy or striated pink/grey cytoplasm.
FIGURE 1-32 A Fite stain show numerous acid-fast organisms in the histiocytes.

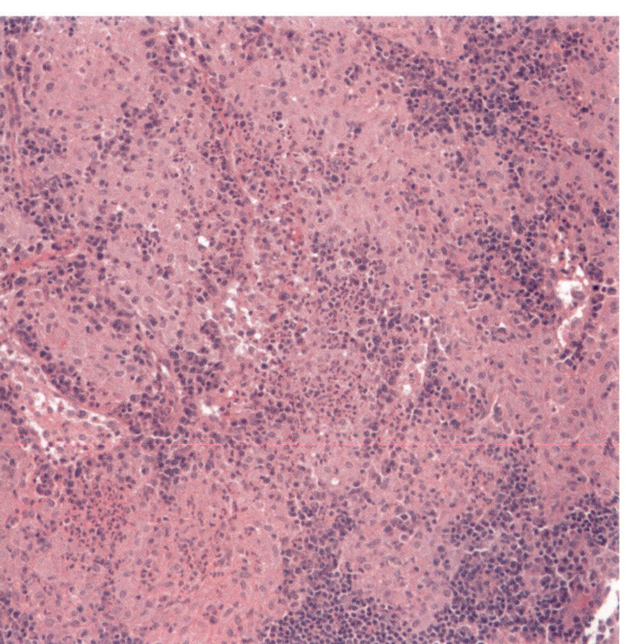

FIGURE 1-30

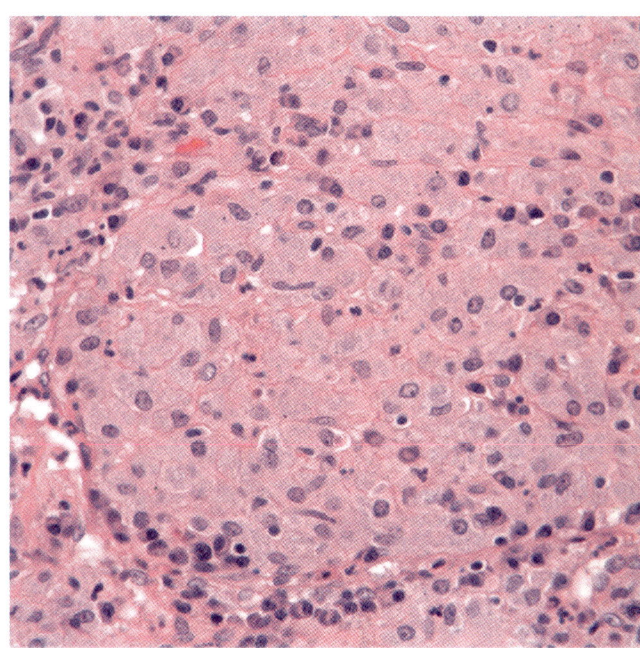

FIGURE 1-31

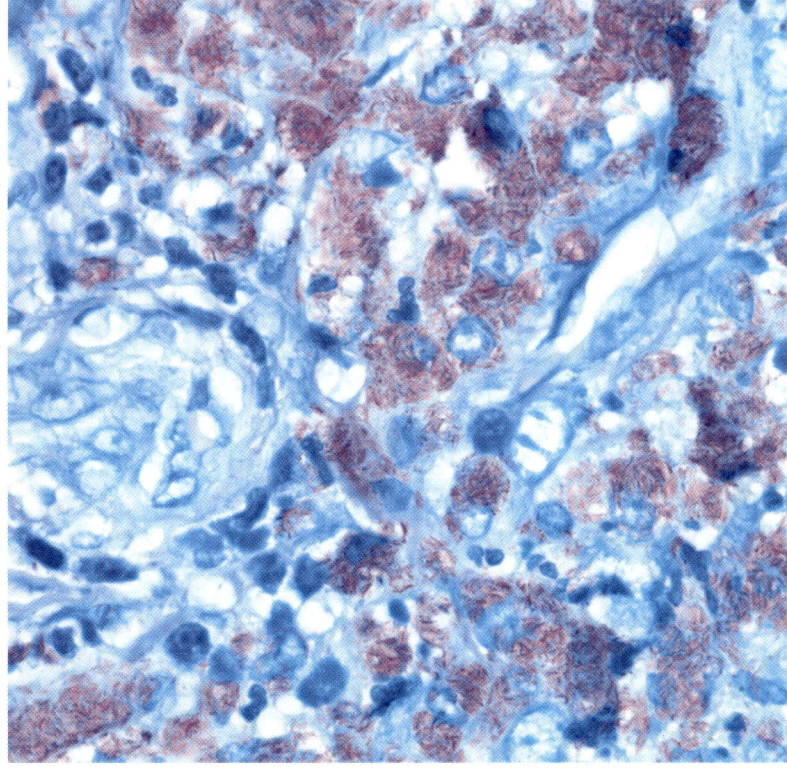

FIGURE 1-32

Histoplasma Lymphadenitis

DEFINITION

Histoplasma lymphadenitis is observed in acute and chronic pulmonary infections and disseminated histoplasmosis caused by the dimorphic fungus, *Histoplasma capsulatum*.

CLINICAL FEATURES

- Most acute *Histoplasma* infections are asymptomatic. Endemic areas include the Ohio and Mississippi River Valleys, Central and South America, and the Caribbean. The organism is inhaled and can disseminate from the lungs through hilar lymph nodes.
- Lymphadenopathy may be observed in acute and chronic pulmonary *Histoplasma* infections and disseminated histoplasmosis. The acute infection presents as a respiratory illness with fever, cough and pleuritic chest pain, while the chronic form shows persistence of these symptoms with/out night sweats and weight loss. The disseminated form presents as sepsis with multiorgan failure following a pneumonia-like illness.
- Hilar and mediastinal lymph nodes are the most commonly affected.
- Disseminated histoplasmosis has an 80% mortality without therapy.

HISTOLOGIC FINDINGS

- The normal lymph node architecture is replaced by geographic areas of necrosis (Figure 1-33) and/or caseating granulomatous inflammation.
- Necrotic areas contain significant nuclear debris and may be devoid of neutrophils.
- If present, granulomas have central areas of necrosis surrounded by palisading histiocytes, giant cells, and lymphocytes.
- Focal calcifications are frequently present in mediastinal lymph nodes of chronically infected patients; yeast organisms may be difficult to identify at this site.
- Yeast organisms are not easily identified on H&E stains and are best visualized with a GMS stain (Figures 1-34 and 1-35).
- Yeast organisms are 2–5 µm, ovoid structures.

DIFFERENTIAL DIAGNOSIS

- Mycobacterial lymphadenitis
- Common bacterial lymphadenitis
- Cat scratch lymphadenitis
- Herpes simplex virus lymphadenitis
- Kikuchi-Fujimoto disease
- Systemic lupus erythematosus
- Wegener's granulomatosis

FIGURE 1-33 This hilar lymph node shows geographic necrosis with minimal residual nodal tissue. The patient died of disseminated histoplasmosis.

FIGURE 1-34 An intermediate magnification of a GMS stain reveals numerous yeast within the necrotic areas.

FIGURE 1-35 High-power examination reveals small, ovoid budding yeast, morphologically consistent with *Histoplasma*. *Histoplasma capsulatum* was cultured from this tissue.

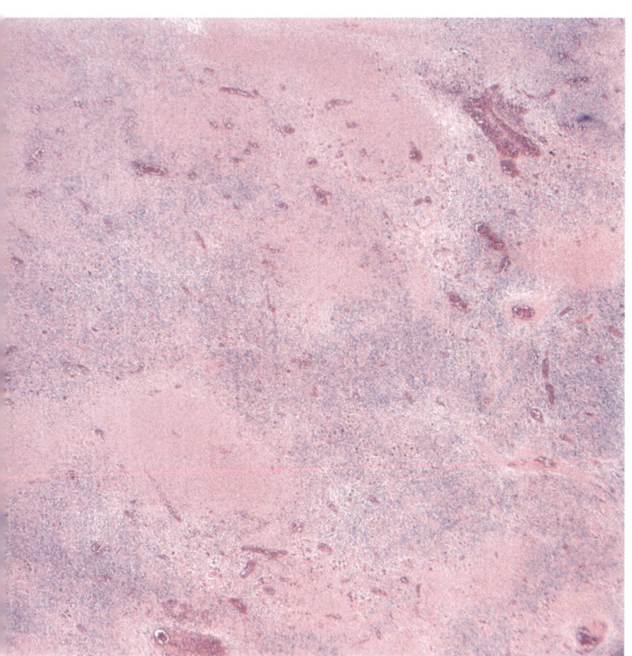

FIGURE 1-33

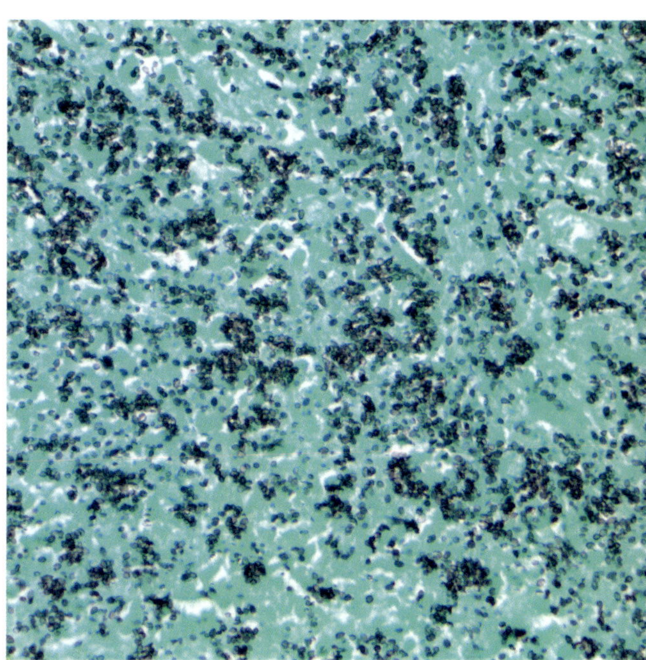

FIGURE 1-34

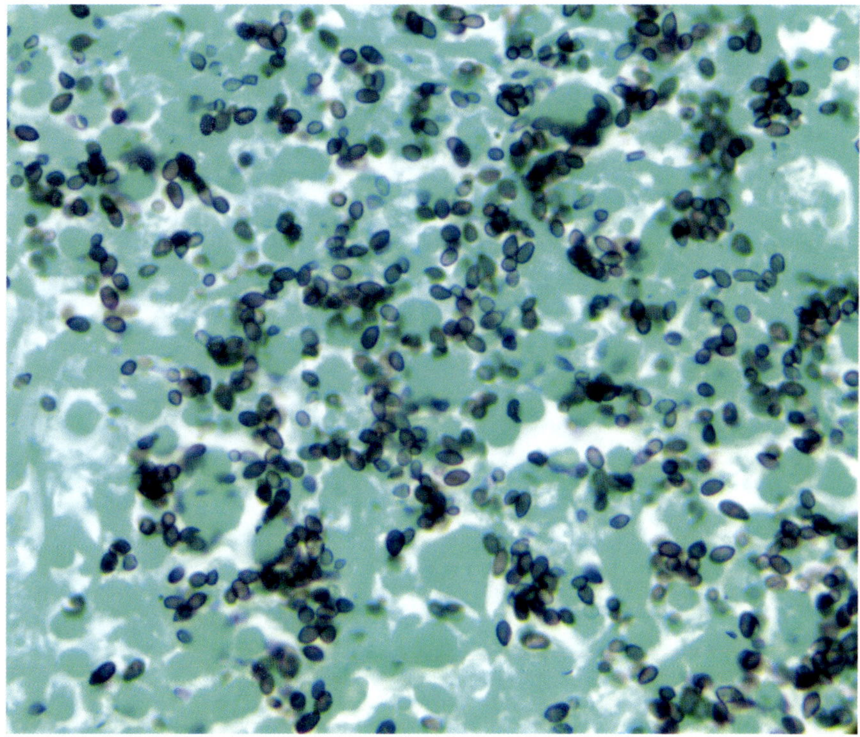

FIGURE 1-35

Coccidioides Lymphadenitis

DEFINITION

Coccidioides lymphadenitis is observed in acute and chronic pulmonary infections and disseminated coccidioidomycosis caused by the dimorphic fungus, *Coccidioides immitis*.

CLINICAL FEATURES

- Most acute *Coccidioides* infections (60%) are asymptomatic. Endemic areas include the southwestern United States, Central America, and Mexico. The organism is highly infectious, inhaled into the lungs, and can disseminate through hilar lymph nodes.
- Lymphadenopathy may be observed in acute and chronic pulmonary *Coccidioides* infections and disseminated coccidioidomycosis. The acute infection presents as a respiratory illness with fever, cough and pleuritic chest pain, while the chronic form shows persistence of these symptoms with night sweats and/or weight loss. The disseminated form is more common in immunosuppressed individuals and certain ethnic groups, namely African Americans and Filipinos; extrapulmonary manifestations, including skin, soft tissue, bone, and meninges involvement, are present in disseminated disease following the pneumonia-like illness.
- Bilateral hilar lymph nodes are enlarged frequently.

HISTOLOGIC FINDINGS

- The normal lymph node architecture is replaced by granulomatous inflammation showing variable caseating necrosis (Figure 1-36). This inflammation may extend into the surrounding perinodal tissue.
- Yeast organisms may be difficult to identify on H&E stains (Figure 1-37) and are best visualized with a Gomori methamine silver stain (Figure 1-38).
- Yeast organisms are 30–100 µm globular spherule structures with thick, refractile walls. They are frequently variable in size within the same biopsy specimen. Occasionally, a spherule may be filled or partially ruptured, revealing multiple 2–5 µm endospores, which may be confused with the yeast form of *Histoplasma*.

DIFFERENTIAL DIAGNOSIS

- *Histoplasma* lymphadenitis
- *Cryptococcus* lymphadenitis
- Mycobacterial lymphadenitis

FIGURE 1-36 This anthracotic hilar lymph node reveals multiple caseating granulomas.

FIGURE 1-37 High-power magnification of a necrotizing granuloma reveals a ruptured spherule with a thick wall (arrow).

FIGURE 1-38 A GMS stain shows multiple ruptured spherules and endospores.

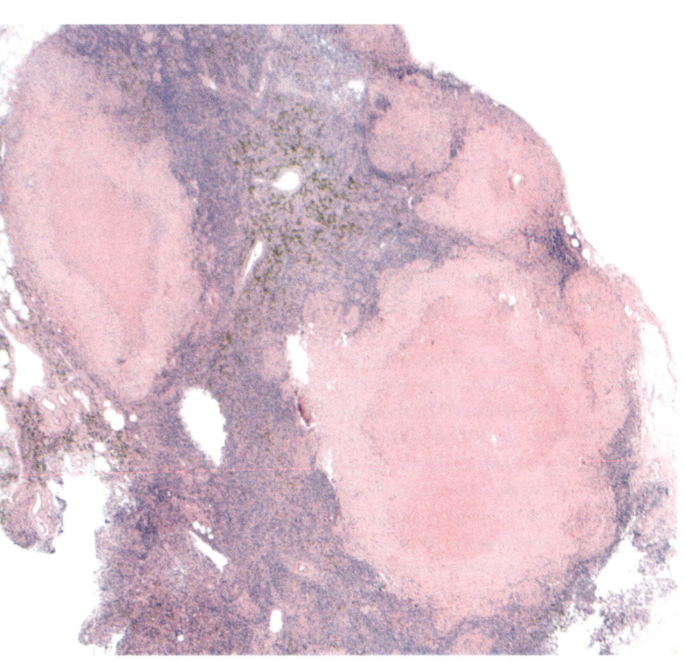

FIGURE 1-36

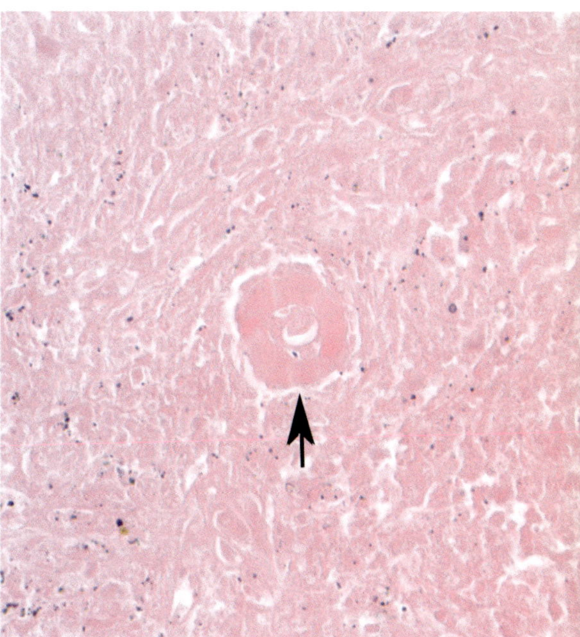

FIGURE 1-37

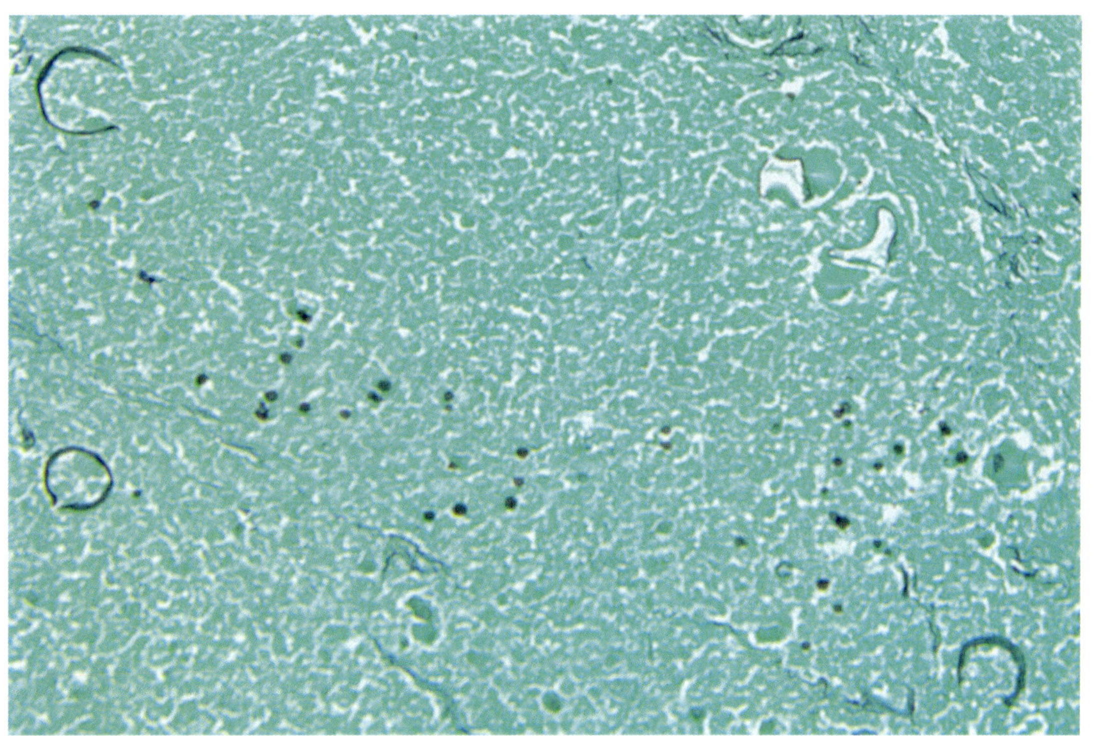

FIGURE 1-38

Filariasis

DEFINITION

Lymphatic filariasis is caused by the roundworms *Wuchereria bancrofti, Brugia malayi* and *Brugia timori.*

CLINICAL FEATURES

- Patients acquire the microfilariae through multiple, repeated mosquito bites in an endemic area, such as central Africa, southern Asia, the Caribbean, and parts of South America.
- The majority of infected patients do not have symptoms.
- Because the microfilariae mature to adult forms in the lymphatics, lymphatic obstruction occurs in some patients, manifesting as swelling in the soft tissues of the extremities, genitals (specifically the epididymis and testes), and/or breasts. The skin undergoes thickening in association with the edema.
- Microfilariae can be identified on peripheral blood smears, most optimally at night and with thick smear preparations.

HISTOLOGIC FINDINGS

- Involved lymph nodes show adult forms within dilated lymphatics (Figures 1-39 and 1-40).
- The lymph node may in addition show variable reactive features, most notably when the parasites degenerate.

FIGURE 1-39 Several adult worms are observed within the lymphatics of this pelvic lymph node.
FIGURE 1-40 High-power view of the adult worms illustrated in Figure 1.39.

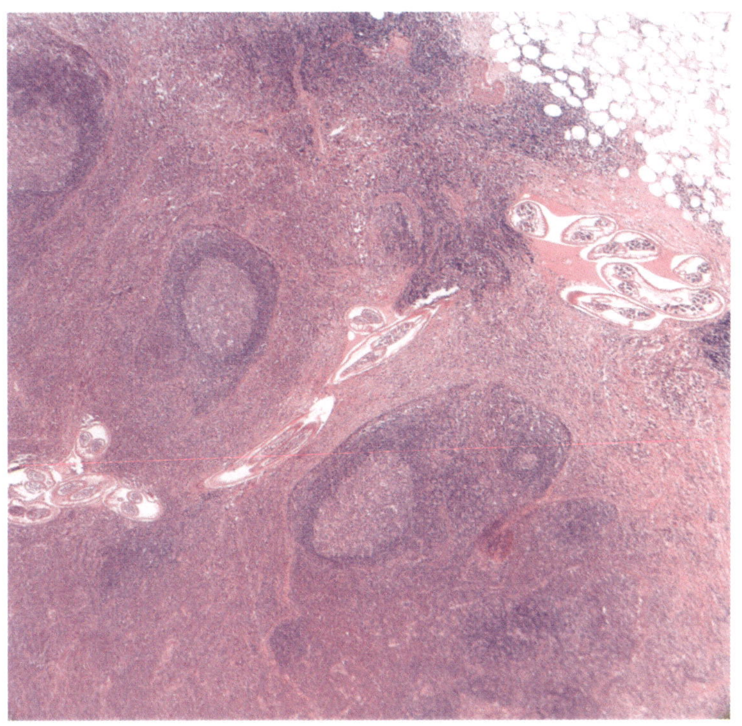

FIGURE 1-39

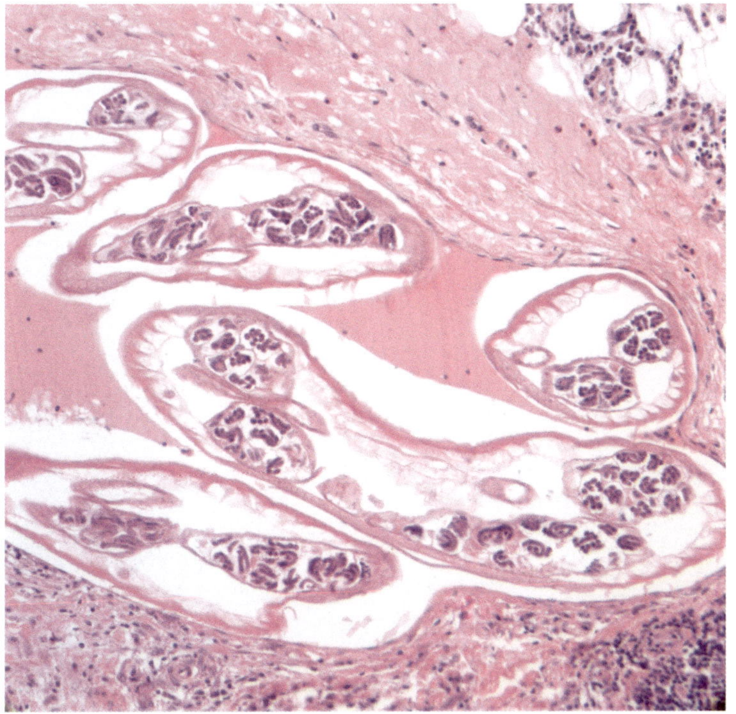

FIGURE 1-40

2

Reactive Lymphadenopathies

FOLLICULAR HYPERPLASIA

PARACORTICAL HYPERPLASIA

SINUS HISTIOCYTOSIS

PROGRESSIVE TRANSFORMATION OF GERMINAL CENTERS (PTGC)

DERMATOPATHIC LYMPHADENOPATHY

Follicular Hyperplasia

DEFINITION

Follicular hyperplasia is a non-specific, benign histologic finding characterized by increased numbers of secondary follicles showing reactive morphologic features. It is a finding observed in various reactive conditions; an etiology usually cannot be ascribed.

CLINICAL FEATURES

- Follicular hyperplasia may present as acute or chronic lymphadenopathy. Associated clinical symptoms are dependent on the underlying cause.
- Enlarged lymph nodes (usually <3 cm in greatest dimension) are most commonly observed in the head, cervical, axillary, and inguinal areas, as these sites are the most subject to repeated antigenic stimulation.
- Follicular hyperplasia is a more frequent histologic finding in pediatric cases of lymphadenopathy compared to adults, as lymphoid hyperplasia accounts for approximately 75% of lymphadenopathy in the pediatric population.

HISTOLOGIC FINDINGS

- Lymph nodes demonstrate intact architecture.
- Follicles with germinal centers are increased in number, variably sized, evenly spaced, and usually retain well-defined mantle zones (Figure 2-1). Follicle shapes vary from round and regular to serpentine.
- Germinal centers are polarized, displaying light and dark zones containing centrocytes and proliferating centroblasts, respectively (Figure 2-2). Centrocytes may be small, medium, or large in size. Frequent tingible body macrophages are observed and often impart a "starry sky" appearance. Mitoses may be abundant.
- Paracortical hyperplasia may be observed in association with the follicular hyperplasia.
- BCL-2 expression is absent in the germinal centers of follicular hyperplasia, except for few BCL2(+) follicular T cells.

DIFFERENTIAL DIAGNOSIS

- Follicular lymphoma
- Angioimmunoblastic T-cell lymphoma with hyperplastic follicles (pattern I)
- Infectious adenopathies: HIV, toxoplasmosis, CMV, EBV
- Castleman lymphadenopathy

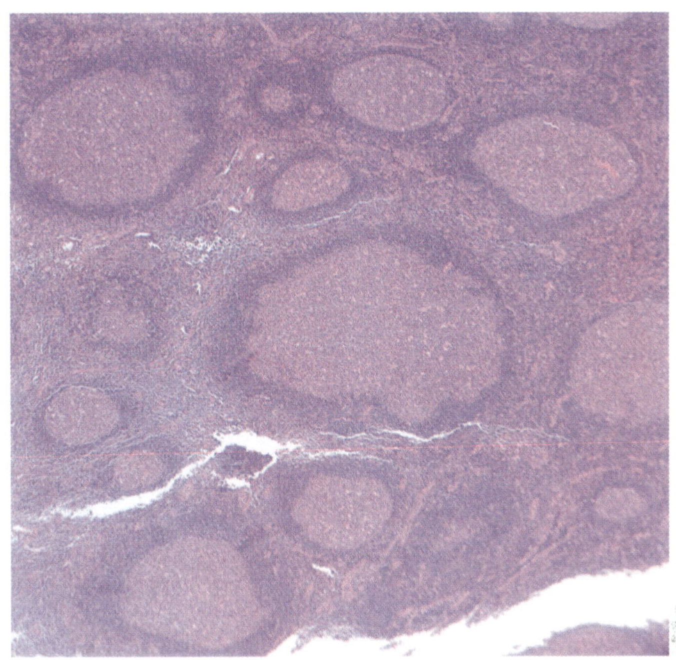

FIGURE 2-1

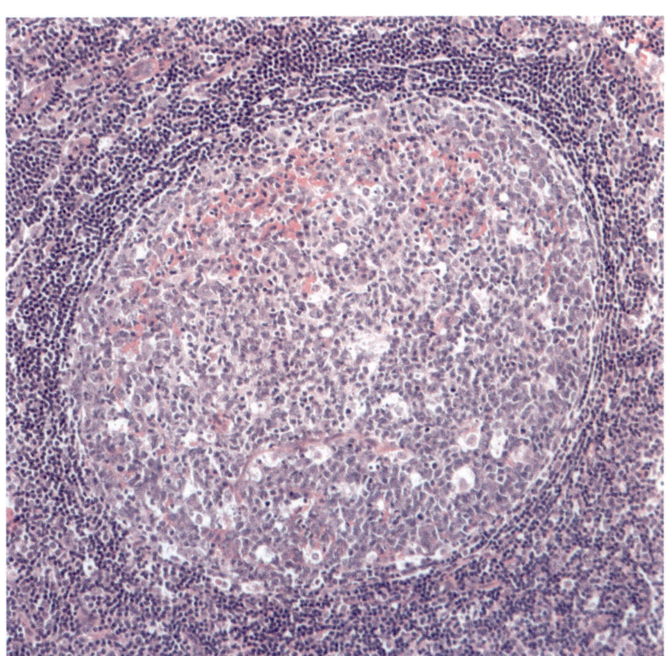

FIGURE 2-2

FIGURE 2-1 Follicles are increased in number, variable in size and shape, and show well-formed mantle zones and polarized germinal centers with tingible body macrophages.

FIGURE 2-2 This reactive follicle shows a polarized germinal center, with light (left) and dark (right) zones and many tingible body macrophages.

Paracortical Hyperplasia

DEFINITION

Paracortical hyperplasia is a non-specific benign histologic finding in reactive lymph nodes. It is a finding observed in various reactive conditions; an etiology usually cannot be ascribed.

CLINICAL FEATURES

- Paracortical hyperplasia may present as acute or chronic lymphadenopathy. Associated clinical symptoms are dependent on the underlying cause.
- Enlarged lymph nodes (usually <3 cm in greatest dimension) are most commonly observed in the head, cervical, axillary, and inguinal areas, as these sites are the most subject to repeat antigenic stimulation.
- Paracortical hyperplasia is a more frequent histologic finding in pediatric cases of lymphadenopathy compared to adults, as lymphoid hyperplasia accounts for approximately 75% of lymphadenopathy in the pediatric population.

HISTOLOGIC FINDINGS

- Lymph nodes demonstrate intact architecture (Figure 2-3).
- The paracortex is expanded by diffuse or vaguely nodular proliferations of small, mature lymphocytes, which lack atypia, and variable numbers of immunoblasts and dendritic cells. Prominent dendritic cells and/or immunoblasts may impart a "starry sky" appearance to the paracortex (Figures 2-4 and 2-5). High endothelial venules may be increased in number.
- Follicular hyperplasia may be present in association with the paracortical expansion.

DIFFERENTIAL DIAGNOSIS

- Angioimmunoblastic T-cell lymphoma (pattern I, II)
- Peripheral T-cell lymphoma, not otherwise specified
- Infectious adenopathies: CMV, EBV, HIV
- Dermatopathic lymphadenopathy

FIGURE 2-3 This low-power image shows an expanded paracortex with few scattered reactive follicles.

FIGURE 2-4 The paracortex is expanded by numerous dendritic cells, imparting a "starry sky" appearance. Increased vascularity is also present.

FIGURE 2-5 The expanded paracortex contains increased numbers of immunoblasts in a background of small lymphocytes, which lack atypia.

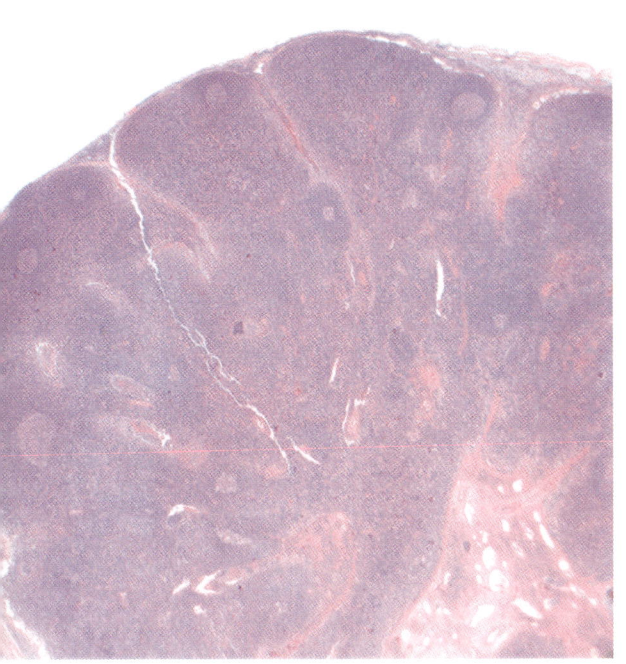

FIGURE 2-3

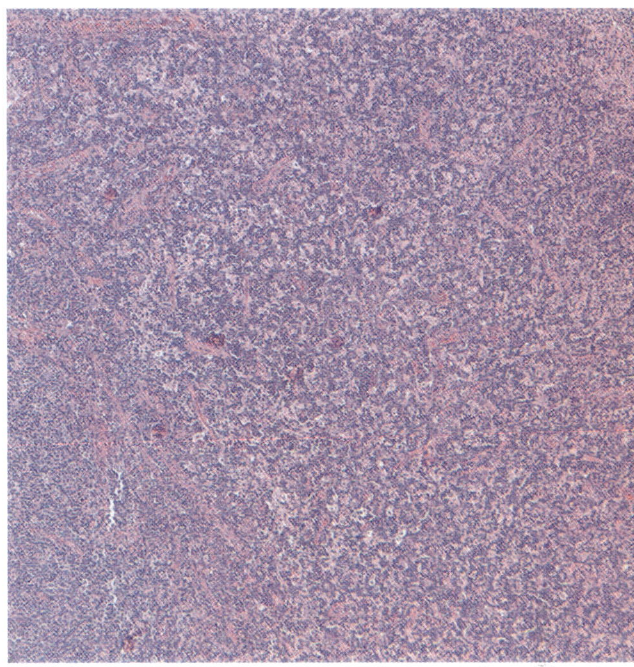

FIGURE 2-4

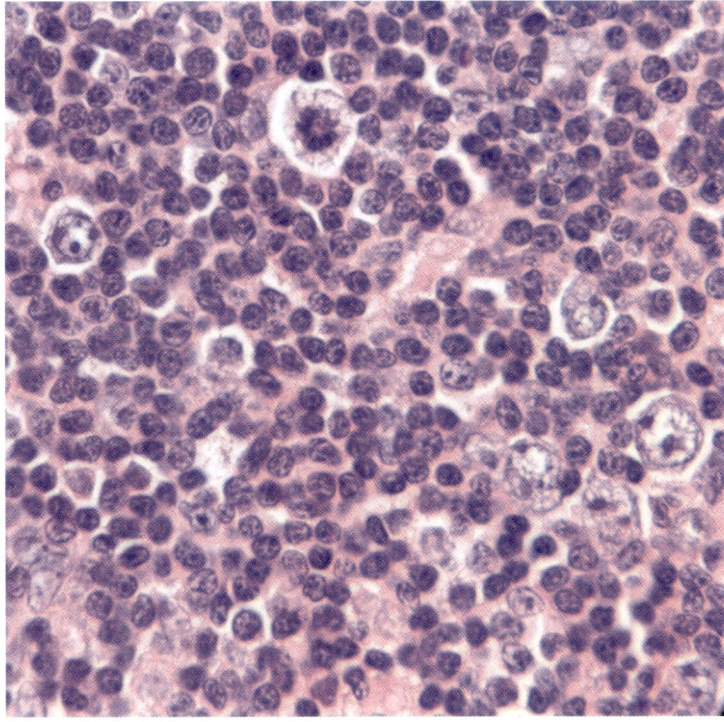

FIGURE 2-5

Sinus Histiocytosis

DEFINITION

Sinus histiocytosis is a non-specific histologic pattern present in lymph nodes of various clinical conditions. It has been most frequently described in lymph nodes draining tumors with or without metastatic disease.

CLINICAL FEATURES

- Associated clinical symptoms are dependent on the underlying cause.
- Lymph nodes may be near normal in size or enlarged.

HISTOLOGIC FINDINGS

- Lymph nodes demonstrate predominantly intact architecture, though cases associated with metastatic disease may have partial effacement.
- Sinuses are dilated and distended with morphologically unremarkable histiocytes (Figures 2-6 and 2-7). Emperipolesis is not present.
- Follicular and/or paracortical hyperplasia are frequently present in association with the sinus histiocytosis.

DIFFERENTIAL DIAGNOSIS

- Rosai-Dorfman lymphadenopathy
- Langerhans cell histiocytosis
- Dermatopathic lymphadenopathy

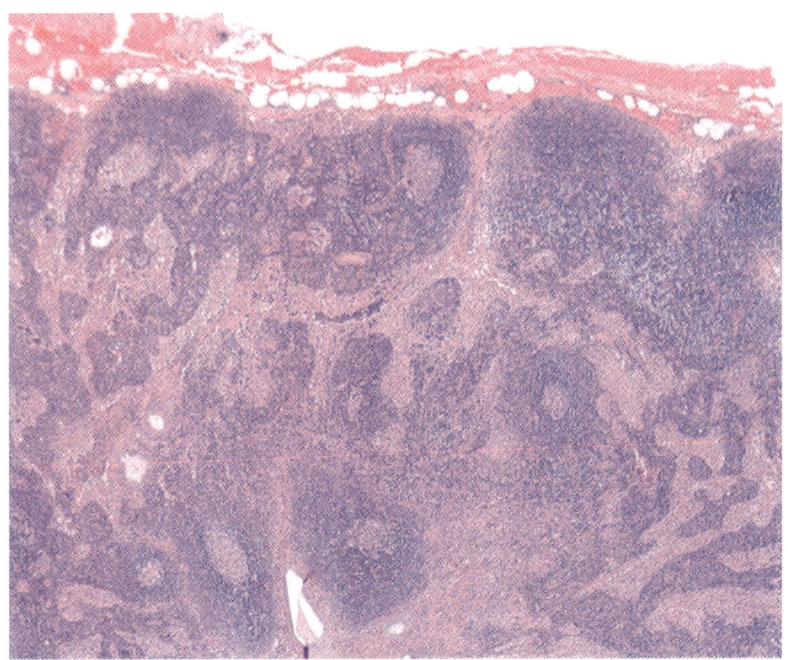

FIGURE 2-6

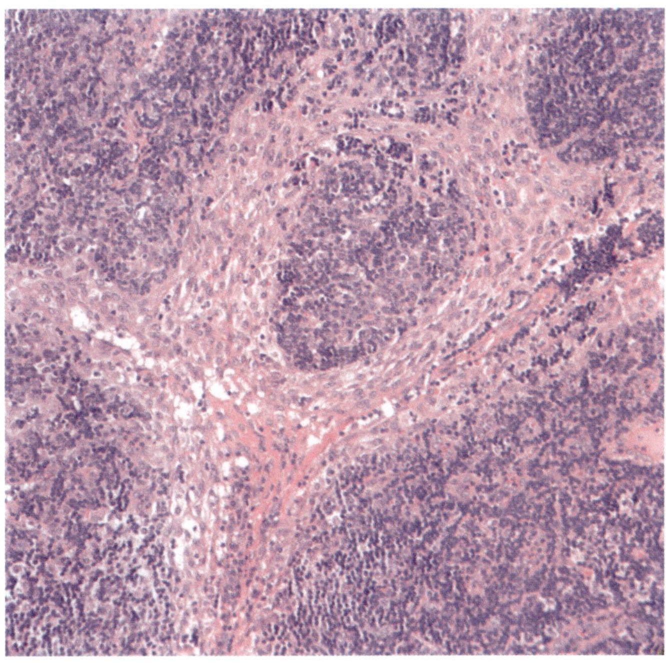

FIGURE 2-7

FIGURE 2-6 Low-power examination reveals many, dilated, branching sinuses.
FIGURE 2-7 The sinuses are distended with bland histiocytes and occasional lymphocytes and eosinophils.

Progressive Transformation of Germinal Centers (PTGC)

DEFINITION

Progressive transformation of germinal centers (PTGC) is a benign histologic finding observed in 3.5–10% of chronic non-specific lymphadenopathies. It is hypothesized to represent a continuum with follicular hyperplasia and follicular lysis and is characterized by the expansion of the follicle accompanied by inward migration of mantle cells and T cells into the germinal center.

CLINICAL FEATURES

- The majority of cases are observed in children or young males in their 20–30s. There is a male predominance (3:1).
- Lymph nodes are non-tender and uniformly enlarged. The lymphadenopathy is not typically accompanied by systemic symptoms.
- Cervical lymph nodes are most commonly affected, though PTGC has been reported in the axillary and inguinal regions as well.
- Approximately 50% of PTGC in children can persist or recur following surgical excision, compared to 25% of PTGCs in adults.
- Up to 35% of adults with florid PTGC (a rare finding) will be diagnosed with nodular lymphocyte predominant Hodgkin lymphoma (NLPHL) either preceding, following, or concomitantly with the PTGC diagnosis. The vast majority of lymph nodes with usual focal PTCG in a background of follicular hyperplasia do not develop Hodgkin lymphoma.

HISTOLOGIC FINDINGS

- PTGC usually occurs in a background of florid follicular hyperplasia (Figure 2-8).
- Follicles show enlargement and variable infiltration by the surrounding mantle zone B cells and T cells (Figure 2-9). Germinal centers range from predominantly intact to irregularly shaped to near completely obliterated (Figure 2-10). The mantle zone cells are monotonous, small in size, and have coarse chromatin with indiscernible cytoplasm.
- Scattered immunoblasts may be observed, but "popcorn" or LP cells should not be present in PTGC without associated NLPHL.
- The transformed follicles of PTGC stain strongly positive for CD20 in confluent aggregates, in contrast to NLPHL wherein CD20 immunostaining imparts a "moth eaten" appearance.
- T-cell rosettes (around immunoblasts) are observed in few cases of PTGC, though this finding is more commonly present around LP cells in NLPHL. T cells tend to be scattered in PTGC, whereas in NLPHL, T cell aggregates are most commonly observed. There is no difference in numbers of CD57(+) T cells observed in PTGC compared to NLPHL.

DIFFERENTIAL DIAGNOSIS

- Nodular lymphocyte predominant Hodgkin lymphoma
- Follicular lymphoma, floral variant
- HIV lymphadenopathy

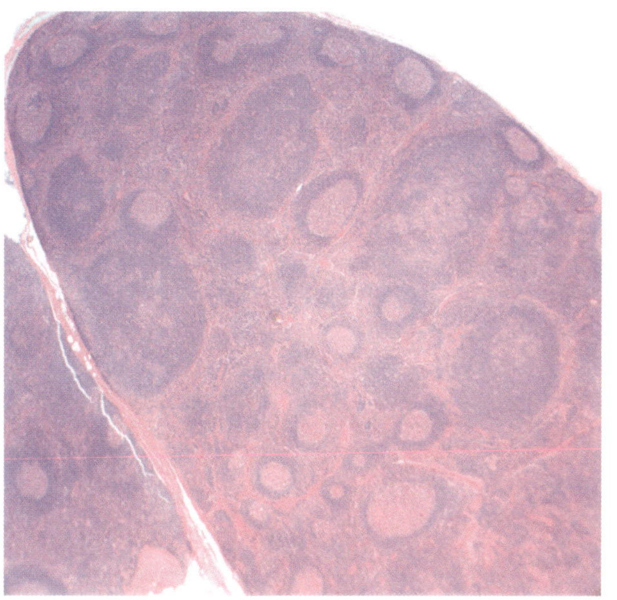

FIGURE 2-8

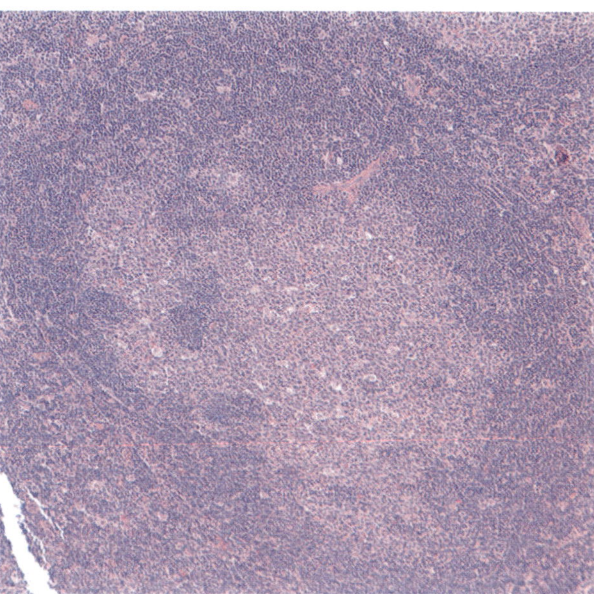

FIGURE 2-9

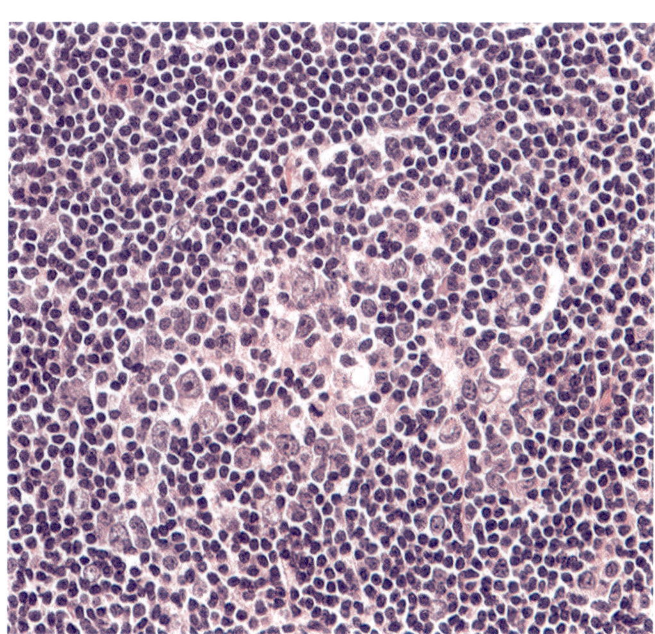

FIGURE 2-10

FIGURE 2-8 This lymph node shows several enlarged follicles with progressive transformation in a background of florid follicular hyperplasia.

FIGURE 2-9 Mantle layer cells haphazardly infiltrate the germinal center, imparting an irregular and disorganized appearance.

FIGURE 2-10 The residual germinal center is small and irregular and infiltrated by monotonous mantle layer cells.

Dermatopathic Lymphadenopathy

DEFINITION

This is a reactive lymph node condition characterized by paracortical infiltrates of interdigitating dendritic cells, Langerhans cells, and pigment- and lipid-laden histiocytes. Dermatopathic lymphadenopathy (DL) is frequently associated with chronic dermatologic conditions.

CLINICAL FEATURES

- DL usually involves axillary and inguinal lymph nodes.
- It is commonly associated with benign (psoriasis, eczema) or malignant (mycosis fungoides/Sezary syndrome) skin conditions.

HISTOLOGIC FINDINGS

- Lymph nodes with DL have preserved architecture with prominent paracortical hyperplasia, which at low-power has the appearance of pale subcapsular nodules (Figure 2-11).
- The paracortex is expanded by dendritic cells (interdigitating dendritic cells and Langerhans cells), which are large cells with delicate nuclear infoldings and grooves and abundant eosinophilic cytoplasm (Figure 2-12).
- Admixed with the dendritic cells are macrophages with foamy, lipid-containing cytoplasm, and pigment-laden histiocytes, usually containing melanin.
- Small, mature T lymphocytes, eosinophils, and plasma cells may also be identified.
- Interdigitating dendritic cells are S100(+), while Langerhans cells are S100(+), CD1a(+), and langerin(+).

DIFFERENTIAL DIAGNOSIS

- Early lymph node involvement by mycosis fungoides/Sezary syndrome
- Classical Hodgkin lymphoma

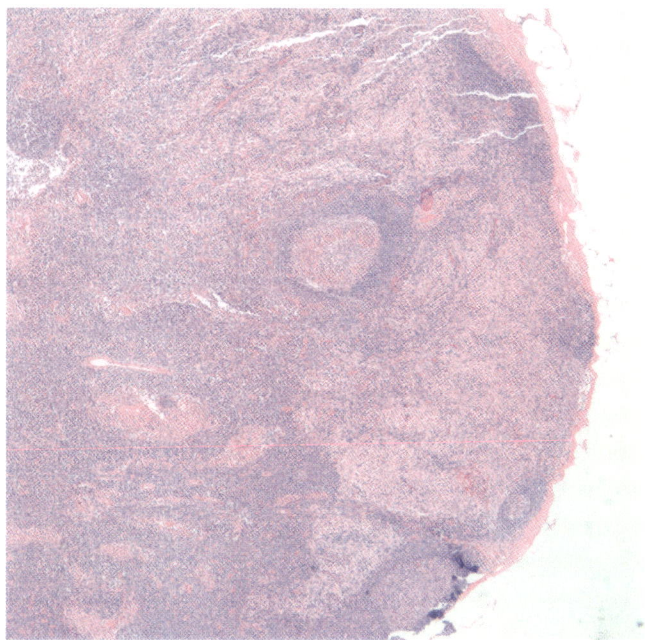

FIGURE 2-11

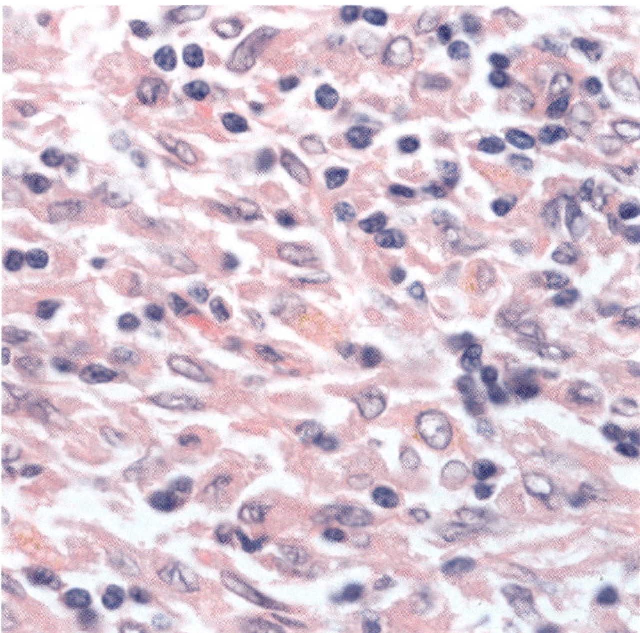

FIGURE 2-12

FIGURE 2-11 This lymph node shows prominent paracortical hyperplasia, consisting of pale-appearing subcortical nodules.

FIGURE 2-12 High-power appearance of a collection of interdigitating dendritic cells, Langerhans cells, and pigment-laden macrophages.

3

Lymphadenopathies Associated With Systemic Disorders

KIMURA LYMPHADENOPATHY

SINUS HISTIOCYTOSIS WITH MASSIVE LYMPHADENOPATHY (ROSAI-DORFMAN DISEASE)

KIKUCHI-FUJIMOTO LYMPHADENOPATHY

SARCOIDOSIS

SYSTEMIC LUPUS ERYTHEMATOSUS LYMPHADENOPATHY

RHEUMATOID LYMPHADENOPATHY

CASTLEMAN DISEASE
- Hyaline Vascular Castleman Disease
- Unicentric Castleman Disease, Plasma Cell Variant
- Multicentric Disease

STILL'S DISEASE

IGG4-RELATED SCLEROSING DISEASE

AUTOIMMUNE LYMPHOPROLIFERATIVE SYNDROME

Kimura Lymphadenopathy

DEFINITION

Also known as eosinophilic lymphogranuloma, Kimura lymphadenopathy is a rare chronic inflammatory disease of the subcutaneous tissue and lymph nodes of the head and neck area characterized by eosinophilic infiltrates with follicular and vascular hyperplasia. Although it is considered to be a benign reactive condition, the etiology and pathogenesis of Kimura lymphadenopathy are unknown.

CLINICAL FEATURES

- Most cases of Kimura's disease are described in Asia (endemic in Japan, China, Taiwan, and Hong Kong)
- This disorder is more common in men than in women (3:1 ratio), with a peak incidence between 27 and 40 years of age.
- Kimura's disease presents with large, painless tumors in the deep subcutaneous tissue of the head and neck, particularly in the infra- and retroauricular areas.
- Other sites of involvement include the axillary, inguinal, and arm regions.
- Peripheral blood eosinophilia and increased levels of serum IgE are present in all cases.
- No skin lesions (ulceration or bleeding) are present, important features for the differential diagnosis with angiolymphoid hyperplasia with eosinophilia.

HISTOLOGIC FINDINGS

- Involved lymph nodes show preserved architecture with prominent follicular hyperplasia, proliferation of postcapillary venules, thickened capsule, and perinodal inflammatory infiltrate (Figures 3-1 and 3-2).
- Paracortical and sinusoidal eosinophilic infiltrates are present, with formation of eosinophilic microabscesses or diffuse eosinophilia (Figures 3-2 and 3-3).
- Follicle lysis, vascularization of germinal centers, and germinal center necrosis can also be seen.
- Warthin-Finkeldey polykaryocytes, though non-specific, are commonly found in the germinal centers or in the paracortex.
- Older lesions may show sclerosis.

DIFFERENTIAL DIAGNOSIS

- Angiolymphoid hyperplasia with eosinophilia
- Classical Hodgkin lymphoma
- Hyaline vascular Castleman disease
- Lymphadenopathy with florid follicular hyperplasia
- Drug-induced lymphadenopathy
- Parasite infections with lymphadenopathy with eosinophilia

FIGURE 3-1 This lymph node displays preserved architecture, thickened capsule, perilymphadenitis, and follicular hyperplasia.

FIGURE 3-2 Lesions demonstrate an eosinophilic infiltrate and vascular proliferation.

FIGURE 3-3 This image demonstrates an eosinophilic microabscess in the paracortex.

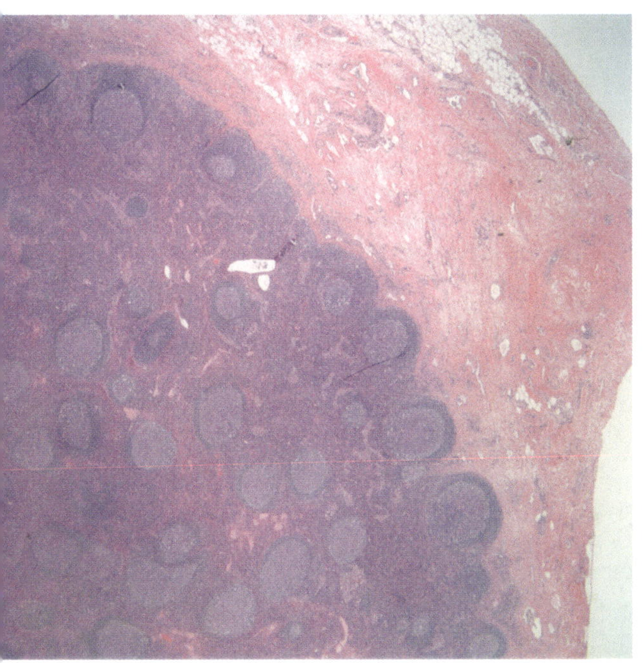

FIGURE 3-1

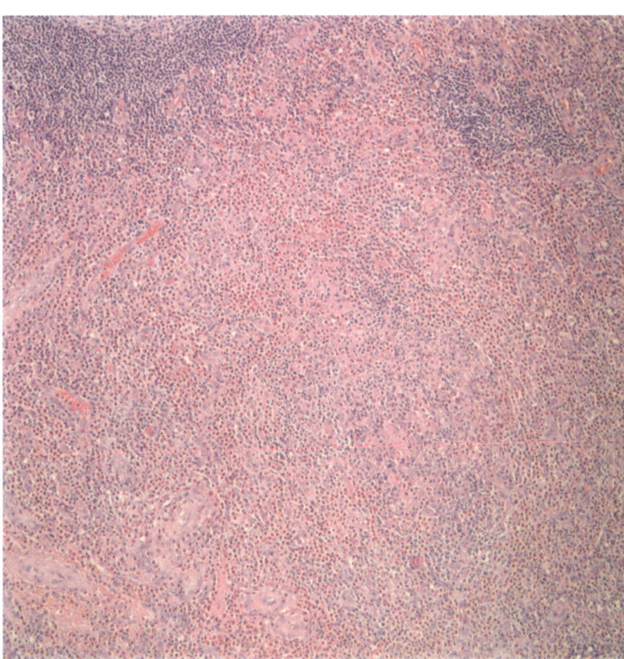

FIGURE 3-2

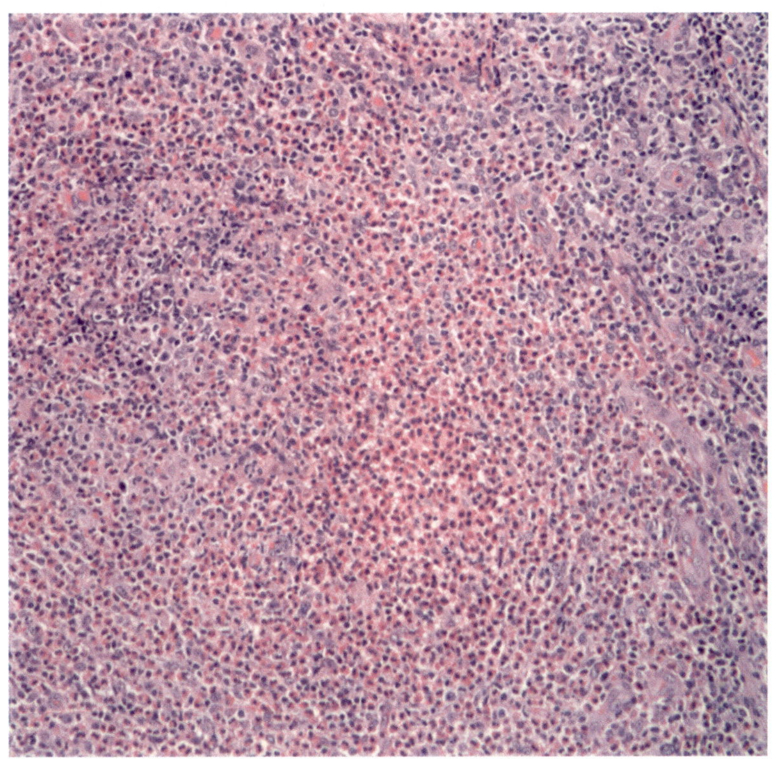

FIGURE 3-3

Sinus Histiocytosis With Massive Lymphadenopathy (Rosai-Dorfman Disease)

DEFINITION

This syndrome represents a benign disorder consisting of lymph node enlargement or extranodal mass lesions produced by a proliferation of characteristic Rosai-Dorfman histiocytes that contain engulfed lymphocytes and other cells (emperipolesis).

CLINICAL FEATURES

- The typical presentation is with prominent bilateral cervical lymphadenopathy.
- Common extranodal sites include head and neck, soft tissue, skin, respiratory and GI tract, breast, bones, and central nervous system.
- The peak incidence is at 21 years (range, 0–74 years), with a higher incidence in men than in women (3:2 ratio).
- Nonspecific symptoms (fever, night sweats, leukocytosis, polyclonal hypergammaglobulinemia) may be encountered in a subset of patients.
- Rare fatal cases occur in patients with involvement of vital organs.
- Association with solid tumors or hematologic neoplasms has been occasionally reported.

HISTOLOGIC FINDINGS

- Involved lymph nodes show effaced architecture with thickened capsule and a prominent dilation of sinuses by histiocytes, lymphocytes and plasma cells (Figures 3-4 and 3-5).
- The histiocytes are large, with regular nuclei, vesicular chromatin, prominent central nucleoli, and abundant pale cytoplasm containing engulfed intact cells (emperipolesis) (Figures 3-5 and 3-6), primarily lymphocytes, but occasionally plasma cells or neutrophils.
- Plasma cell infiltrates are prominent between the aggregates of histiocytes.
- Rosai-Dorfman disease associated with follicular lymphoma or nodular lymphocyte-predominant Hodgkin lymphoma usually presents as limited areas of sinusoidal involvement.
- Rosai-Dorfman histiocytes are positive for S100 and the monocyte/macrophage-associated antigens CD11b, CD14, CD68, CD163, but are CD1a(−).

DIFFERENTIAL DIAGNOSIS

- Nonspecific sinus histiocytosis
- Granulomatous lymphadenitis
- Langerhans cell histiocytosis
- Classical Hodgkin lymphoma

FIGURE 3-4 This lymph node shows a thickened capsule and florid sinus histiocytosis.

FIGURE 3-5 This dilated sinus shows histiocytosis and emperipolesis. The surrounding parenchyma contains numerous plasma cells.

FIGURE 3-6 Characteristic Rosai-Dorfman histiocytes show round nuclei, distinct central nucleoli, and abundant, finely granular cytoplasm, with emperipolesis.

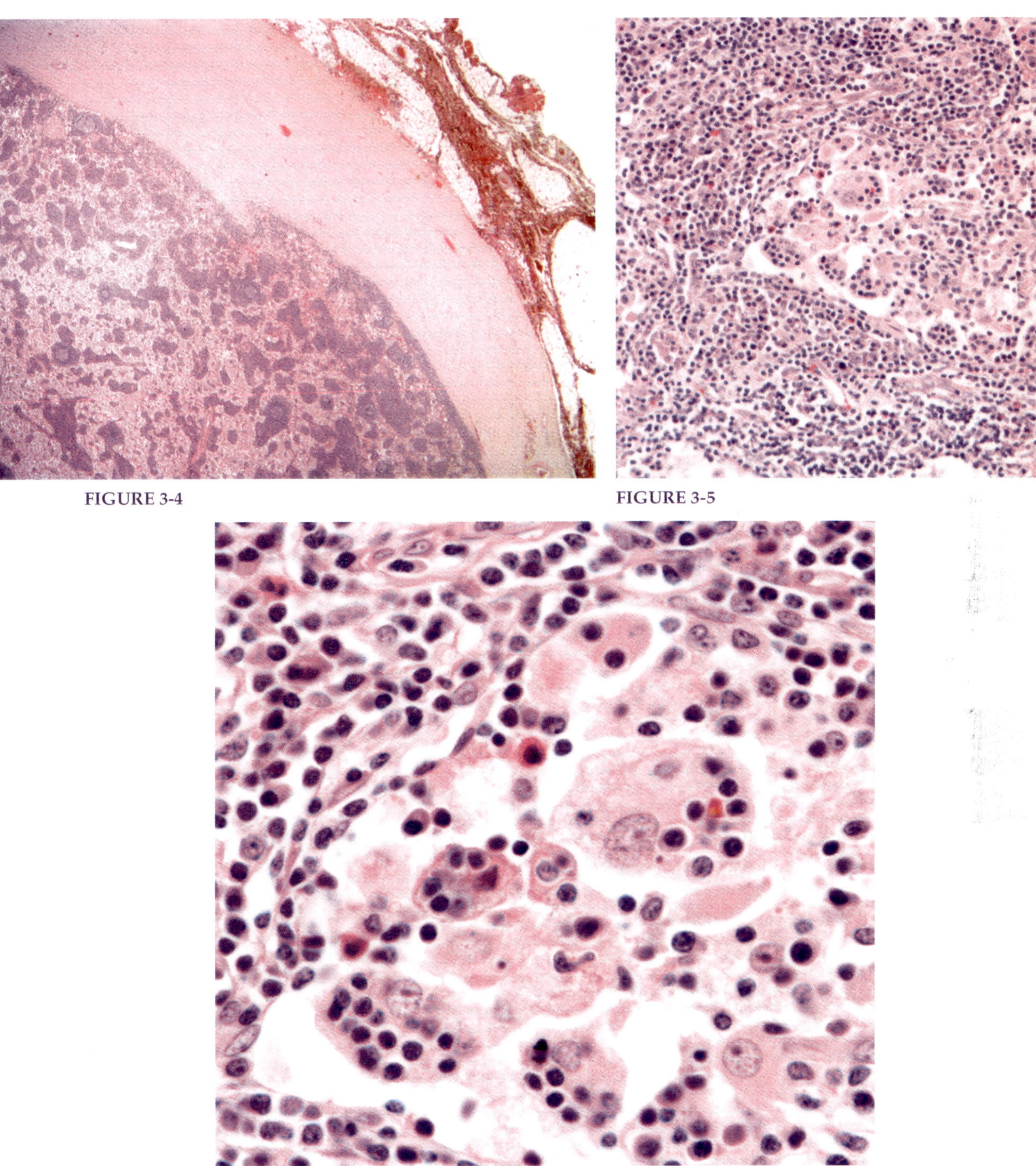

FIGURE 3-4

FIGURE 3-5

FIGURE 3-6

Kikuchi-Fujimoto Lymphadenopathy

DEFINITION

Also known as histiocytic necrotizing lymphadenitis, Kikuchi-Fujimoto lymphadenopathy is a relatively uncommon febrile condition associated with subacute necrotizing lymphadenitis.

CLINICAL FEATURES

- Most cases are described in young Asian patients; this demographic preponderance may be related to certain HLA class II genes.
- This disorder is more common in women than in men (3–4:1 ratio), with a peak incidence between 25–29 years (range, 2–75 years).
- Kikuchi-Fujimoto disease usually presents with subacute (2–3 weeks), occasionally tender, cervical lymphadenopathy; generalized lymphadenopathy can occur in 20% of cases.
- Nonspecific symptoms include fever, night sweats, weight loss, and nausea.
- Other sites of involvement include the skin, bone marrow, or multiple organ systems (in solid organ transplant recipients).

HISTOLOGIC FINDINGS

- The morphologic triad of karyorrhectic debris, crescentic histiocytes, and paracortical clusters of plasmacytoid monocytes represents a minimal diagnostic criterion.
- The lymph node shows partially preserved architecture with reactive follicles, paracortical hyperplasia, and wedge-shaped areas of fibrinoid necrosis with a paracortical distribution (Figure 3-7).
- The necrotic areas consist of karyorrhectic debris with a conspicuous lack of neutrophils, with frequent phagocytic histiocytes with abundant, pale cytoplasm, and eccentrically displaced nuclei (crescentic histiocytes) (Figure 3-8).
- Clusters of plasmacytoid monocytes surround areas of necrosis (Figure 3-9); these are admixed with histiocytes, immunoblasts, and small lymphocytes.
- Occasional immunoblasts and/or plasmacytoid monocytes may show cytologic atypia.
- Three histologic types have been described: proliferative (29% of cases), necrotizing (53% of cases), and xanthomatous (18% cases).
- Immunohistochemistry shows a predominance of CD3(+)/CD8(+) cytotoxic T lymphocytes; histiocytes are CD68(+) and myeloperoxidase(+); plasmacytoid monocytes are CD123(+) and MPO(−); immunoblasts are CD30(+), CD45(+), CD15(−).

DIFFERENTIAL DIAGNOSIS

- Lymph node infarction
- Systemic lupus erythematosus lymphadenitis
- Necrotizing lymphadenitis due to specific agents (tuberculosis, histoplasmosis, syphilis, bacteria, or viruses: HSV and EBV)
- Cat-scratch lymphadenitis
- Large cell lymphoma

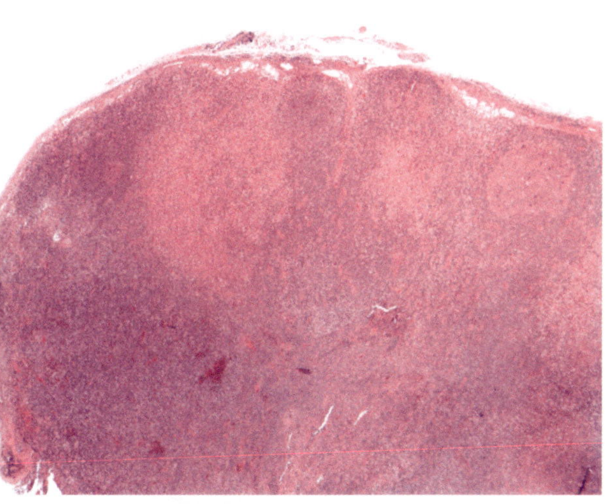

FIGURE 3-7

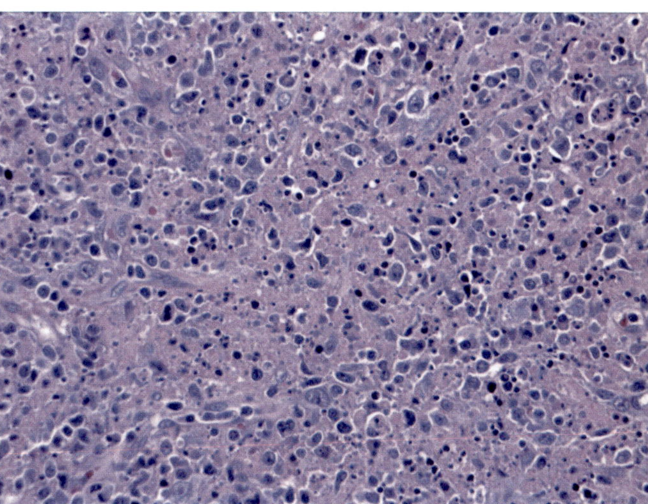

FIGURE 3-8

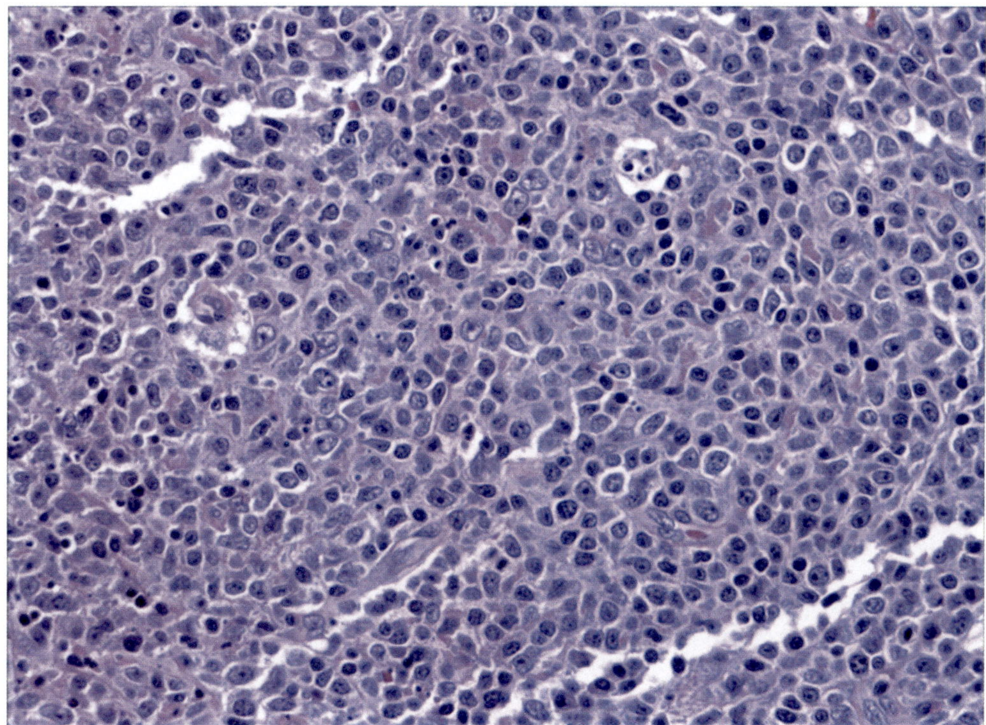

FIGURE 3-9

FIGURE 3-7 This example shows partially effaced architecture, reactive follicles, paracortical hyperplasia, and pale, wedge-shaped areas of paracortical necrosis.

FIGURE 3-8 Necrotic areas contain abundant apoptotic debris with an absence of neutrophils and heterogeneous mononuclear cells, including crescentic histiocytes.

FIGURE 3-9 This cellular area shows abundant plasmacytoid dendritic cells and scattered immunoblasts.

Sarcoidosis

DEFINITION

This is a condition of unknown etiology characterized by granulomatous inflammation involving multiple organ systems.

CLINICAL FEATURES

- Sarcoidosis has a worldwide distribution, with Northern Europeans and African Americans demonstrating a particularly high risk. In the US, the incidence is 10 times higher in African-Americans than in Caucasians.
- The peak incidence in the U.S. is in the 3rd decade (Caucasians) or 4th decade (African-Americans).
- Women are affected more commonly than men.
- Sarcoidosis presents in 90% of patients with a combination of hilar lymphadenopathy, pulmonary, skin, or ocular involvement.
- The onset of sarcoidosis is typically gradual. Acute presentation (Lofgren's syndrome) is less common and consists of fever, hilar lymphadenopathy, erythema nodosum, and lower extremity arthritis.
- An elevated CD4/CD8 ratio in bronchoaleveolar lavage fluid has high specificity, but low sensitivity for sarcoidosis.
- Hypercalciuria and increased serum ACE and lysozyme are present in 40–80% of patients.

HISTOLOGIC FINDINGS

- Lymph nodes show diffuse or partial replacement by non-caseating granulomatous inflammation (Figures 3-10 and 3-11).
- Non-necrotizing granulomas are composed of epithelioid histiocytes and multinucleated giant cells (Figures 3-11–3-13).
- Schaumann bodies, asteroid bodies, birefringent crystals, and Hamazaki-Wesenberg bodies can also be seen (Figures 3-12 and 3-13).
- Acid-fast and fungal special stains are negative. Of note, acid-fast stains (Ziehl-Neelsen, Kinyoun, and auramine O) have low sensitivity in tissues for microorganisms.

DIFFERENTIAL DIAGNOSIS

- Mycobacterial, fungal, and parasitic granulomatous lymphadenitides
- Berylliosis (and other pneumoconioses)
- Classical Hodgkin lymphoma
- Lymphoepithelioid peripheral T-cell lymphoma (Lennert lymphoma)

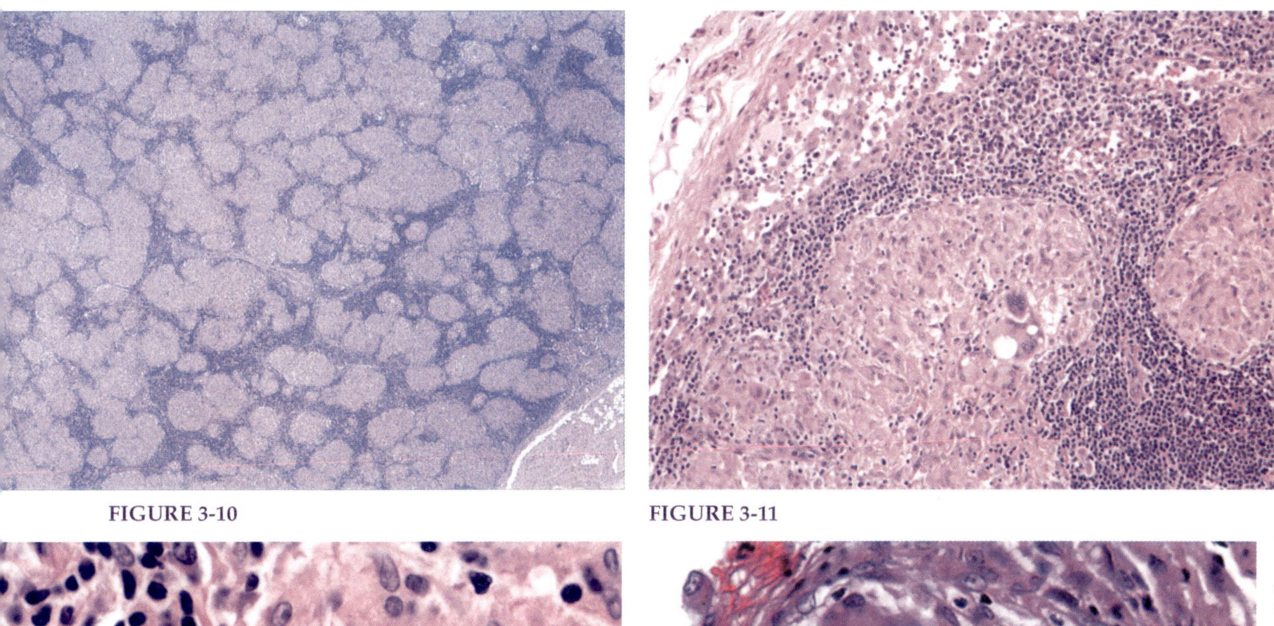

FIGURE 3-10

FIGURE 3-11

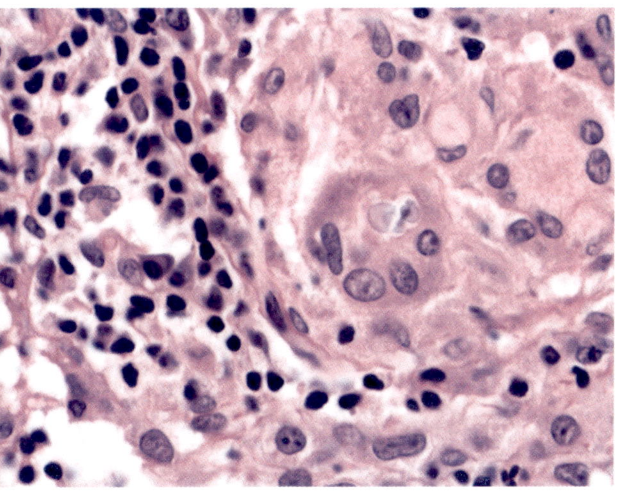

FIGURE 3-12

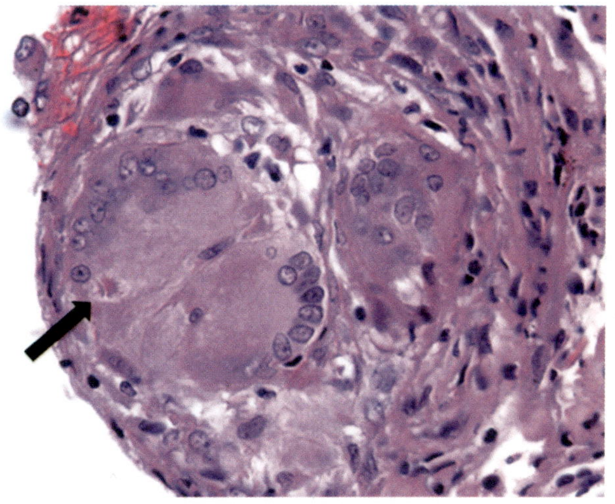

FIGURE 3-13

FIGURE 3-10 This lymph node is largely replaced by innumerable, well-formed, non-necrotizing granulomas.

FIGURE 3-11 Medium-power reveals that the granulomas are composed of epithelioid histiocytes and multinucleated giant cells.

FIGURE 3-12 This multinucleated giant cell contains a Schaumann body (calcified, concentrically lamellar, intracytoplasmic inclusion).

FIGURE 3-13 Asteroid bodies (arrow) may occasionally be seen within multinucleated giant cells.

Systemic Lupus Erythematosus Lymphadenopathy

DEFINITION

This represents reactive lymph node enlargement associated with systemic lupus erythematosus (SLE).

CLINICAL FEATURES

- In the U.S., SLE is 3–4 times more common in African Americans than in Caucasians, and is more common in women than in men (3.5:1 ratio).
- The median age of incidence is between 20 and 30 years.
- The clinical course is highly variable, with episodes of exacerbation alternating with quiescent periods.
- Constitutional symptoms (fever, weight loss, fatigue) are present in 100% of patients.
- Skin rash and musculoskeletal symptoms (arthritis, myalgia) are seen in 75–100% of patients.
- Cytopenias, pleuritis, pericarditis, neurologic and renal symptoms are present in 50–60% of patients.
- Lymphadenopathy is more common in active disease and in the presence of high titers of anti-double stranded DNA antibodies.
- Cervical lymphadenopathy is most common; mesenteric, axillary, inguinal, and retroperitoneal lymph nodes can also be involved.

HISTOLOGIC FINDINGS

- The classic histologic findings of lupus lymphadenopathy occur in patients with acute disease.
- Lymph nodes show prominent necrotic areas in the paracortex, without neutrophils or eosinophils (Figures 3-14 and 3-15).
- In a subset of cases, the areas of necrosis contain hematoxylin bodies, consisting of amorphous, deeply basophilic extracellular material, and blood vessels with fibrinoid necrosis and deposits of basophilic nuclear debris (Azzopardi phenomenon) (Figure 3-15).
- Follicular and paracortical hyperplasia are present in the viable portions of the lymph node.

DIFFERENTIAL DIAGNOSIS

- Kikuchi-Fujimoto lymphadenopathy
- Infectious mononucleosis

FIGURE 3-14 This lymph node contains extensive areas of geographic necrosis.

FIGURE 3-15 High-power magnification demonstrates prominent apoptotic debris without neutrophils or eosinophils, adjacent to a vessel with fibrinoid necrosis.

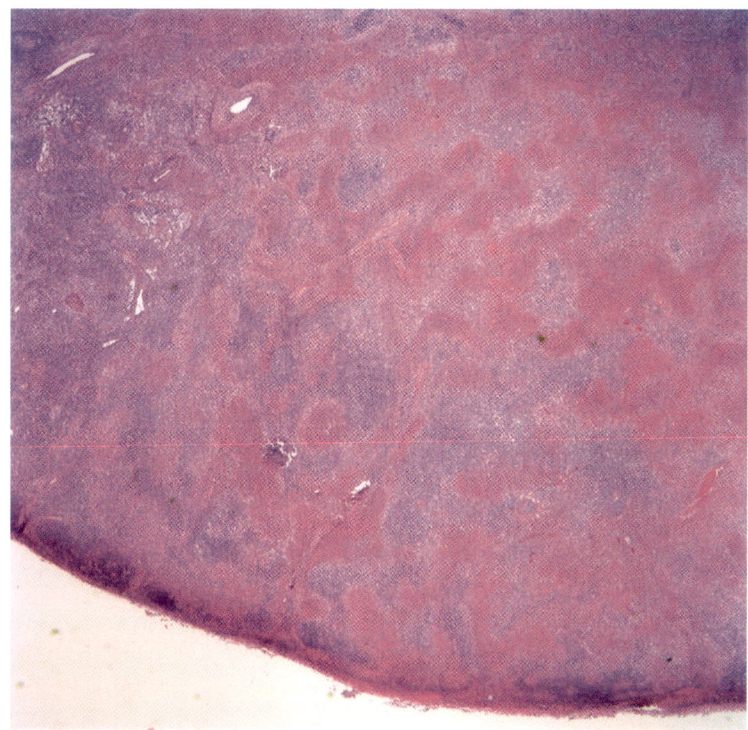

FIGURE 3-14

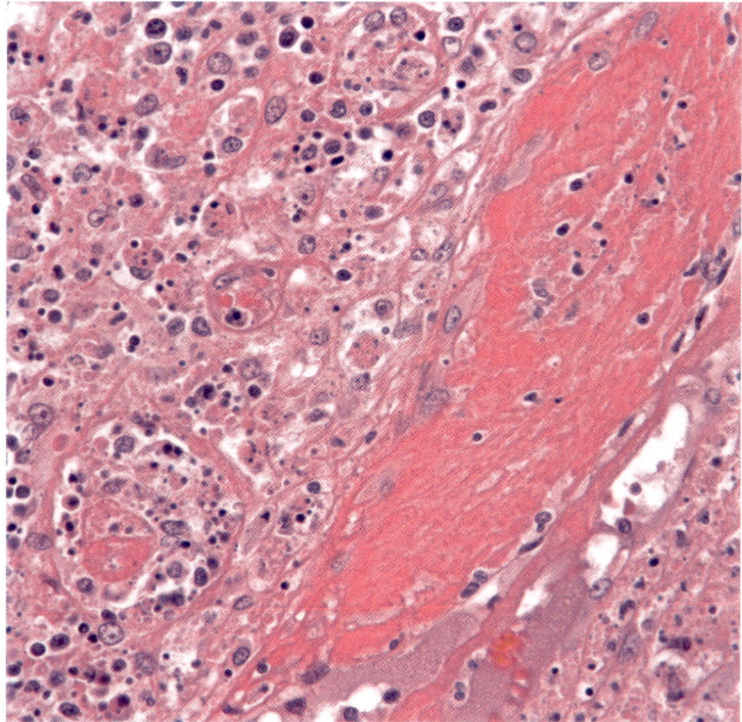

FIGURE 3-15

Rheumatoid Lymphadenopathy

DEFINITION

This entity consists of reactive lymph node enlargement associated with rheumatoid arthritis (RA).

CLINICAL FEATURES

- RA is an autoimmune disease with systemic manifestations, primarily presenting with symmetric arthritis.
- RA is more common in women than in men (4:1 ratio), with a peak incidence between 35 and 50 years.
- Lymphadenopathy occurs in 50–75% of patients, most often involving axillary, cervical and supraclavicular lymph nodes.
- Nonspecific symptoms (fever, weight loss, fatigue), polyclonal hypergammaglobulinemia, and cryoglobulinemia are common.
- Serology (rheumatoid factor) is positive in 75% of patients.
- Some patients have splenomegaly and cytopenias (Felty syndrome).

HISTOLOGIC FINDINGS

- The lymph node shows striking follicular and paracortical hyperplasia (Figures 3-16 and 3-17).
- The reactive follicles show variable shape and size and have well-defined mantle zones and prominent germinal centers with tingible body macrophages (Figure 3-17).
- Paracortical hyperplasia is due to clusters of plasma cells, immunoblasts, and vascular proliferation (Figure 3-17).
- Perilymphadenitis, with inflammatory cells disrupting the capsule and spilling over into the extranodal fat is frequently present.
- Focal areas of necrosis and hyaline material may be encountered.

DIFFERENTIAL DIAGNOSIS

- Syphilis lymphadenitis
- Multicentric Castleman disease
- Angioimmunoblastic T-cell lymphoma (AITL)

FIGURE 3-16 This lymph node shows prominent follicular and paracortical hyperplasia.

FIGURE 3-17 This secondary follicle demonstrates a reactive germinal center with polarization and well circumscribed mantle zone, adjacent to an area of paracortical expansion with increased vascular proliferation and frequent tingible body macrophages.

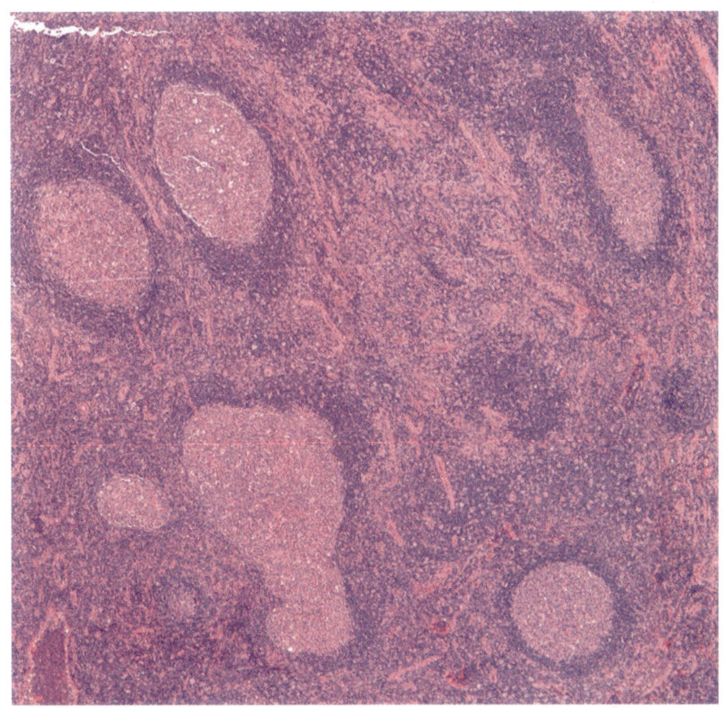

FIGURE 3-16

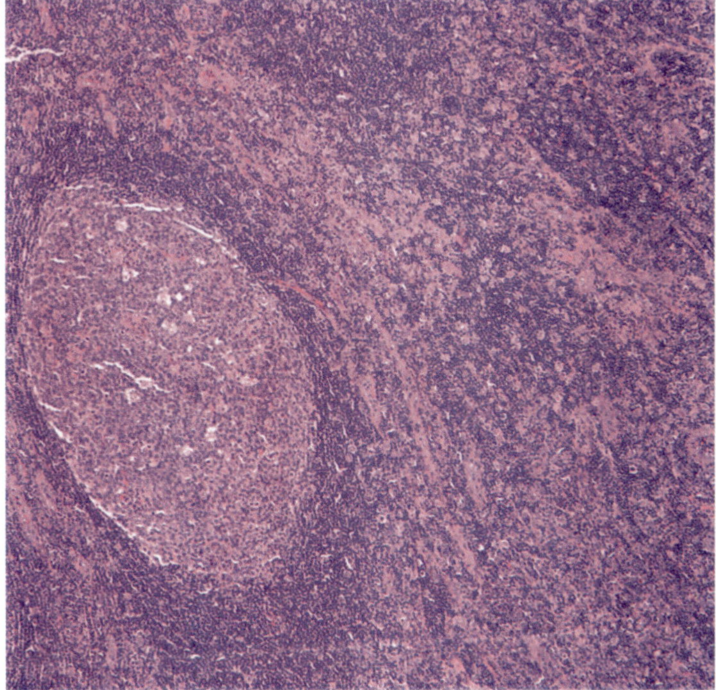

FIGURE 3-17

Castleman Disease

DEFINITION

Castleman disease is the term used to describe a group of lymphoproliferative disorders with heterogeneous clinical (unicentric and multicentric variant) and morphologic features (hyaline vascular and plasma cell variant).

HYALINE VASCULAR CASTLEMAN DISEASE

CLINICAL FEATURES

- Hyaline vascular Castleman disease is essentially always unicentric, and comprises 80–90% of unicentric Castleman disease cases.
- This disorder shows no gender predilection, and has a peak incidence in the 4th decade.
- The typical presentation is with mediastinal lymphadenopathy; other sites of involvement include the axillary, cervical, and abdominal regions.

HISTOLOGIC FINDINGS

- The capsule is often thickened and fibrotic.
- The lymph node shows distorted architecture, with loss of normal cortical and medullary differentiation and obliterated sinuses in most cases.
- There are numerous, variably sized follicles (Figure 3-18) containing involuted germinal centers and hyaline deposits; some follicles are confluent and share multiple germinal centers (Figure 3-19).
- Involuted germinal centers contain few lymphocytes, and consist of flattened, concentrically layered follicular dendritic cells and endothelial cells, and are surrounded by broad mantle zones with "onion skin" patterned small lymphocytes (Figure 3-20).
- Some follicles show "lollipop" lesions (radially penetrating arterioles with sclerotic walls) (Figure 3-20).
- The interfollicular areas are occupied and expanded by a proliferation of small vessels with variable hyaline change (Figure 3-21). Endothelial cells are usually flattened, but are occasionally plump.
- Larger muscular vessels may undergo progressive sclerosis, with resultant fibrotic nodules.

DIFFERENTIAL DIAGNOSIS

- Reactive lymphadenopathy
- HIV lymphadenopathy
- Follicular lymphoma
- Mantle cell lymphoma
- Marginal zone lymphoma

(continued)

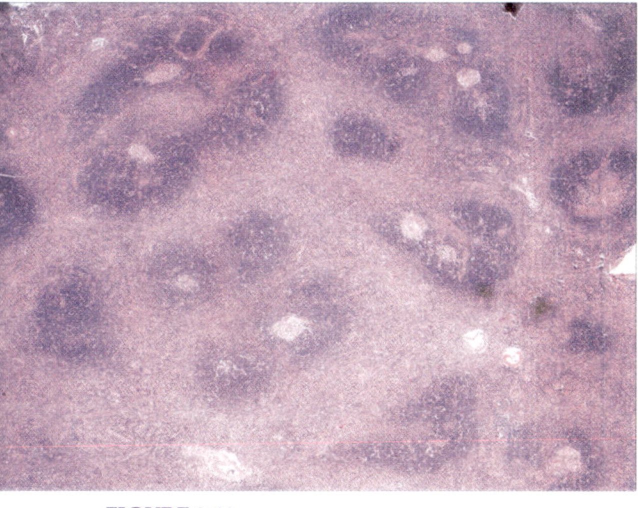

FIGURE 3-18

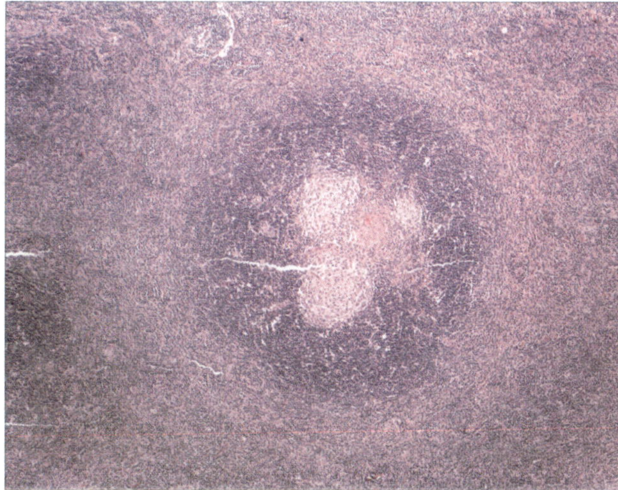

FIGURE 3-19

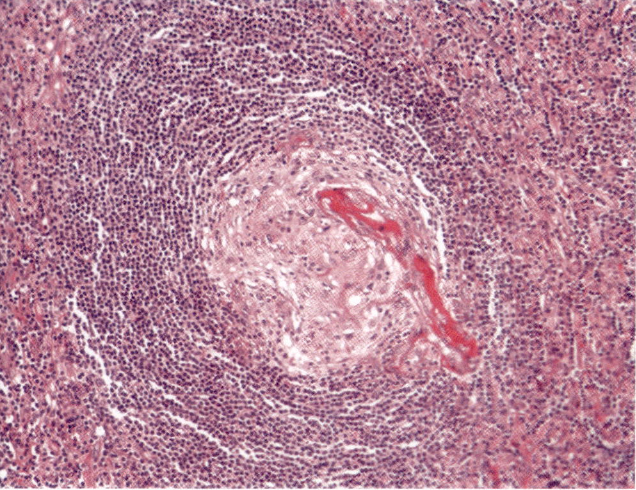

FIGURE 3-20

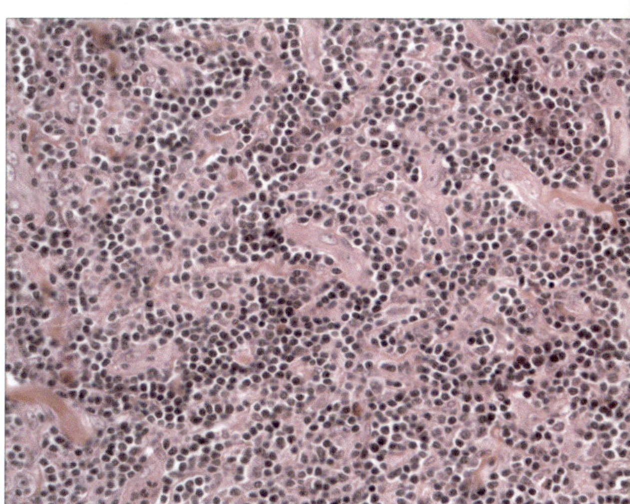

FIGURE 3-21

FIGURE 3-18 This low-power image demonstrates follicles with regressed germinal centers and broad mantle zones.

FIGURE 3-19 This field demonstrates an enlarged follicle with multiple germinal centers and increased vascularity.

FIGURE 3-20 Involuted follicle often have an "onion skin" expanded mantle zone and "lollipop" lesion.

FIGURE 3-21 There is a paracortical proliferation of small vessels evident, several with hyaline change.

Castleman Disease *(continued)*

UNICENTRIC CASTLEMAN DISEASE, PLASMA CELL VARIANT

CLINICAL FEATURES

- Unicentric plasma cell variant of Castleman disease comprises 10–20% of unicentric Castleman disease.
- This disorder shows a similar age and gender distribution as hyaline vascular variant.
- Plasma cell Castleman disease most often present in the abdomen (56%), followed by anterior mediastinum (38%).
- Some patients present with constitutional symptoms.

HISTOLOGIC FINDINGS

- The lymph node shows preserved architecture with follicular hyperplasia and prominent interfollicular plasma cell infiltrates (Figures 3-22 and 3-23). Follicles are not regressed, but instead display banal hyperplastic features.

DIFFERENTIAL DIAGNOSIS

- Rheumatoid lymphadenopathy
- Lymphoplasmacytic lymphoma
- Plasmacytoma

(continued)

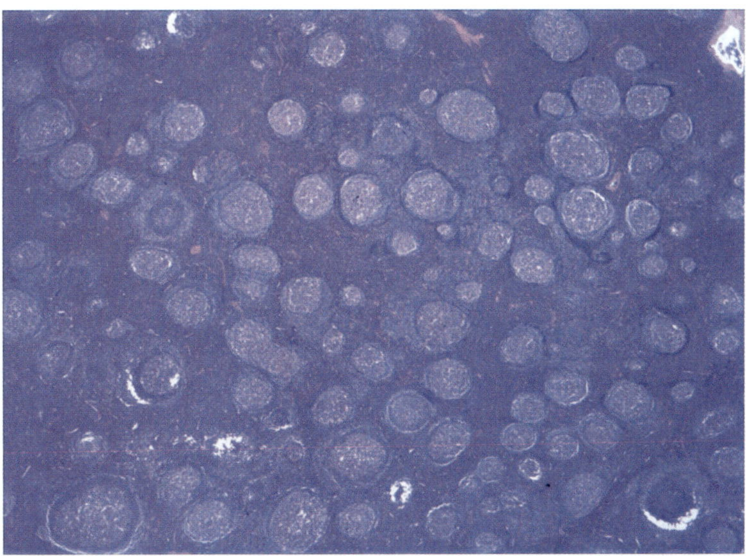

FIGURE 3-22

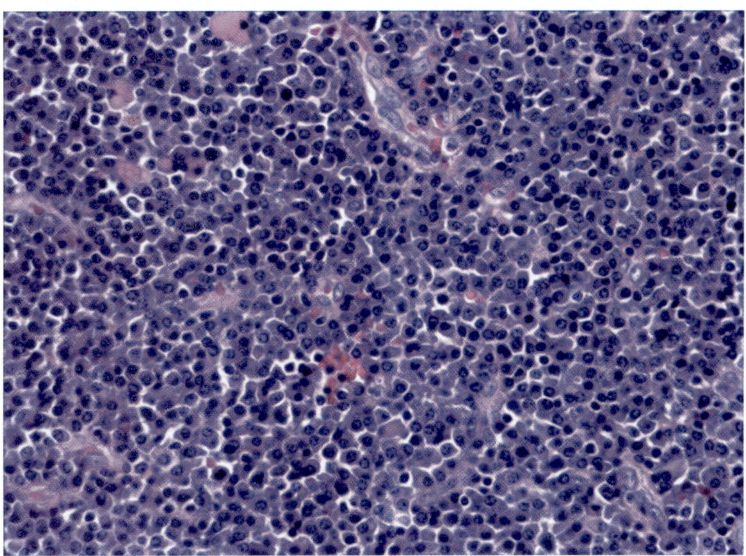

FIGURE 3-23

FIGURE 3-22 This low-power image of a lymph node shows striking follicular hyperplasia.
FIGURE 3-23 Interfollicular sheets of mature plasma cells are present.

Castleman Disease *(continued)*

MULTICENTRIC CASTLEMAN DISEASE

CLINICAL FEATURES

- Multicentric Castleman disease is most common in HIV-infected individuals.
- This disorder demonstrates a male predilection with a peak incidence at age 40 in HIV positive individuals and age 50–60 in the non-HIV population.
- By definition, multicentric Castleman disease presents with extensive lymphadenopathy and organomegaly.
- Constitutional symptoms (fever, night sweats, weight loss), cytopenias, polyclonal hypergammaglobulinemia, and elevated LDH are common features.
- Multicentric Castleman disease shows a strong association with Kaposi's sarcoma (Figure 3-24).
- Some cases are associated with POEMS syndrome (Polyneuropathy, organomegaly, endocrinopathy, edema, M-protein, and skin lesions).
- Multicentric Castleman disease is associated with HHV-8 infection in many cases [HIV-associated cases are uniformly HHV-8(+)].

HISTOLOGIC FINDINGS

- The histologic findings are similar to unicentric Castleman disease, plasma cell variant, although follicles show a morphologic spectrum from hyperplastic to regressed, and interfollicular vascularity is more prominent.
- Interfollicular mature plasmacytosis is a feature of both HHV-8(−) and HHV-8(+) cases. HHV-8(+) cases are additionally characterized by varying numbers of HHV-8(+) "plasmablasts" in the mantle zones of follicles (Figures 3-25 and 3-26).

DIFFERENTIAL DIAGNOSIS

Similar to unicentric Castleman disease, plasma cell variant

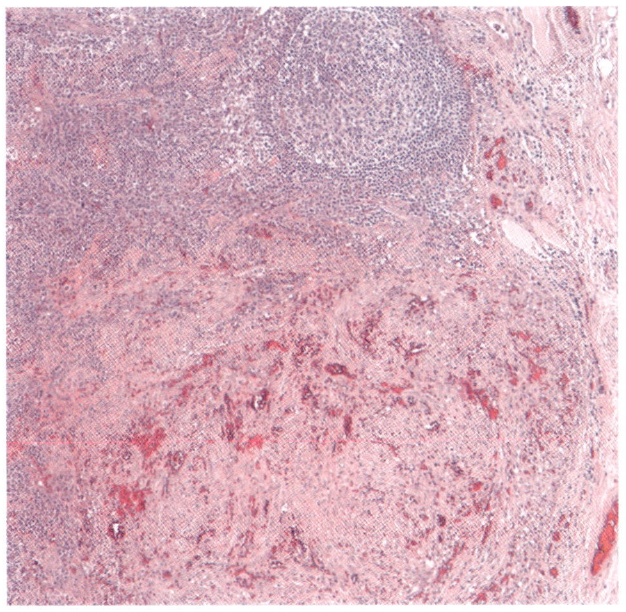

FIGURE 3-24

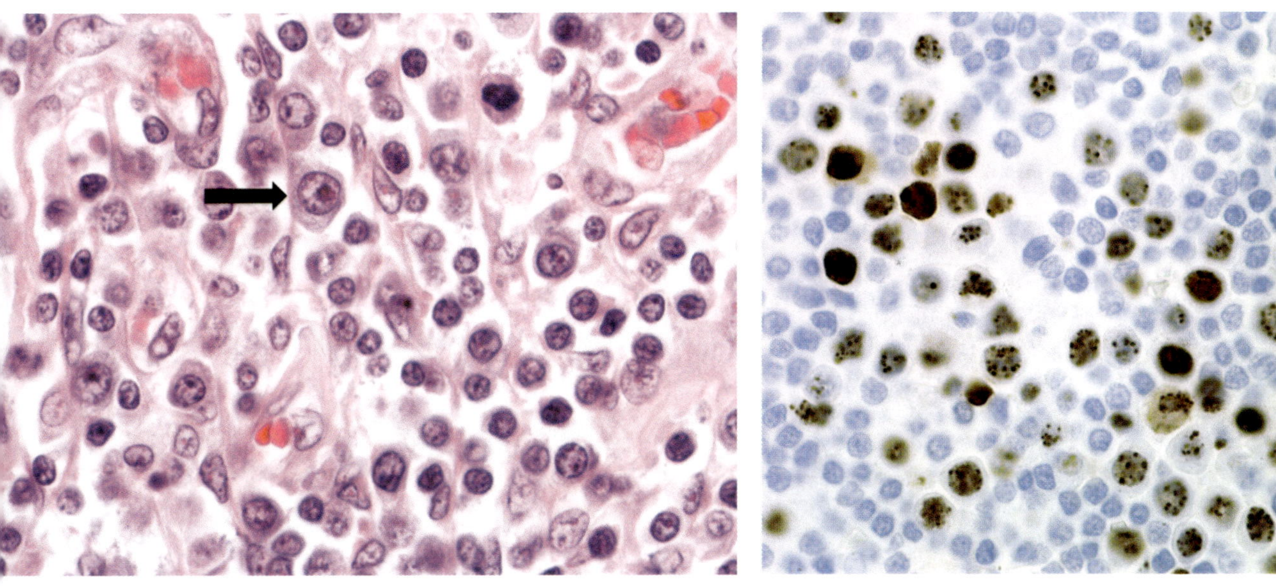

FIGURE 3-25

FIGURE 3-26

FIGURE 3-24 Kaposi's sarcoma (lower half of field) associated with multicentric Castleman disease.

FIGURE 3-25 Plasmablasts with prominent central nucleoli and dispersed chromatin (arrow) in the mantle zone of a follicle.

FIGURE 3-26 HHV8 immunohistochemistry in an HIV patient with multicentric Castleman disease demonstrates HHV8 expression in plasmablasts.

Still's Disease

DEFINITION

Still's disease is a systemic form of the chronic inflammatory disorder juvenile rheumatoid arthritis. The etiology is unknown.

CLINICAL FEATURES

- Most patients present by age 16; presentation in adulthood is rare. The peak incidence in adult onset Still's disease (AOSD) is between 15–25 years and 36–46 years. Males and females are affected equally.
- Patients have the following constellation of findings: high fever, rash, arthralgias, and organomegaly.
- Lymphadenopathy is present in 44–90% of patients with AOSD.

HISTOLOGIC FINDINGS

- Several histologic patterns have been described in Still's disease, including paracortical hyperplasia with and without florid immunoblastic reactions, follicular hyperplasia, and sinus histiocytosis.
- Most cases show paracortical hyperplasia (Figure 3-27), with the paracortex distorted and expanded by a heterogeneous infiltrate of small and medium-sized lymphocytes that lack atypia, immunoblasts, high endothelial venules, and scattered plasma cells and eosinophils (Figure 3-28). The majority of the paracortical infiltrate consists of T cells, with slightly more CD4(+) T cells than CD8(+) T cells.
- Immunoblasts may be present in significantly increased numbers, causing potential diagnostic confusion with lymphoma (Figure 3-29). Both T- and B immunoblasts are present.
- Sinuses are usually patent and may show variable sinus histiocytosis.
- Nonspecific follicular hyperplasia is less commonly observed. Atrophic, hyalinized germinal centers have been described in few cases.
- Monocytoid B cell collections may also be observed.
- Areas closely resembling Kikuchi-Fujimoto lymphadenitis may also be observed.

DIFFERENTIAL DIAGNOSIS

- Viral-associated lymphadenopathy, including infectious mononucleosis and cytomegalovirus lymphadenitis
- Angioimmunoblastic T-cell lymphoma
- Peripheral T-cell lymphoma, not otherwise specified
- Castleman disease

FIGURE 3-27

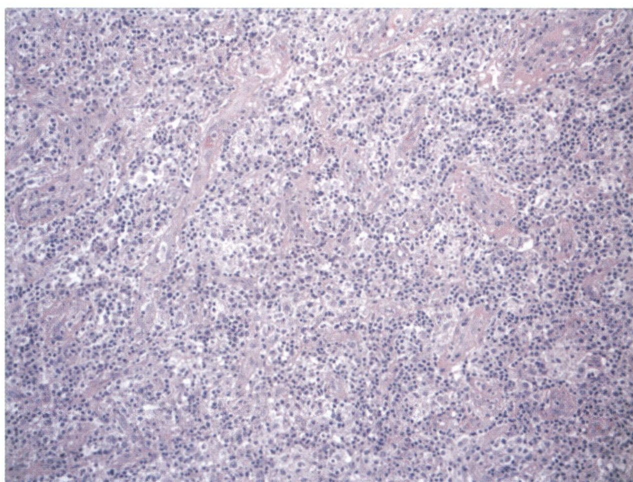

FIGURE 3-28

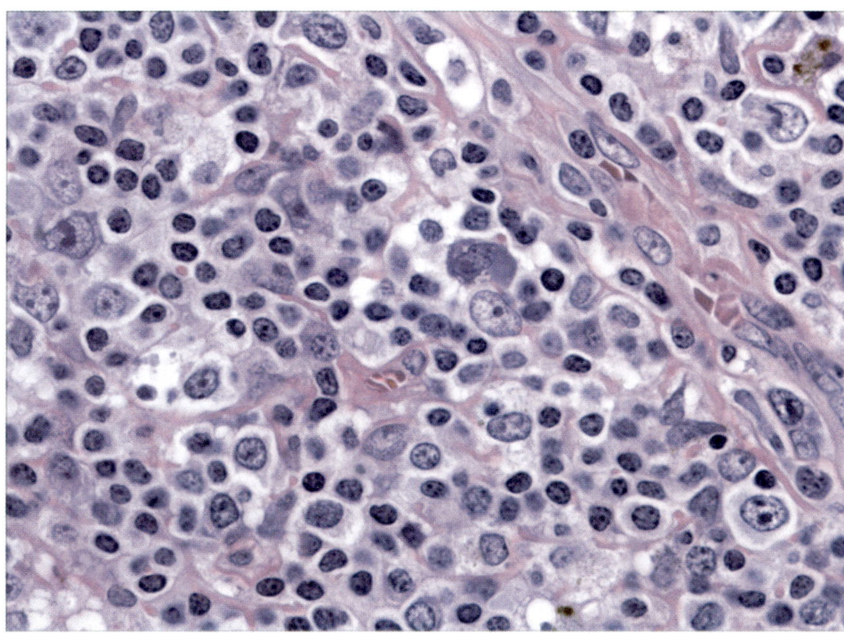

FIGURE 3-29

FIGURE 3-27 Low-power examination reveals a prominent paracortical expansion with few scattered reactive follicles.

FIGURE 3-28 This intermediate power image demonstrates a prominent increase in paracortical vascularity.

FIGURE 3-29 High-power reveals a heterogeneous cellular infiltrate, including increased immunoblasts.

IgG4-Related Sclerosing Disease

DEFINITION

IgG4-related sclerosing disease is a newly described entity characterized by lymphoplasmacytic infiltrates with dense sclerosis forming mass lesions, most frequently in exocrine organs, particularly the pancreas and salivary glands. Involvement of many other tissue sites has been described, including the lung, kidney, lymph node, retroperitoneum, and aorta.

CLINICAL FEATURES

- The majority of patients present with variable patterns of pancreatitis, sialadenititis, dacryoadenitis, and/or cholangitis. 80% of patients also have lymphadenopathy, and small case series exist of isolated primary lymph node involvement.
- The median age range for patients with lymphadenopathy is 57–69 years old. There is a male predominance.
- Elevated serum IgG4 levels are frequently observed in cases, but this is not required for the diagnosis.
- The syndrome shows excellent clinical response to corticosteroid therapy.

HISTOLOGIC FINDINGS

- Several patterns have been described in lymph nodes including: follicular hyperplasia, Castleman disease-like changes, interfollicular expansion by plasma cells, and angioimmunoblastic T-cell lymphoma-like. Sclerosis is present in approximately one-third of involved lymph nodes.
- Castleman disease-like changes consist of hyalinized, atrophic germinal centers with mantle zones showing onion-skinning and variable numbers of interfollicular plasma cells.
- The ratio of IgG4(+) plasma cells to overall IgG(+) plasma cells is >40%.
- Plasma cells show normal, mature morphology and are polytypic.

DIFFERENTIAL DIAGNOSIS

- Reactive follicular and/or paracortical hyperplasia
- Castleman disease, hyaline vascular or plasma cell variant
- Syphilis
- Autoimmune lymphadenopathy
- B-cell non-Hodgkin lymphoma with plasmacytic differentiation
- Nodal plasmacytoma

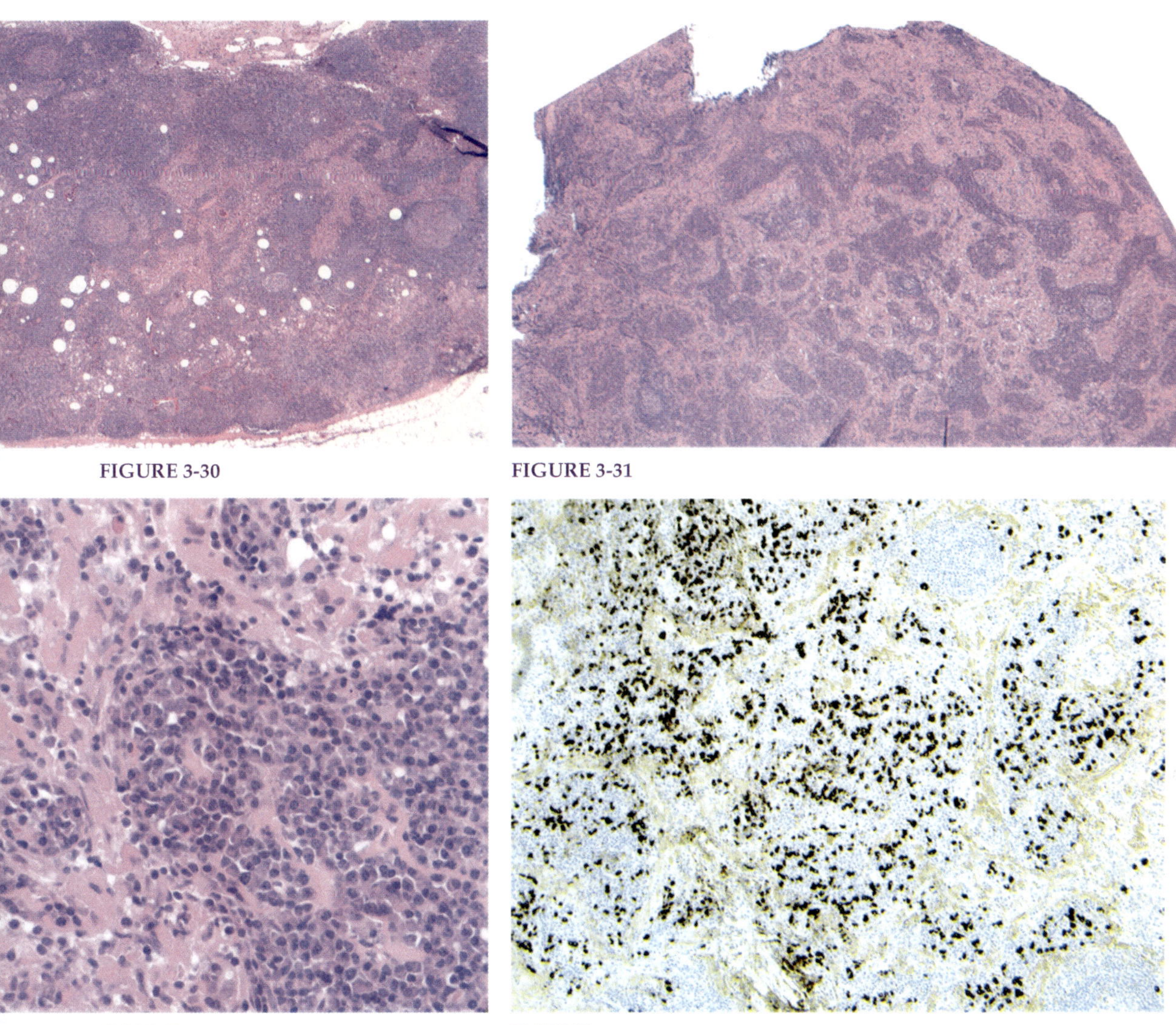

FIGURE 3-30

FIGURE 3-31

FIGURE 3-32

FIGURE 3-33

FIGURE 3-30 This peripancreatic lymph node shows both follicular hyperplasia and sinus histiocytosis.

FIGURE 3-31 The architecture is effaced with bands of sclerosis dividing dense plasma cell aggregates and follicles.

FIGURE 3-32 High-power magnification reveals morphologically unremarkable plasma cells, which were polytypic by immunohistochemistry.

FIGURE 3-33 An IgG4 stain reveals increased numbers of IgG4-expressing plasma cells (representing >40% of IgG(+) cells).

Autoimmune Lymphoproliferative Syndrome

DEFINITION

Autoimmune lymphoproliferative syndrome (ALPS) is a congenital disorder caused by gene mutations resulting in defective Fas-mediated cellular apoptosis.

CLINICAL FEATURES

- The median age at diagnosis is 24 months; it is uncommonly diagnosed in adults with autoimmune manifestations.
- ALPS is characterized clinically by lymphadenopathy, splenomegaly, and hypergammaglobulinemia.
- Autoimmune complications are seen in 50–70% of patients, most often manifesting as immune-mediated cytopenias. Various other organ-based autoimmune phenomena are seen uncommonly.
- Hodgkin or non-Hodgkin lymphomas occur in about 10% of ALPS patients (relative risks of 51x and 14x, respectively, compared to the general population).

HISTOLOGIC FINDINGS

- ALPS lymph nodes demonstrate an intact architecture with a typically marked paracortical hyperplasia with prominently increased immunoblasts and increased blood vessels (Figures 3-34 and 3-35).
- Variable follicular hyperplasia is present, sometimes florid. Regressed follicles and progressive transformation of germinal centers may each be seen in a minority of cases.
- The cardinal immunophenotypic feature of ALPS is increased numbers of non-clonal CD4/CD8 double negative T cells in both tissue and blood. These express the alpha/beta T-cell receptor.

DIFFERENTIAL DIAGNOSIS

- Non-specific reactive paracortical hyperplasia
- Infectious mononucleosis
- Still's disease
- Peripheral T-cell lymphoma

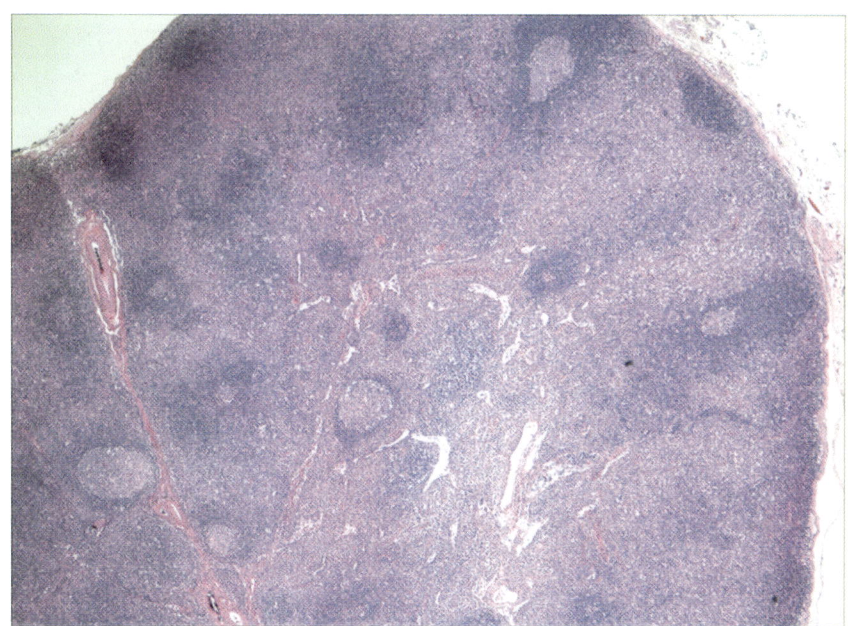

FIGURE 3-34

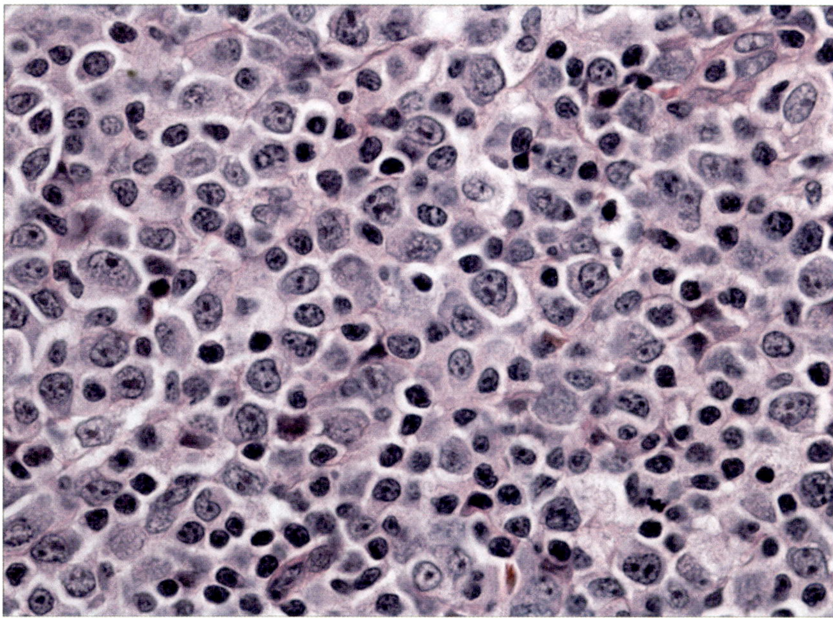

FIGURE 3-35

FIGURE 3-34 This low-power image demonstrates an expanded paracortex with scattered reactive follicles.

FIGURE 3-35 High-power of the paracortex demonstrates a prominent increase in immunoblasts.

4

Lymph Node Inclusions

EPITHELIAL CELL INCLUSIONS IN LYMPH NODES

NEVUS CELL INCLUSIONS IN LYMPH NODES

Epithelial Cell Inclusions in Lymph Nodes

DEFINITION

These processes represent benign clusters of mature epithelial cells in lymph nodes.

CLINICAL FEATURES

- This is a relatively rare finding, and is thought to be secondary to developmental heterotopia or metaplastic changes.
- Depending on the anatomic site, these may represent salivary gland structures (cervical lymph nodes), thyroid follicles (cervical lymph nodes), mammary glands and ducts (axillary lymph nodes), colonic glandular epithelium (mesenteric lymph nodes), or endosalpingiosis (pelvic lymph nodes).

HISTOLOGIC FINDINGS

- Lymph nodes show preserved architecture and contain glandular or epithelial structures without significant atypia or desmoplastic reaction (Figures 4-1 and 4-2).

DIFFERENTIAL DIAGNOSIS

- Metastatic carcinoma

FIGURE 4-1 Axillary lymph node with subcapsular mammary gland inclusion.

FIGURE 4-2 High-power view of the same case, showing benign ductal epithelium without desmoplastic reaction.

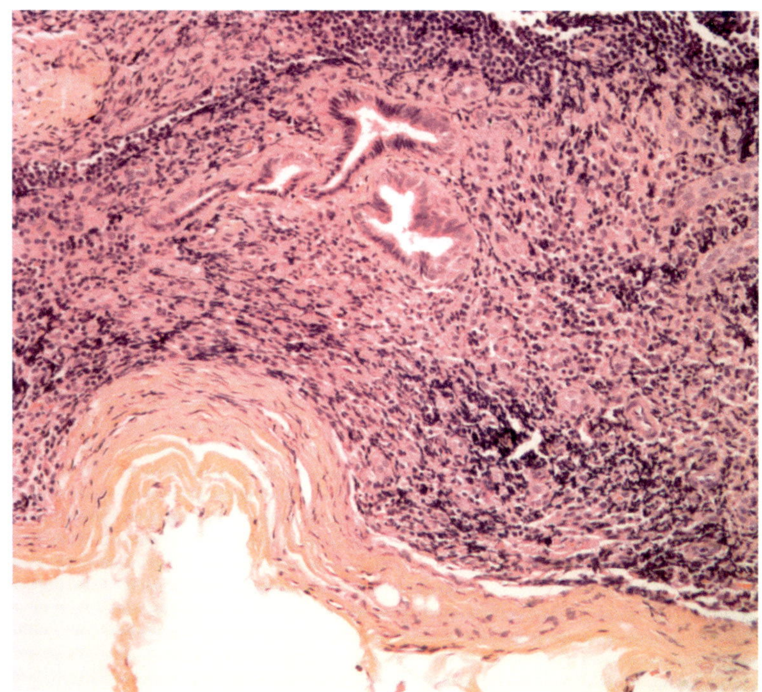

FIGURE 4-1

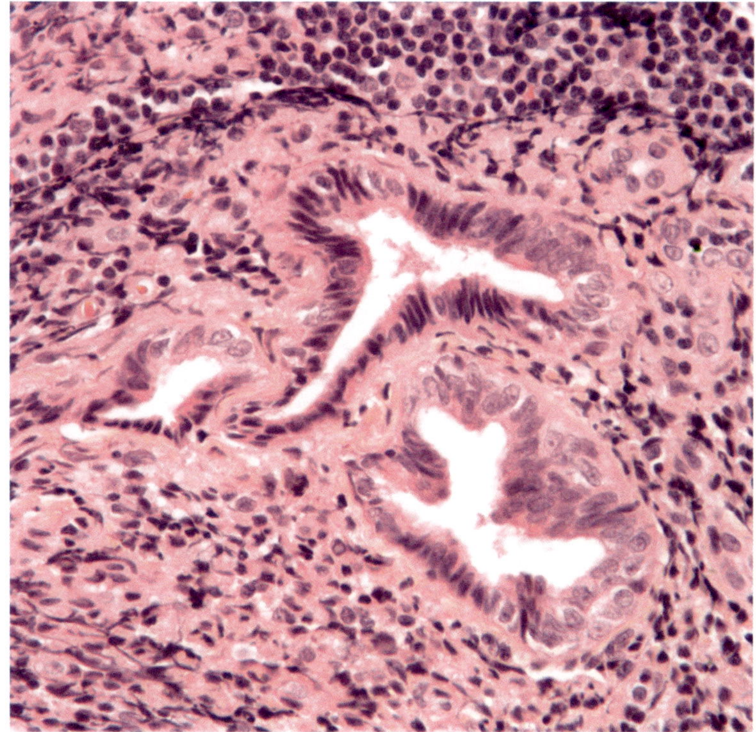

FIGURE 4-2

Nevus Cell Inclusions in Lymph Nodes

DEFINITION

This entity consists of clusters of nevus cells in lymph nodes.

CLINICAL FEATURES

- This is a relatively rare finding, most commonly seen in sentinel lymph nodes removed for breast carcinoma or melanoma surgery.
- Nevus cell inclusions may arise due to developmental heterotopia or "benign metastatic" displacement of nevus cells from cutaneous sites.
- They are most frequently seen in superficial lymph nodes (axillary, cervical), as opposed to visceral lymph nodes.

HISTOLOGIC FINDINGS

- Lymph nodes show preserved architecture, with aggregates of benign-appearing nevus cells, most commonly located in the capsular connective tissue, lymph node hilum or trabeculae (Figures 4-3 and 4-4).
- Infrequently, blue nevus cell clusters may be seen in the lymph node capsule (Figure 4-5).
- Nevus cells are positive for S100, tyrosinase, and melan-A.

DIFFERENTIAL DIAGNOSIS

- Metastatic melanoma

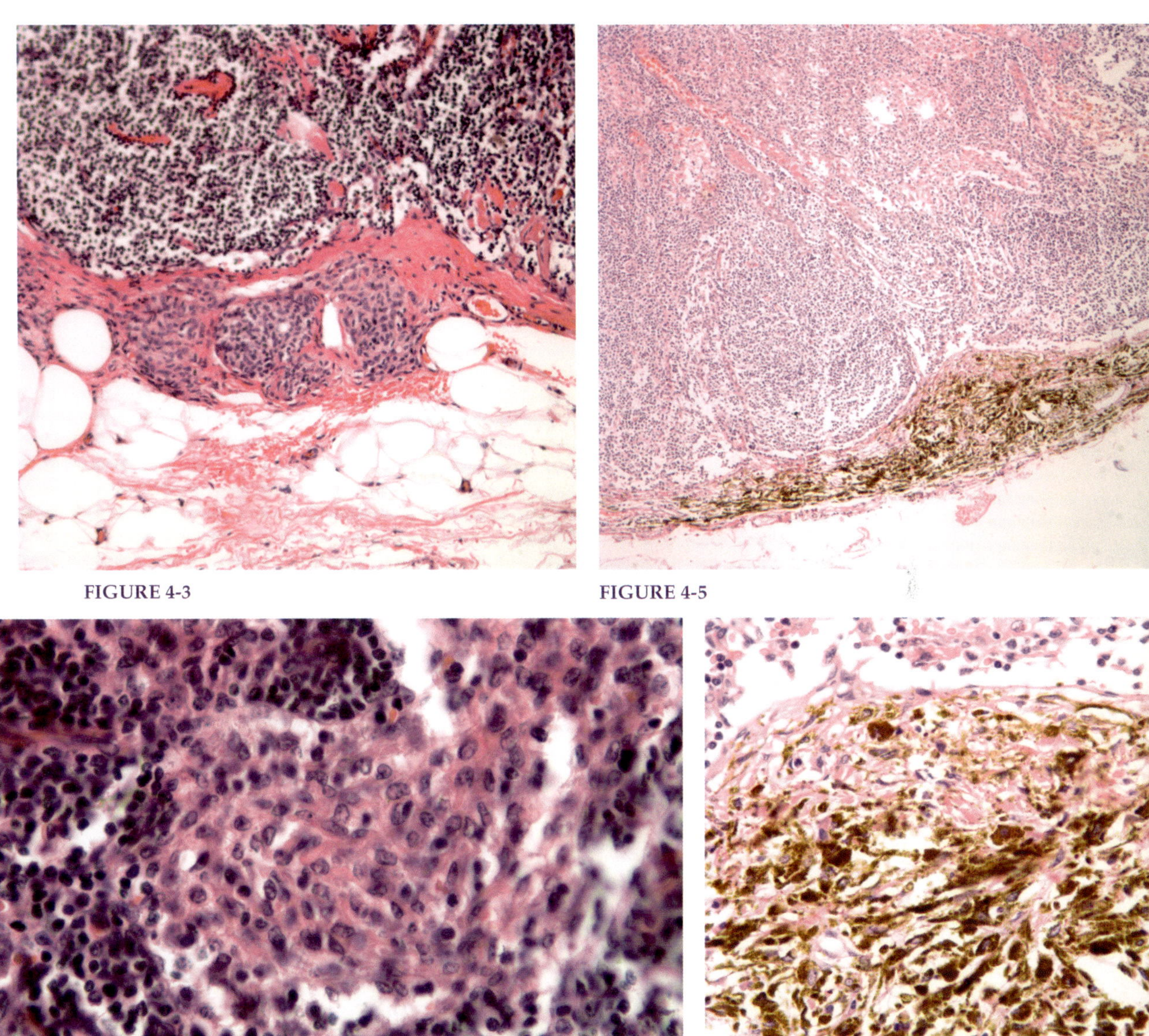

FIGURE 4-3

FIGURE 4-5

FIGURE 4-4

FIGURE 4-6

FIGURE 4-3 This lymph node contains a cluster of nevus cells in the capsule.
FIGURE 4-4 A high-power view demonstrates a nest of benign nevus cells with eosinophilic cytoplasm and indistinct cellular borders.
FIGURE 4-5 This lymph node contains a capsular blue nevus aggregate.
FIGURE 4-6 At high-power, capsular blue nevus cells with abundant melanin pigment are evident.

Spindle Cell Neoplasms of Lymph Nodes

5

PALISADED MYOFIBROBLASTOMA

INFLAMMATORY PSEUDOTUMOR OF LYMPH NODE

Palisaded Myofibroblastoma

DEFINITION

There is a benign mesenchymal neoplasm composed of palisading spindle cells, amianthoid fibers, and areas of hemorrhage.

CLINICAL FEATURES

- This lesion is more common in adults (6th decade) and in men.
- Patients present with a solitary, asymptomatic, inguinal mass.

HISTOLOGIC FINDINGS

- Palisaded myofibroblastoma consists of a nodular proliferation of spindle-shaped cells with slender, elongated nuclei, and eosinophilic cytoplasm, arranged in a palisading pattern (Figures 5-1 and 5-2).
- The fascicles of spindle cells are separated by amianthoid bodies, which are stellate deposits of hair-like collagen fibers, surrounded by granular, proteinaceous material at the periphery (Figure 5-3).
- Scattered hemorrhagic foci are also present.
- The spindle cells are positive for smooth muscle actin, myosin, vimentin, and negative for: desmin, factor VIII, S100, synaptophysin, and cytokeratin.
- Amianthoid fibers stain dark blue with a trichrome stain.

DIFFERENTIAL DIAGNOSIS

- Kaposi sarcoma
- Inflammatory pseudotumor of lymph node

FIGURE 5-1 This lymph node show effaced architecture and dense fascicles of spindle cells.

FIGURE 5-2 Medium-power view demonstrates a band of degenerated collagen fibers (amianthoid body) surrounded by spindle cells with a parallel or intersecting orientation.

FIGURE 5-3 High-power view of an amianthoid body reveals fine, hair-like collagen fibers. The cellular infiltrate consists of bland spindle cells with oval or tapered nuclei and eosinophilic cytoplasm.

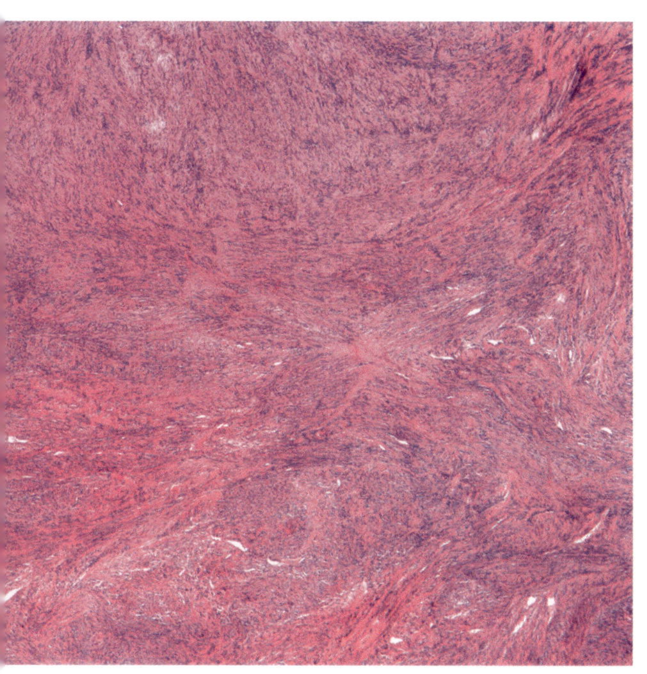

FIGURE 5-1

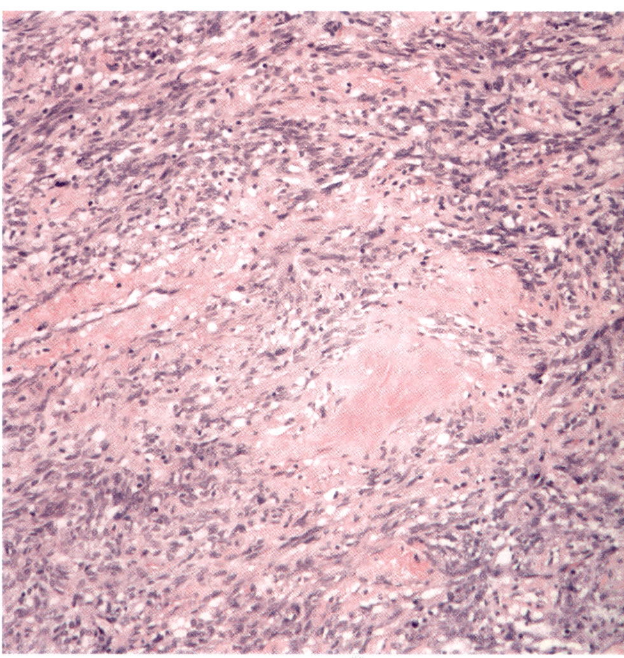

FIGURE 5-2

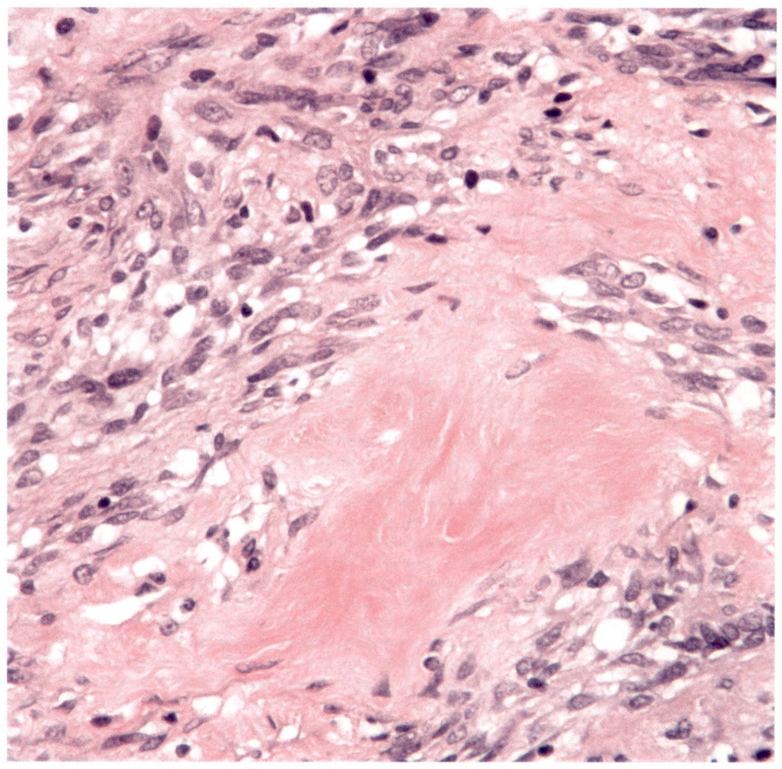

FIGURE 5-3

Inflammatory Pseudotumor of Lymph Node

DEFINITION

This entity consists of a histiocytic and fibroblastic non-neoplastic proliferation, involving the lymph node connective tissue framework and associated with vascular proliferation.

CLINICAL FEATURES

- Inflammatory pseudotumor of lymph node occurs across a broad age range (median, 33 years); male:female = 1:1.
- Patients present with fever, night sweats, fatigue, anemia, hypergammaglobulinemia, and lymphadenopathy.

HISTOLOGIC FINDINGS

- Cases may show morphologic heterogeneity, ranging from stage I (small localized nodule, with preservation of the nodal architecture, through stage II (more extensive involvement with marked distortion of the fibrovascular framework), to stage III (diffuse architectural effacement with complete sclerosis).
- Lesions contain an admixture of bland myofibroblastic and/or histiocytic spindle cells (Figures 5-4 and 5-5) and a polymorphic inflammatory cell infiltrate (Figure 5-6).
- The spindle cells are vimentin(+), smooth muscle actin(+), and CD68(+), and are negative for desmin, factor XIII, and CD34.

DIFFERENTIAL DIAGNOSIS

- Palisaded myofibroblastoma
- Mycobacterial spindle cell pseudotumor
- Follicular dendritic cell sarcoma

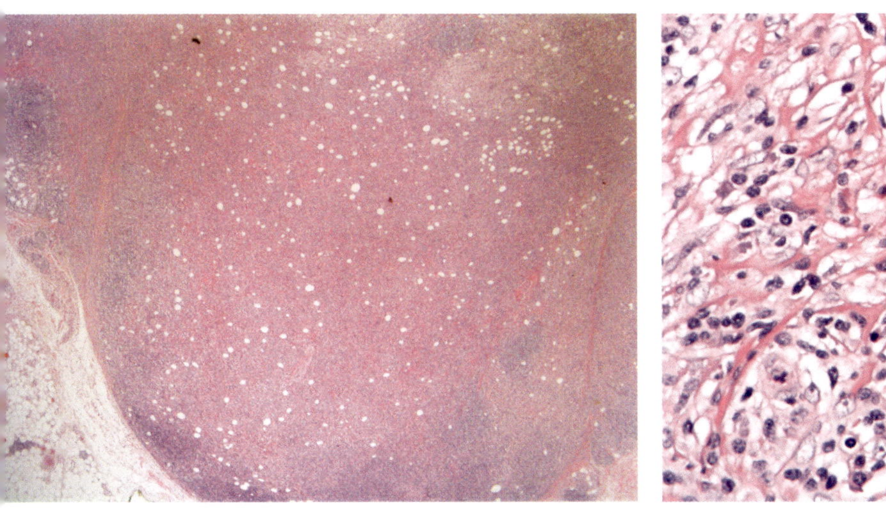

FIGURE 5-4

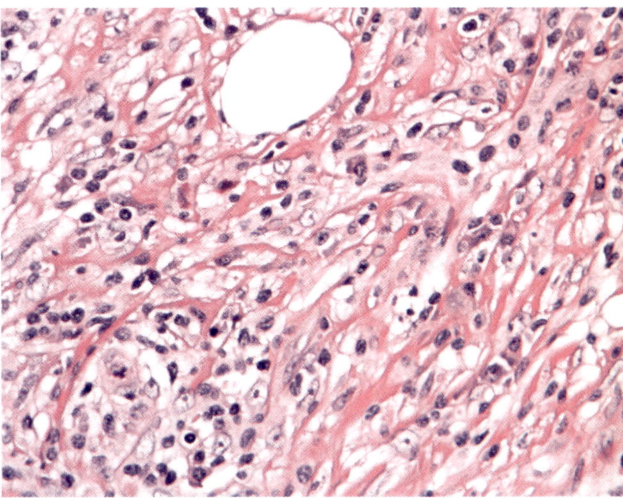

FIGURE 5-5

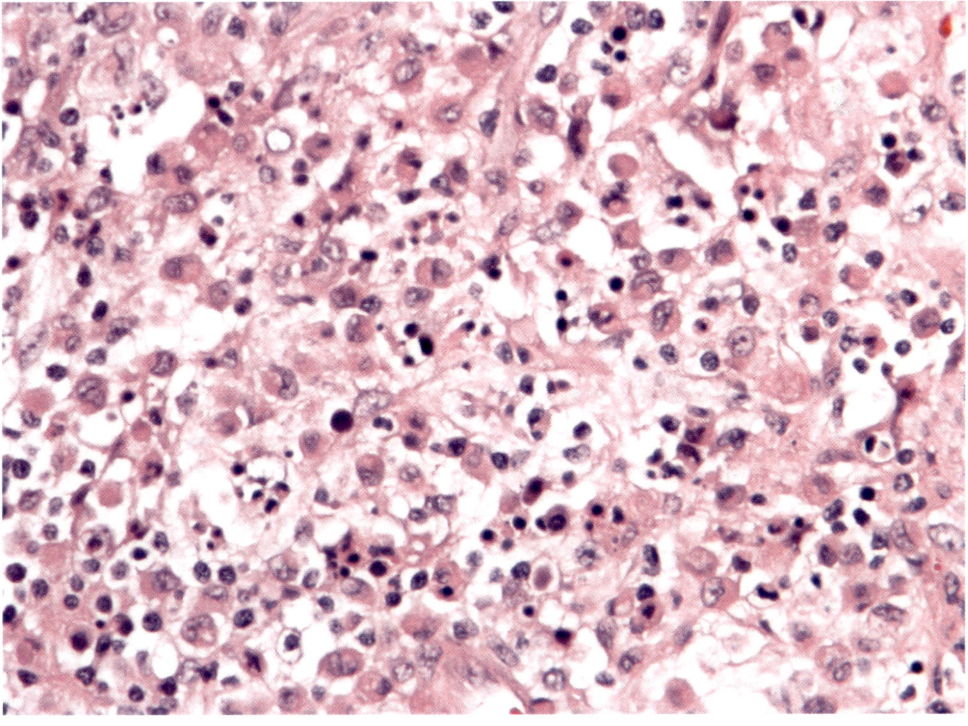

FIGURE 5-6

FIGURE 5-4 The lymph node shows a partially effaced architecture with an infiltrate composed of spindle cells and myofibroblasts.

FIGURE 5-5 This high-power view reveals a proliferation of myofibroblasts admixed with occasional inflammatory cells.

FIGURE 5-6 Another high-power view shows an area of mixed inflammatory infiltrate, composed of frequent plasma cells, and occasional small lymphocytes and neutrophils.

6

Vascular Lymphadenopathies and Neoplasms of Lymph Nodes

VASCULAR TRANSFORMATION OF LYMPH NODE SINUSES

ANGIOMYMATOUS HAMARTOMA

HEMANGIOMAS AND HEMANGIOENDOTHELIOMAS

KAPOSI SARCOMA

Vascular Transformation of Lymph Node Sinuses

DEFINITION

Vascular transformation of lymph node sinuses (VTS) is a benign vasoproliferative finding in lymph nodes that may be observed in association with regional carcinoma and/or thrombosis.

CLINICAL FEATURES

- Most VTS are incidental findings discovered in staging lymph node dissections.
- Rarely, VTS presents as isolated lymphadenopathy.

HISTOLOGIC FINDINGS

- The lymph node may show a focal or diffuse pattern of VTS.
- Subcapsular, cortical and intramedullary sinuses are affected. The lymph node capsule is spared, in contrast to Kaposi's sarcoma.
- The vascular proliferation may show four histologic patterns: cleft-like sinuses, rounded vascular spaces, solid, and plexiform sinuses. Most VTS cases show a combination of these patterns. A nodular variant has also been described in retroperitoneal nodes.
- Vascular spaces are variably formed and show maturation heterogeneity within each lesion, ranging from ill-formed, narrow, slit-like spaces to mature, round or ovoid, patent structures (Figure 6-1). The spaces are lined by flattened or cuboidal, plump endothelium without atypia (Figure 6-2). Mitoses are rare. Lymphocytes, histiocytes, eosinophils, and red blood cells are present within the sinuses in variable numbers.
- There is variable stromal fibrosis. Inflammatory cells are not characteristic in the stroma.
- Adjacent nodal parenchyma shows atrophy with lymphoid depletion.
- Eosinophilic hyaline globules are unusual.
- HHV-8 staining is negative, in contrast to Kaposi's sarcoma.

DIFFERENTIAL DIAGNOSIS

- Kaposi's sarcoma
- Epithelioid hemangioma/hemangioendothelioma
- Angiosarcoma
- Nodal hemangioma
- Bacillary angiomatosis
- Inflammatory pseudotumor

FIGURE 6-1 The vaso-proliferative component of this lesion starts in the subcapsular sinus and is characterized by ill-formed and round vascular spaces lined by bland endothelial cells. The sinuses contain few histiocytes, eosinophils, and lymphocytes. Note that the capsule (left) is not involved.

FIGURE 6-2 The sinuses show a focal, nodular architecture with vessels lined by bland endothelial cells; these vessels show maturation heterogeneity, and some contain red blood cells. There is additionally increased sclerosis within the stroma.

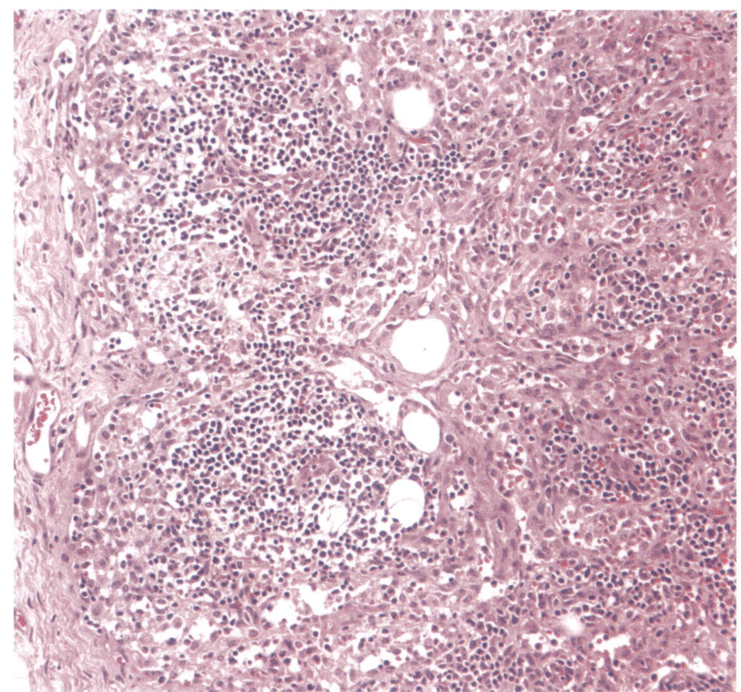

FIGURE 6-1

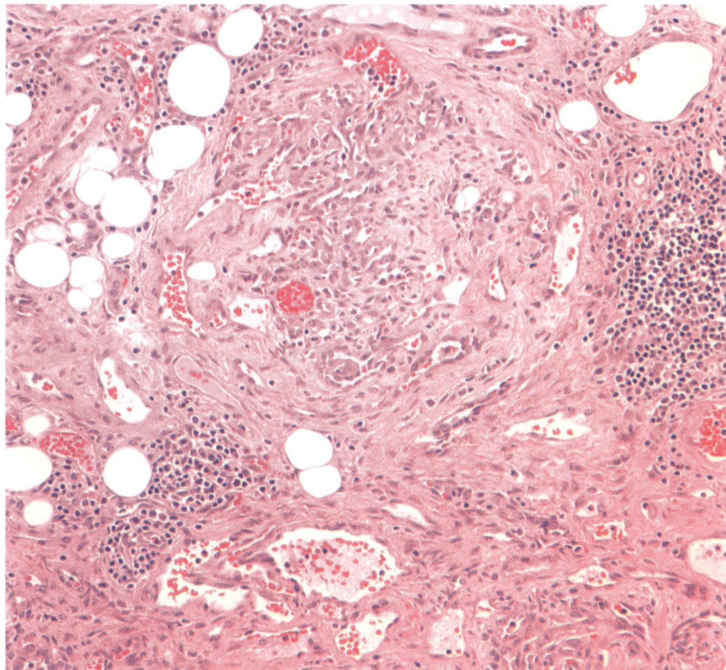

FIGURE 6-2

Angiomymatous Hamartoma

DEFINITION

This is a hamartomatous lesion composed of blood vessels, smooth muscle, and fibrous tissue, in the absence of cellular fascicle formation.

CLINICAL FEATURES

- Angiomyomatous hamartoma is seen in adults (mean age, 42 years), with a male to female ratio of 5:1.
- These typically present with painless, unilateral inguinal lymphadenopathy; rarely they may involve other anatomic sites.

HISTOLOGIC FINDINGS

- The lesion originates in the hilum as a proliferation of thick-walled vessels distributed in a collagenous stroma (Figures 6-3 and 6-4).
- As it extends into the parenchyma and towards the periphery of the lymph node, the vascular proliferation becomes less discernible in a background of sclerotic stroma and smooth muscle cells with elongated nuclei and eosinophilic cytoplasm (Figure 6-5).

DIFFERENTIAL DIAGNOSIS

- Kaposi sarcoma
- Vascular transformation of sinuses
- Palisaded myofibroblastoma
- Inflammatory pseudotumor of lymph node
- Hemangioma/hemagioendothelioma

FIGURE 6-3 Low-power view demonstrates a hilar lesion, extending into the parenchyma.

FIGURE 6-4 Medium-sized, thick-walled vessel proliferation and collagenous stroma are evident in the hilar region.

FIGURE 6-5 High-power reveals sclerotic stroma with a haphazard distribution of occasional smooth muscle cells.

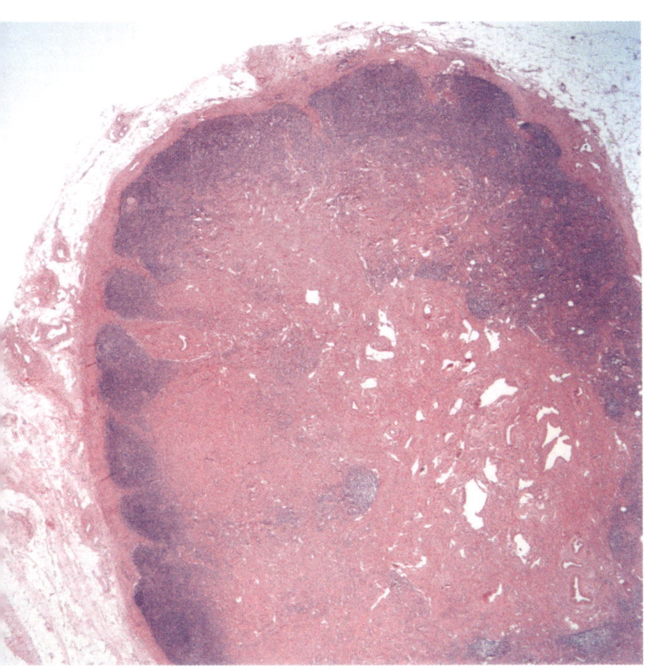
FIGURE 6-3

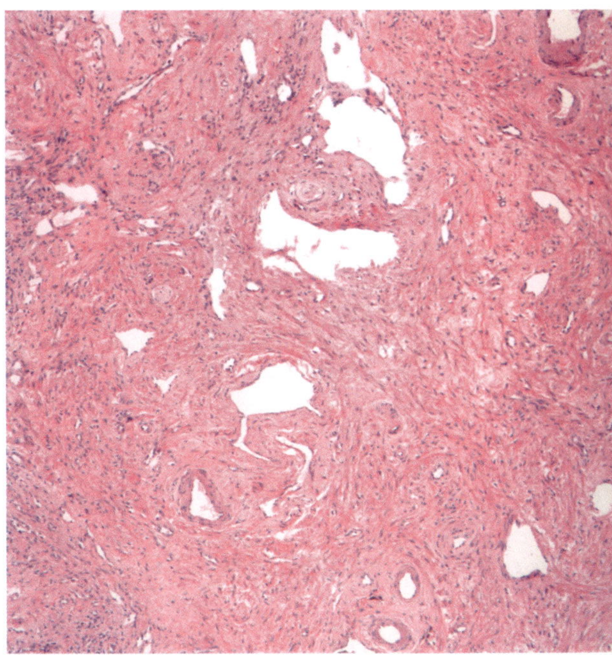
FIGURE 6-4

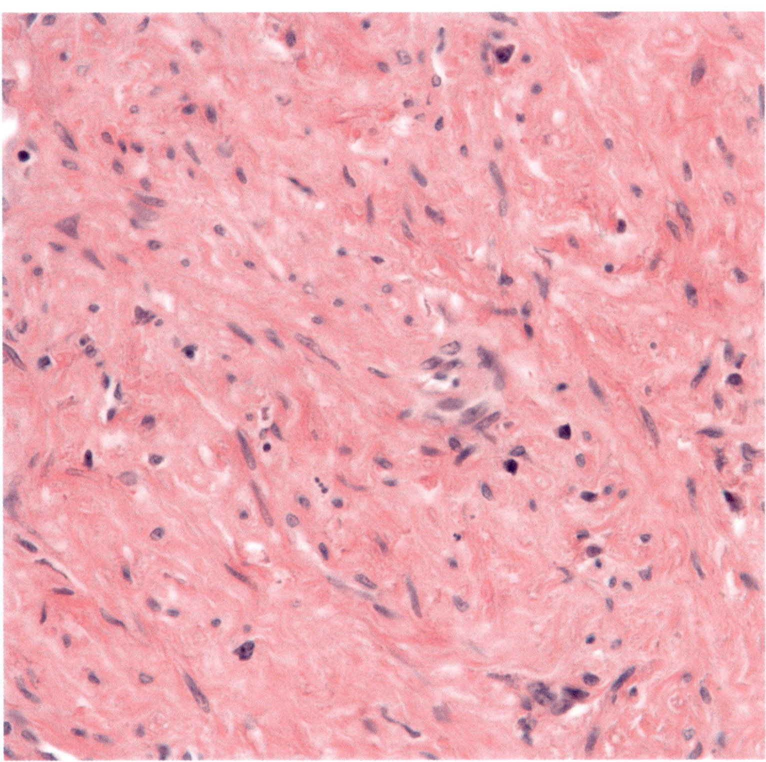
FIGURE 6-5

Hemangiomas and Hemangioendotheliomas

DEFINITION

Hemangiomas and Hemangioendotheliomas comprise a set of benign vascular tumors of lymph nodes.

CLINICAL FEATURES

- These rare lymph node tumors occur mostly in adults; hemangiomas have a female predominance, while hemagioendotheliomas are more common in males.
- These lesions present with asymptomatic lymphadenopathy or are incidentally discovered.

HISTOLOGIC FINDINGS

- Hemangiomas form a distinct mass lesion and otherwise show similar morphology to those found in soft tissue. They fall into three histologic types: capillary, cavernous, and mixed (Figures 6-6 and 6-7).
- Capillary hemangiomas consist of closely packed capillaries lined by flat endothelial cells.
- Cavernous hemangiomas show a conglomerate of congested cavernous spaces with occasional thrombin.
- Hemangioendotheliomas are comprised by blood vessels and aggregates of polygonal, plump or spindle-shaped cells with abundant eosinophilic cytoplasm and bland nuclei (Figures 6-8 and 6-9).

DIFFERENTIAL DIAGNOSIS

- Kaposi sarcoma
- Vascular transformation of sinuses
- Bacillary angiomatosis
- Metastatic angiosarcoma

FIGURE 6-6 This lymph node containing a hemangioma shows replacement by a conglomerate of vascular spaces.

FIGURE 6-7 High-power view shows vascular spaces of various shapes and sizes, lined by generally flat endothelial cells.

FIGURE 6-8 This lymph node involved by an epithelioid hemangioendothelioma is effaced with only a thin rim of preserved lymphoid parenchyma.

FIGURE 6-9 A high-power view shows polygonal cells with abundant eosinophilic cytoplasm, surrounding occasional vascular spaces.

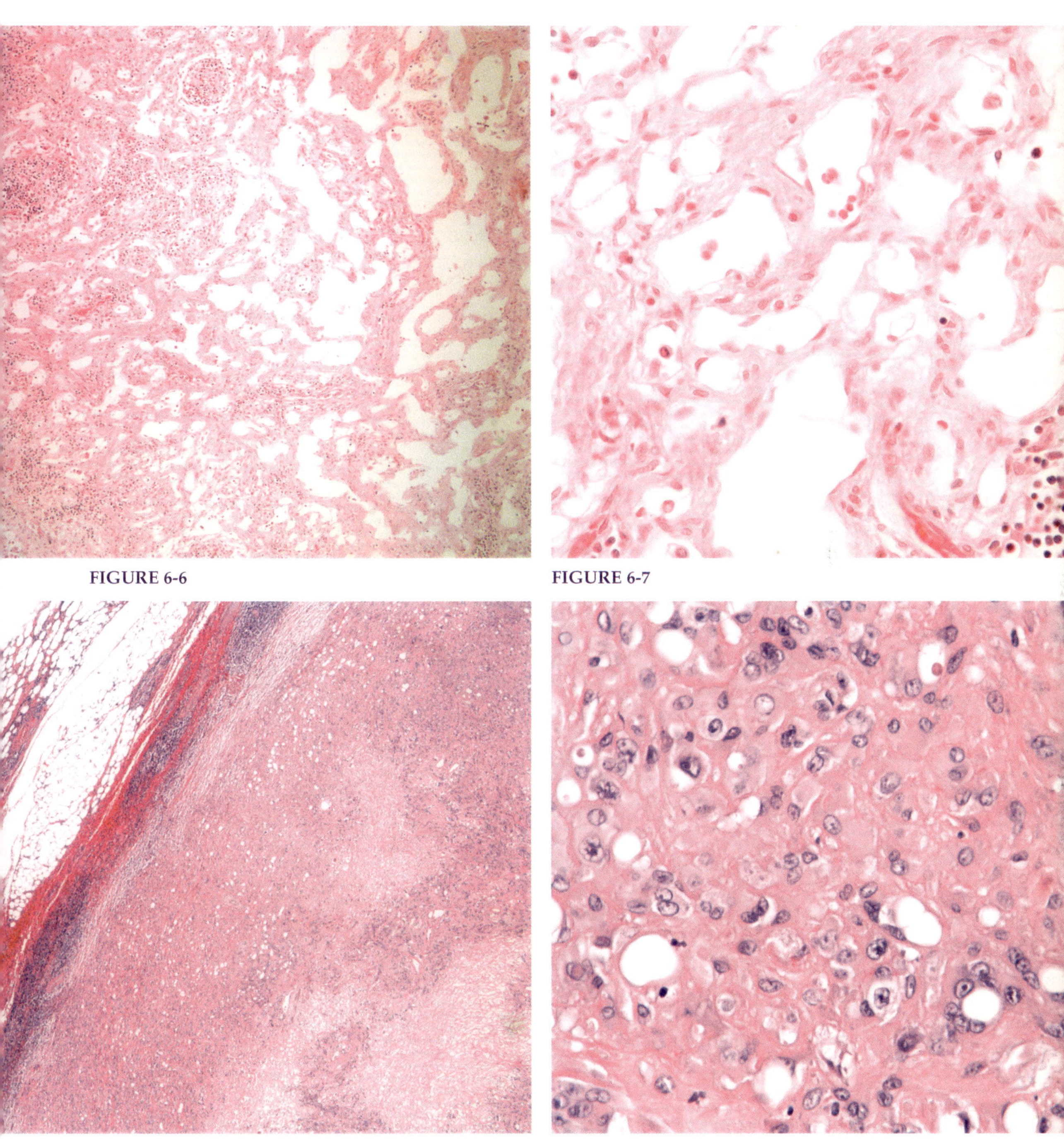

FIGURE 6-6

FIGURE 6-7

FIGURE 6-8

FIGURE 6-9

Kaposi Sarcoma

DEFINITION

Kaposi sarcoma represents a vascular and spindle cell neoplasm caused by human herpesvirus-8.

CLINICAL FEATURES

- Kaposi sarcoma is most commonly seen patients with AIDS, with a male predominance.
- Sporadic cases in immunocompetent individuals are rarely encountered, usually in elderly men.
- The typical presentation is with cutaneous and mucosal lesions; lymph nodes may also be involved.

HISTOLOGIC FINDINGS

- Lymph nodes typically contain distinct nodular aggregates of tumor cells with a whorled appearance (Figures 6-10 and 6-11). Early involvement may manifest as subtle infiltration of the capsule or trabeculae.
- Neoplastic spindle cells are distributed around vascular clefts that contain red blood cells; extravasated red cells are also typically seen (Figure 6-12). Plasma cells and small lymphocytes are also present.
- The neoplastic cells are positive for CD31, CD34 and HHV-8 LNA-1.

DIFFERENTIAL DIAGNOSIS

- Bacillary angiomatosis
- Metastatic angiosarcoma

FIGURE 6-10 This lymph node shows follicular and paracortical hyperplasia, and a distinct tumor nodule in the hilum.

FIGURE 6-11 There is a Proliferation of slit-like vascular spaces, surrounded by whorles and bundles of elongated cells with eosinophilic cytoplasm.

FIGURE 6-12 High-power reveals spindle-shaped neoplastic cells with abundant eosinophilic cytoplasm and bland nuclei. Cleft-like capillaries contain variable numbers of red blood cells. Extravasated red cells are present, as well.

FIGURE 6-13 The neoplastic spindle cells show strong reactivity for HHV-8 LNA-1.

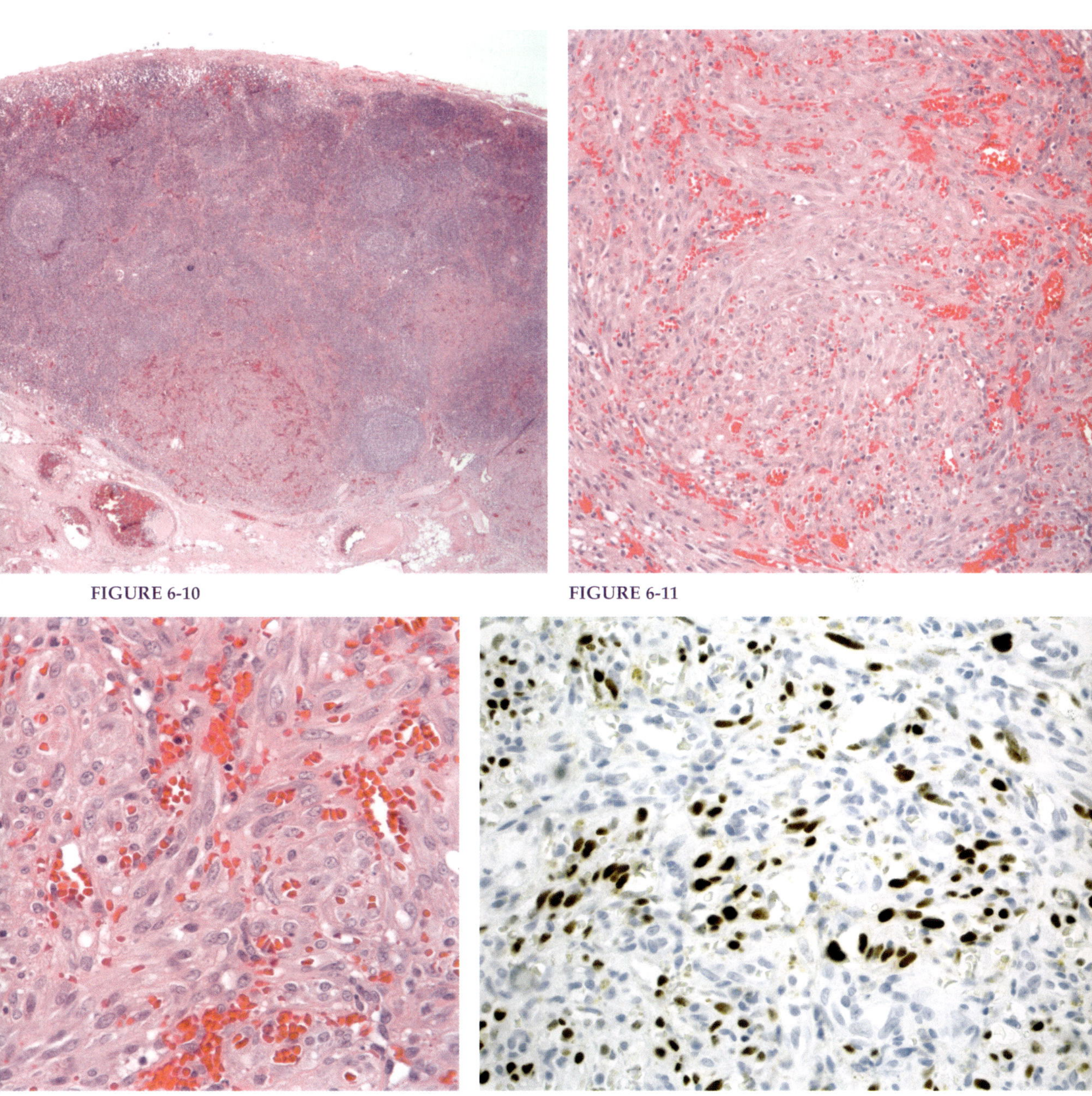

FIGURE 6-10

FIGURE 6-11

FIGURE 6-12

FIGURE 6-13

7

Foreign Body Lymphadenopathies

METAL DEBRIS-ASSOCIATED LYMPHADENOPATHY

LYMPHANGIOGRAPHY-ASSOCIATED LYMPHADENOPATHY

Metal Debris-Associated Lymphadenopathy

DEFINITION

This represents lymphadenopathy caused by histiocytic proliferations and metal debris deposition, secondary to lymph node drainage of an anatomic area associated with joint prosthesis.

CLINICAL FEATURES

- This finding commonly occurs in pelvic lymph nodes of individuals with a hip prosthesis.

HISTOLOGIC FINDINGS

- Lymph nodes show architectural effacement and a sinusoidal infiltrate of large, foamy histiocytes (Figure 7-1).
- The histiocytes contain needle-shaped, black metal particles (Figure 7-2) that show strong birefringence under polarized light.

DIFFERENTIAL DIAGNOSIS

- Sinus histiocytosis of other etiology
- Granulomatous inflammation due to fungal and acid-fast organisms
- Metastatic carcinoma

FIGURE 7-1 An axillary lymph node from a patient with shoulder joint prosthesis shows an abundant infiltrate of foamy histiocytes, admixed with scattered multinucleated foreign-body giant cells.

FIGURE 7-2 High-power magnification of the same case shows histiocytes with ample foamy cytoplasm, containing black flakes or needle-shaped metal debris.

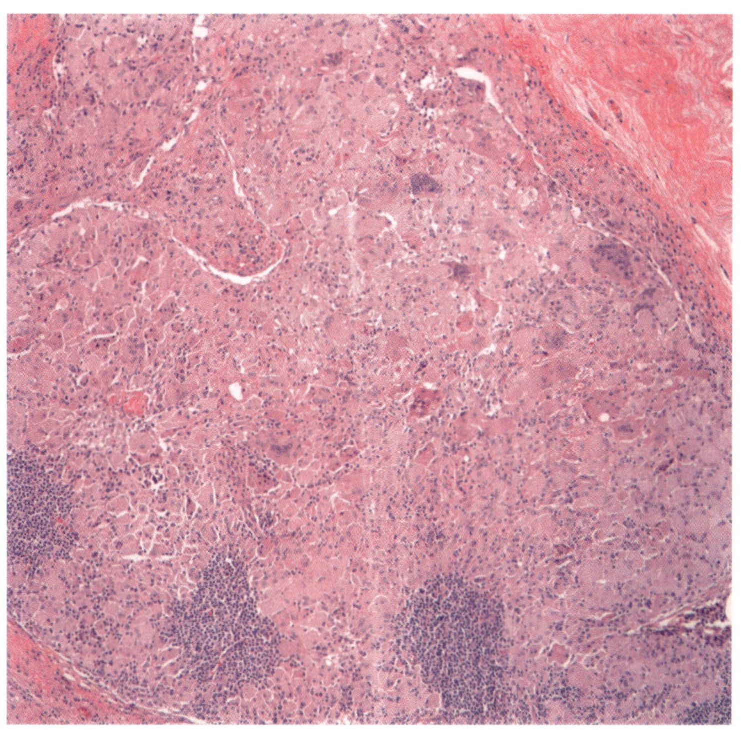
FIGURE 7-1

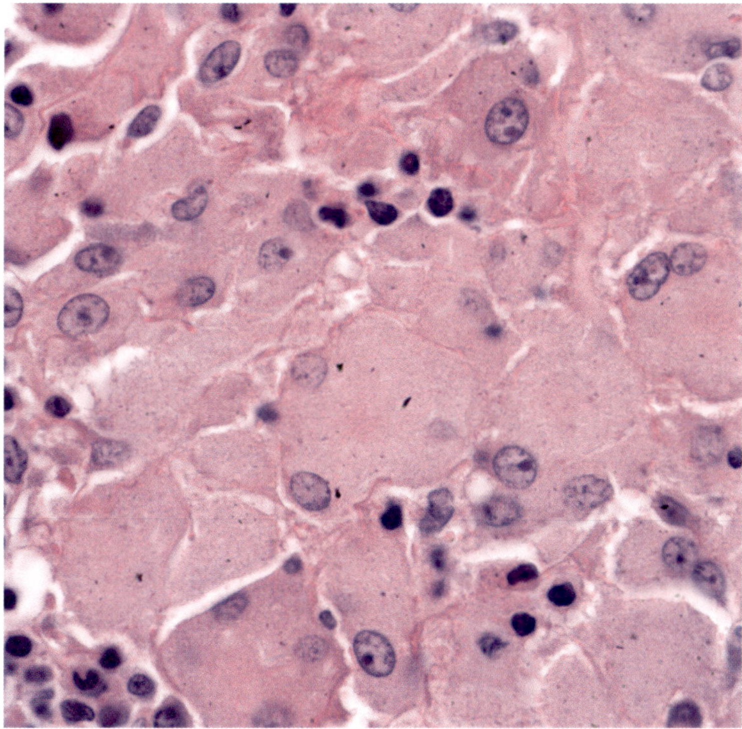
FIGURE 7-2

Lymphangiography-Associated Lymphadenopathy

DEFINITION

Lymphadenopathy secondary to lymphangiograms results from foreign body reaction to lipid material present in lymphangiography contrast medium.

CLINICAL FEATURES

- Lymphangiography is used to visualize the lymphatic system and identify blockages in lymph drainage. It currently has only limited use due to the widespread use of more advanced imaging techniques. The contrast medium from lymphangiography may be retained in lymph nodes for up to two years.

HISTOLOGIC FINDINGS

- Lymphangiography lymphadenopathy is characterized by numerous vacuoles of varying size throughout the lymph node with resultant reduction in normal lymphoid tissue (Figure 7-3). The vacuoles are surrounded by epithelioid histiocytes and foreign body giant cells (Figure 7-4). The vacuoles appear to be devoid of contents because the lipid material is lost in processing.

DIFFERENTIAL DIAGNOSIS

- Lipid granulomas due to other exogenous or endogenous sources of lipid
- Whipple disease

FIGURE 7-3 This low-power image demonstrates numerous vacuoles of varying size partially replacing a lymph node, with consequent diminution of lymphoid tissue.

FIGURE 7-4 High-power demonstrates a foreign body reaction rimming the vacuoles, with epithelioid histiocytes and foreign body giant cells. Eosinophils are also present.

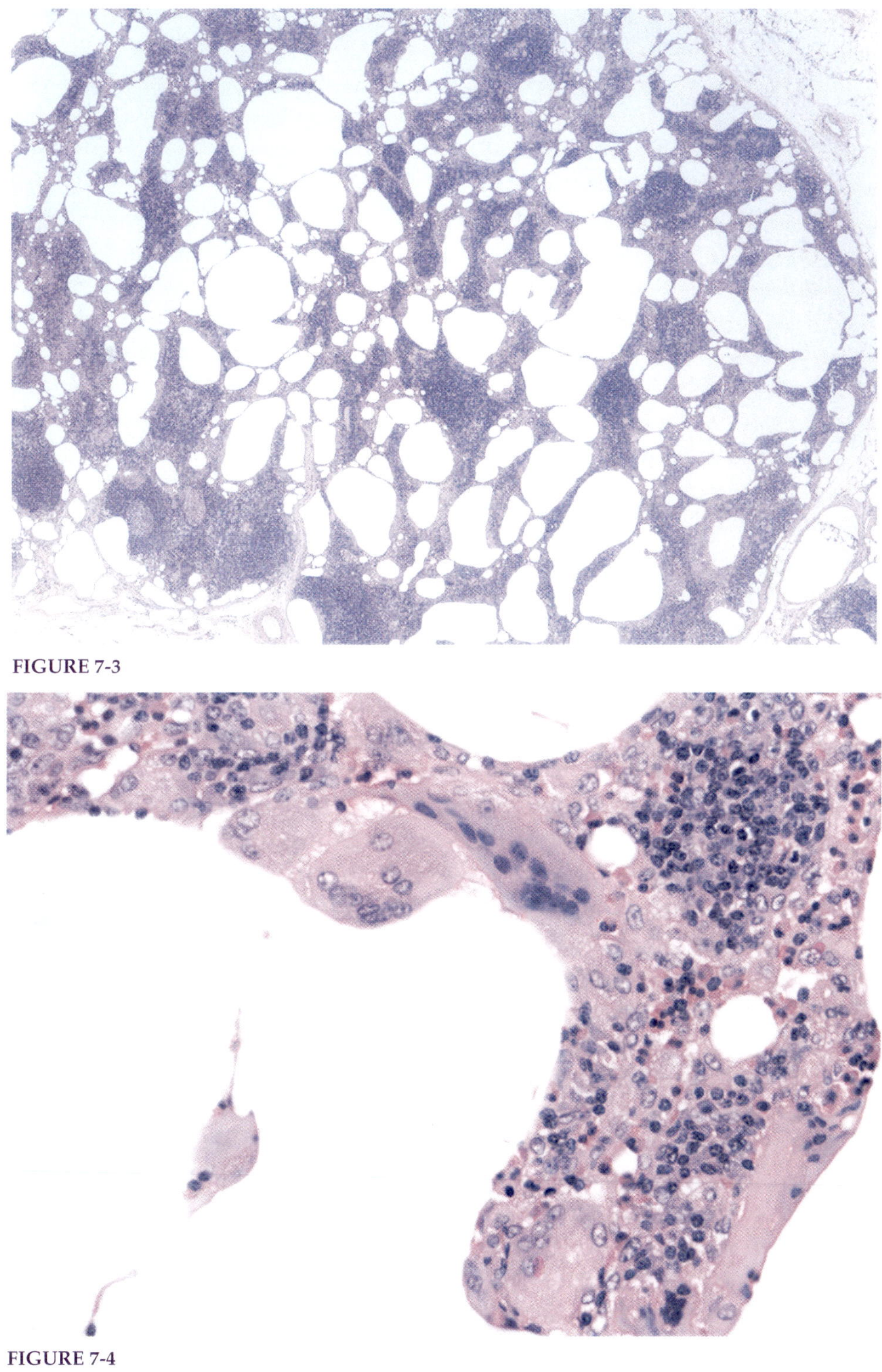

FIGURE 7-3

FIGURE 7-4

8

Mature B-Cell Neoplasms

NOMENCLATURE AND CLASSIFICATION

CHRONIC LYMPHOCYTIC LEUKEMIA/SMALL LYMPHOCYTIC LYMPHOMA (CLL/SLL)

SPLENIC B-CELL MARGINAL ZONE LYMPHOMA (SMZL)

HAIRY CELL LEUKEMIA (HCL)

LYMPHOPLASMACYTIC LYMPHOMA (LPL)

HEAVY CHAIN DISEASES (HCDS)

EXTRAOSSEOUS PLASMACYTOMA

NODAL MARGINAL ZONE LYMPHOMA (MZL)

FOLLICULAR LYMPHOMA (FL)

MANTLE CELL LYMPHOMA (MCL)

DIFFUSE LARGE B-CELL LYMPHOMA, NOT OTHERWISE SPECIFIED (DLBCL, NOS)

DLBCL SUBTYPES

PRIMARY MEDIASTINAL LARGE B-CELL LYMPHOMA (PMLBCL)

ALK POSITIVE LARGE B-CELL LYMPHOMA

PLASMABLASTIC LYMPHOMA (PBL)

LARGE B-CELL LYMPHOMA ARISING IN HHV8-ASSOCIATED MULTICENTRIC CASTLEMAN DISEASE

BURKITT LYMPHOMA (BL)

B-CELL LYMPHOMA, UNCLASSIFIABLE, WITH FEATURES INTERMEDIATE BETWEEN DIFFUSE LARGE B-CELL LYMPHOMA AND BURKITT LYMPHOMA

B-CELL LYMPHOMA, UNCLASSIFIABLE, WITH FEATURES INTERMEDIATE BETWEEN DIFFUSE LARGE B-CELL LYMPHOMA AND CLASSICAL HODGKIN LYMPHOMA

Nomenclature and Classification

Mature B-cell neoplasms represent >80% of non-Hodgkin lymphomas and are a heterogeneous group of conditions that originate from cells at various stages of differentiation beyond the progenitor cell state. The 2008 WHO classification of tumors of hematopoietic and lymphoid tissues lists many types of mature B-cell neoplasms (Table 8-1). The following chapter will cover in detail most of the lymphomas that occur primarily in, or commonly affect lymph nodes, in addition to other anatomic sites.

Nomenclature and Classification

TABLE 8-1 WHO 2008 Classification of Mature B-Cell Neoplasms

Chronic lymphocytic leukemia/small lymphocytic lymphoma
B-cell prolymphocytic leukemia
Splenic B-cell marginal zone lymphoma
Hairy cell leukemia
Splenic B-cell lymphoma/leukemia, unclassifiable
Splenic diffuse red pulp B-cell lymphoma
Hairy cell leukemia – variant
Lymphoplasmacytic lymphoma
Heavy chain disease
Gamma heavy chain disease
Mu heavy chain disease
Alpha heavy chain disease
Plasma cell neoplasms
Monoclonal gammopathy of undetermined significance (MGUS)
Plasma cell myeloma
Solitary plasmacytoma of bone
Extraosseous plasmacytoma
Monoclonal immunoglobulin deposition disease
Extranodal marginal zone lymphoma of mucosa-associated lymphoid tissue (MALT lymphoma)
Nodal marginal zone lymphoma
Follicular lymphoma
Primary cutaneous follicle center cell lymphoma
Mantle cell lymphoma
Diffuse large B-cell lymphoma (DLBCL), NOS
T cell/histiocyte–rich large B-cell lymphoma
Primary DLBCL of CNS
Primary cutaneous DLBCL, leg type
EBV positive DLBCL of the elderly
DLBCL associated with chronic inflammation
Lymphomatoid granulomatosis
Primary mediastinal (thymic) large B-cell lymphoma
Intravascular large B-cell lymphoma
ALK positive large B-cell lymphoma
Plasmablastic lymphoma
Large B-cell lymphoma arising in HHV8-associated multicentric Castleman disease
Primary effusion lymphoma
Burkitt lymphoma
B-cell lymphoma, unclassifiable, with feature intermediate between DLBCL and Burkitt lymphoma
B-cell lymphoma, unclassifiable, with feature intermediate between DLBCL and classical Hodgkin lymphoma

Chronic Lymphocytic Leukemia/Small Lymphocytic Lymphoma (CLL/SLL)

DEFINITION

CLL/SLL is a mature B-cell neoplasm composed of predominantly small cells with regular nuclei, involving the peripheral blood, bone marrow, spleen, and lymph nodes. By definition, in the absence of extramedullary tissue involvement, a diagnosis of CLL requires the presence of ≥5,000 PB neoplastic cells/µl in the blood. SLL is diagnosed in non-leukemic patients with typical tissue histology and immunophenotype.

CLINICAL FEATURES

- CLL/SLL is the most common leukemia in Western countries.
- The mean age is 65 years, with a male:female ratio of 1.5–2:1.
- Peripheral blood, bone marrow, spleen, and lymph nodes are typically involved, depending on disease stage.
- Most patients are asymptomatic; some present with nonspecific symptoms (fatigue, infections, anemia) and/or lymphadenopathy/organomegaly.

HISTOLOGIC FINDINGS

- The lymph node architecture is effaced by a vaguely nodular infiltrate composed of monotonous small cells with mostly regular nuclei, clumped chromatin, and scant cytoplasm (Figures 8-1 and 8-2).
- Variable numbers of larger cells (prolymphocytes and paraimmunoblasts) are present, usually concentrated in nodular collections known as proliferation centers or pseudofollicles. Prolymphocytes are medium-sized cells with clumped chromatin and small nucleoli, whereas paraimmunoblasts are large cells with round to oval nuclei, vesicular chromatin, and prominent central nucleoli (Figures 8-1 to 8-3).

(*continued*)

FIGURE 8-1 This lymph node shows effaced architecture and a diffuse infiltrate with vague nodularity, corresponding to proliferation centers.

FIGURE 8-2 Typical CLL/SLL cells are small in size, with regular nuclei, clumped chromatin, and scant cytoplasm.

FIGURE 8-3 This high-power magnification of a proliferation center shows frequent paraimmunoblasts (arrows) and prolymphocytes (arrow heads), admixed with small CLL/SLL cells.

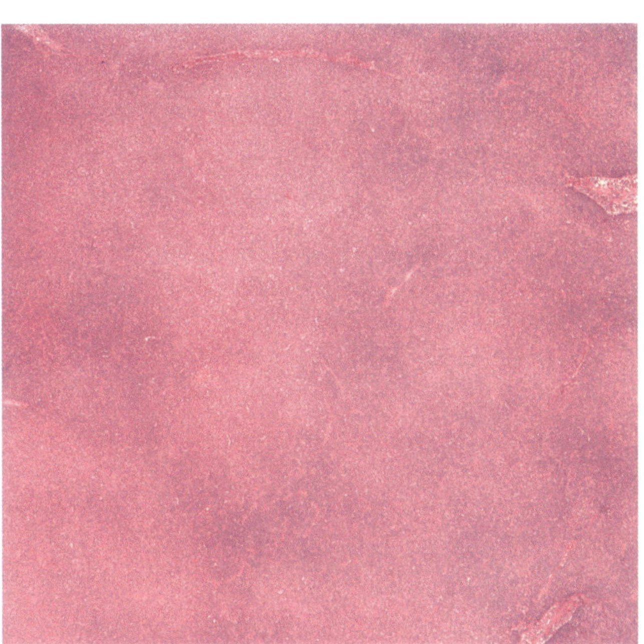

FIGURE 8-1

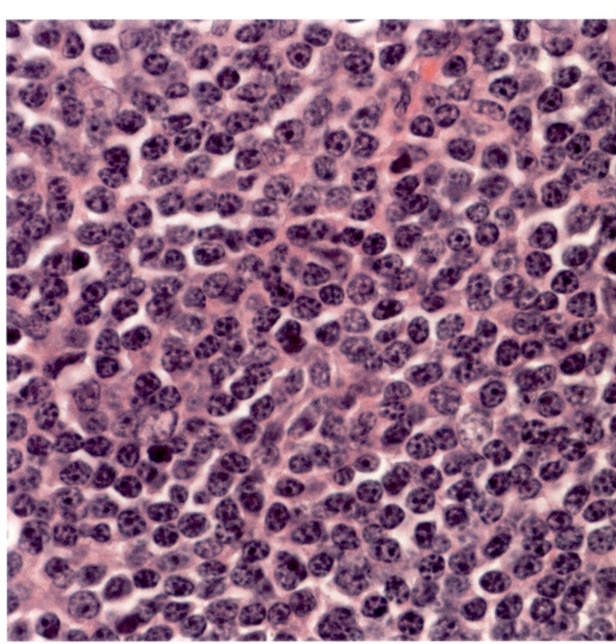

FIGURE 8-2

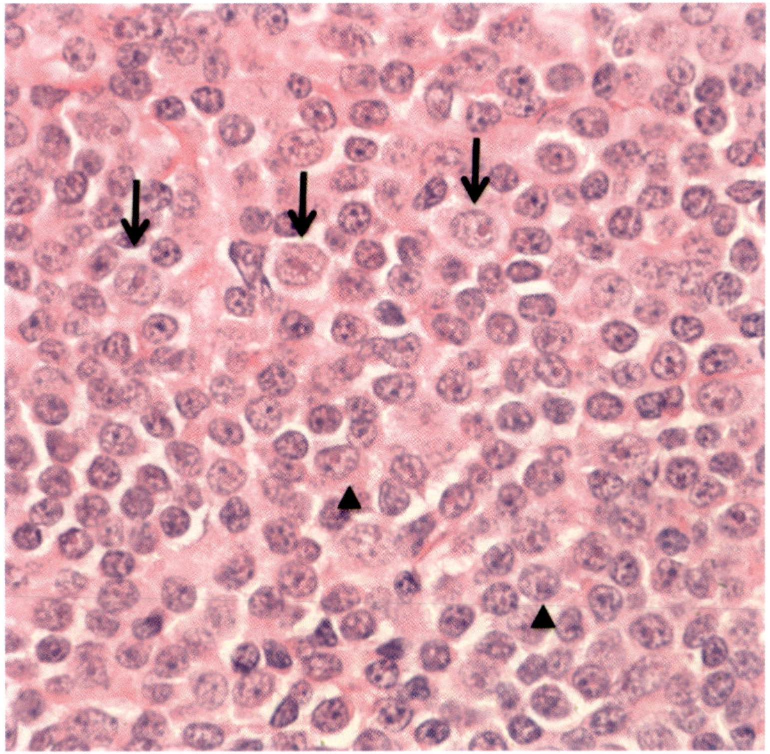

FIGURE 8-3

Chronic Lymphocytic Leukemia/Small Lymphocytic Lymphoma (CLL/SLL) *(continued)*

- CLL/SLL is comprised by clonal, light chain-restricted B cells that are CD19(+), CD20(dim +), CD22(dim+), CD5(+), CD10(−), CD23(+), FMC-7(−), CD38(variably +), surface immunoglobulin(dim +).
- Large cell (Richter's) transformation morphologically manifests as a pleomorphic diffuse large B-cell lymphoma (Figure 8-4).
- Occasionally, Reed-Sternberg-like cells may be present in CLL/SLL (Figure 8-5); if they are present in an appropriate background milieu, a diagnosis of classical Hodgkin lymphoma arising in CLL/SLL may be rendered.

DIFFERENTIAL DIAGNOSIS

- Mantle cell lymphoma
- Follicular lymphoma
- Marginal zone lymphoma
- Lymphoplasmacytic lymphoma

FIGURE 8-4 This image demonstrates a large cell (Richter's) transformation of CLL/SLL. The inset demonstrates focal CD5 positivity in the large neoplastic cells.

FIGURE 8-5 This high-power image shows large atypical cells with vesicular chromatin and prominent central nucleolus (Reed-Sternberg-like cells), in a background of small CLL/SLL cells. Without an appropriate Hodgkin lymphoma milieu surrounding the Reed-Sternberg-like cells, this is not diagnosed as Hodgkin lymphoma.

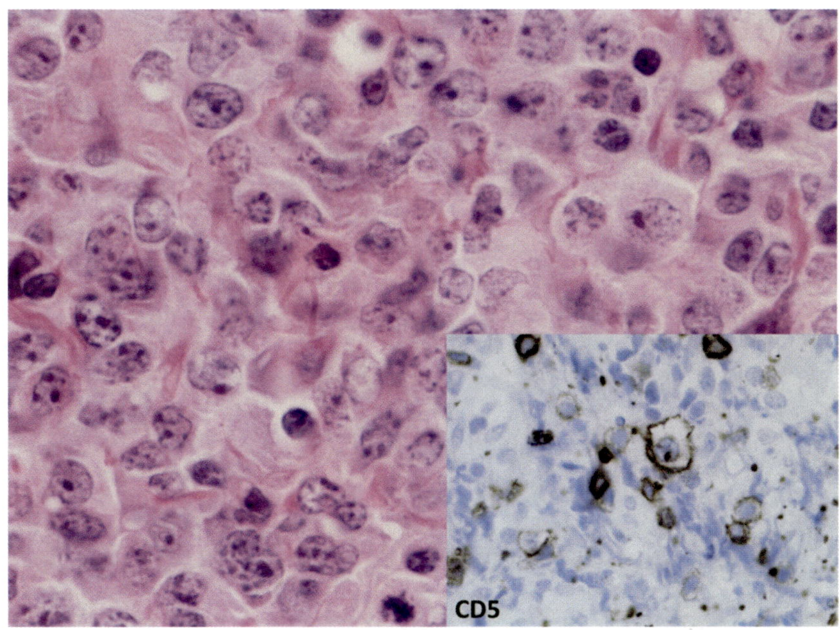

FIGURE 8-4

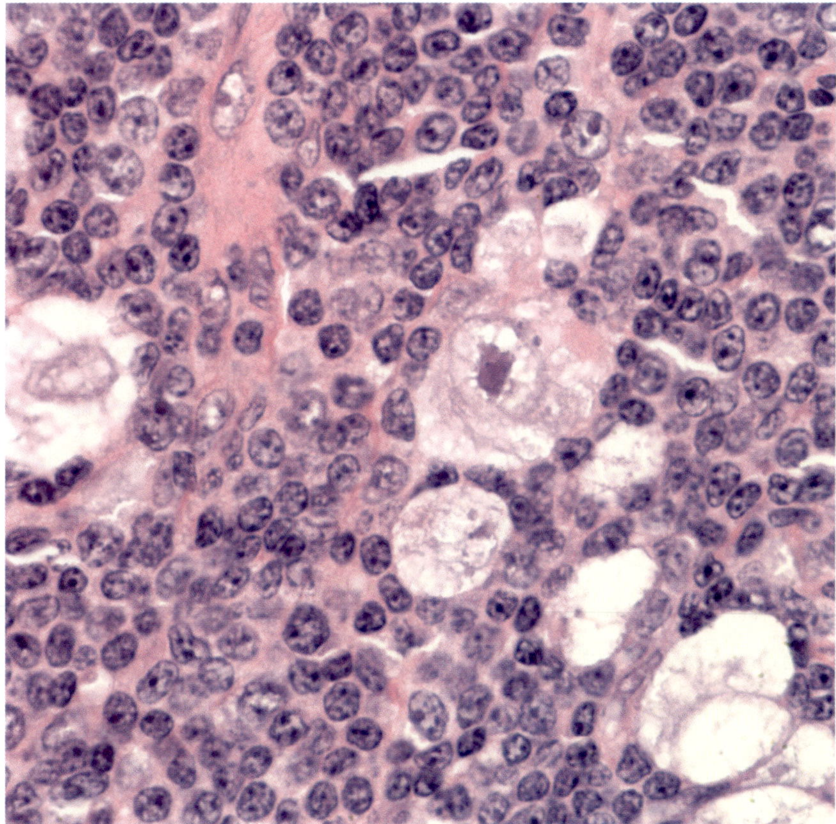

FIGURE 8-5

Splenic B-Cell Marginal Zone Lymphoma (SMZL)

DEFINITION

Splenic marginal zone lymphoma is a B-cell lymphoma arising in splenic white pulp with morphologic features that recapitulate normal splenic marginal zone cells.

CLINICAL FEATURES

- SMZL is a rare lymphoma (<2% of lymphoid neoplasm).
- It typically presents in patients over 50 years of age, with no gender predilection.
- In addition to spleen and splenic hilar lymph nodes, bone marrow and peripheral blood are often involved.
- Patients present with splenomegaly and cytopenias (anemia and/or thrombocytopenia).

HISTOLOGIC FINDINGS

- Splenic hilar lymph nodes show mostly preserved architecture, dilated sinuses, and a nodular infiltrate composed of small to medium-sized lymphocytes with regular to mildly irregular nuclei, slightly open chromatin, scattered small nucleoli, and moderate amounts of pale cytoplasm (Figures 8-6 and 8-7).
- The clonal B cells are characteristically CD19(+), CD20(+), CD5(−), CD10(−), CD23(−), CD103(−), IgM(+), IgD(+), and surface light chain restricted.

DIFFERENTIAL DIAGNOSIS

- Lymphoplasmacytic lymphoma
- Nodal marginal zone lymphoma
- Chronic lymphocytic leukemia/small lymphocytic lymphoma
- Mantle cell lymphoma
- Follicular lymphoma

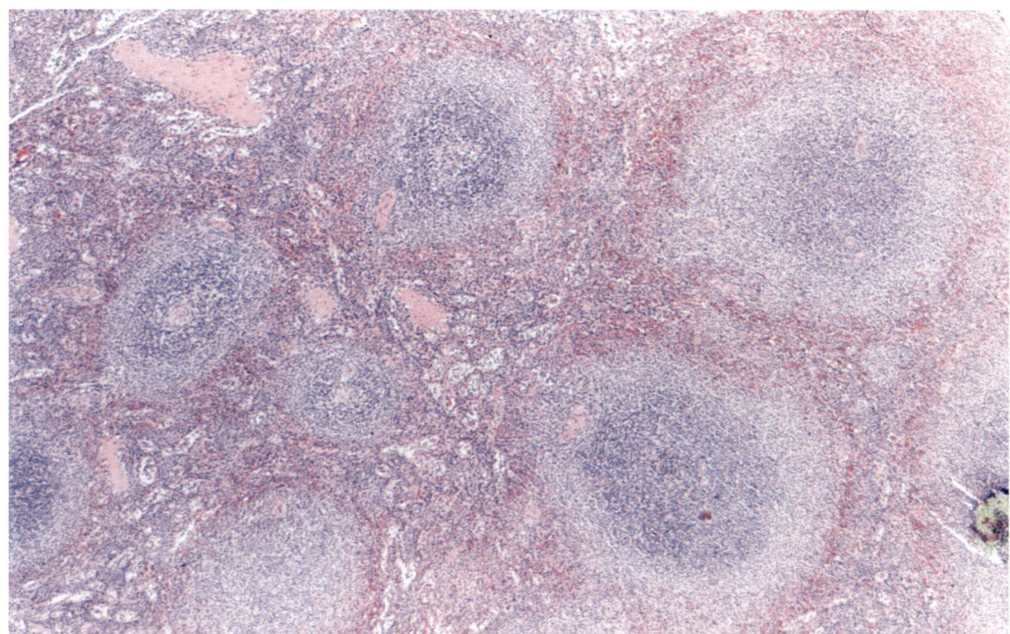

FIGURE 8-6

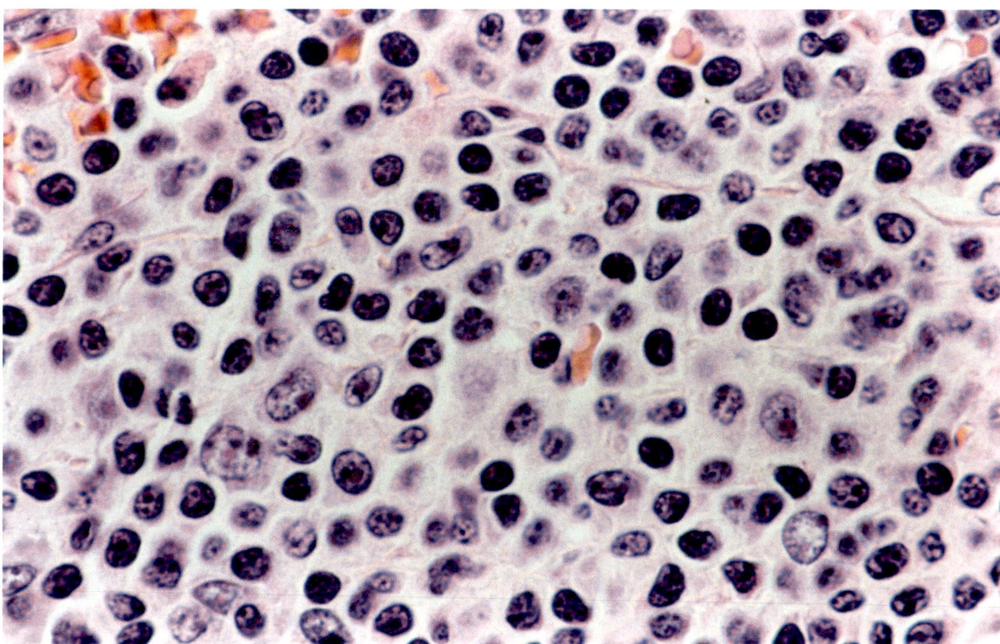

FIGURE 8-7

FIGURE 8-6 These white pulp follicles in the spleen have expanded, pale marginal zones.

FIGURE 8-7 This high-power view of the neoplastic cells reveals small lymphocytes and frequent medium-sized cells with mild nuclear irregularities, slightly open chromatin, and moderately abundant pale cytoplasm. Occasional transformed cells are also present.

Hairy Cell Leukemia (HCL)

DEFINITION

HCL is a mature B-cell neoplasm consisting of medium-sized cells with oval nuclei, reticular chromatin, and abundant cytoplasm with characteristic "hairy" projections. Peripheral blood, bone marrow, and splenic red pulp are consistently involved; occasionally, lymph nodes demonstrate hairy cell infiltrates.

CLINICAL FEATURES

- HCL is a rare neoplasm (2% of lymphoid leukemias) with median age of diagnosis of 50 years and a striking male predominance (male:female = 5:1).
- Patients present with splenomegaly, nonspecific symptoms (weakness, fatigue), and cytopenias (including monocytopenia in nearly all cases).

HISTOLOGIC FINDINGS

- In peripheral blood, typical hairy cells are medium in size, with oval or indented nuclei, smooth chromatin, occasional inconspicuous nucleoli, and abundant pale cytoplasm with characteristic "hairy" projections (Figure 8-8).
- Lymph nodes may show partially effaced architecture with an infiltrate composed of medium-sized cells with regular to mildly irregular nuclei and abundant pale cytoplasm ("fried egg" appearance) (Figures 8-9 and 8-10).
- The typical immunophenotype of HCL is CD19(+), CD20(+), CD5(−), CD10(−), CD22(bright +), CD11c(bright +), CD103(+), CD25(+), CD123(+), annexin A1(+).

DIFFERENTIAL DIAGNOSIS

- Marginal zone lymphoma

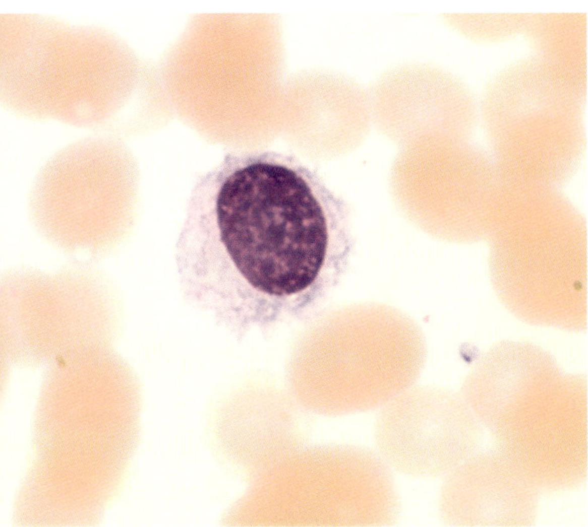

FIGURE 8-8

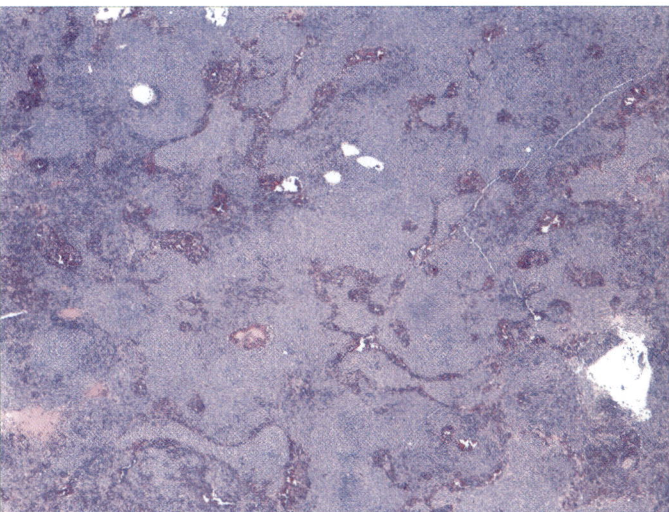

FIGURE 8-9

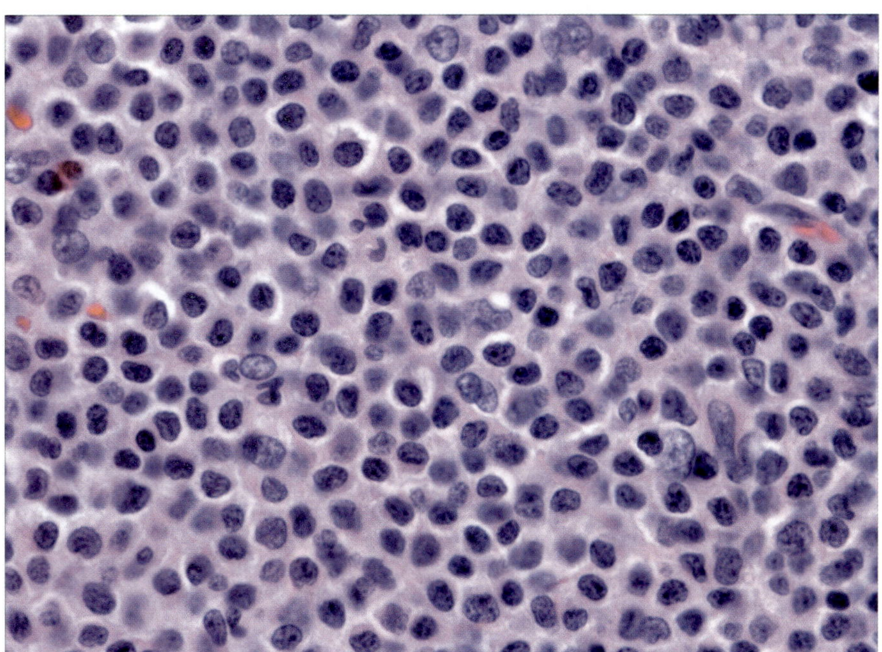

FIGURE 8-10

FIGURE 8-8 This is a typical neoplastic cell in HCL. It is medium in size, with an oval nucleus, smooth chromatin, and abundant pale cytoplasm with characteristic "hairy" projections.

FIGURE 8-9 This unusual example of lymph node enlargement by HCL demonstrates patent sinuses, but otherwise effaced architecture.

FIGURE 8-10 High-power of the lymph node infiltrate demonstrates small to medium-sized cells with mildly irregular nuclei, mature chromatin, absent nucleoli, and moderately abundant cytoplasm.

Lymphoplasmacytic Lymphoma (LPL)

DEFINITION

LPL is a neoplasm of small B cells, plasmacytoid lymphocytes, and plasma cells, that usually involves the bone marrow, lymph nodes, and spleen. Waldenstrom macroglobulinemia is defined as the combination of LPL with bone marrow involvement and a serum IgM paraprotein.

CLINICAL FEATURES

- LPL occurs at a median age of 60 years, with a male to female ratio of 2:1.
- Patients may present with nonspecific symptoms (weakness, fatigue), anemia, hyperviscosity (30%), or cryoglobulinemia.

HISTOLOGIC FINDINGS

- Involved lymph nodes are diffusely or partially effaced, although sinuses are characteristically patent. The infiltrate is composed of an admixture of small lymphocytes, plasmacytoid lymphocytes, and mature plasma cells; occasional transformed cells may be present (Figures 8-11 and 8-12).
- The characteristic immunophenotype of the clonal B cells is CD19(+), CD20(+), CD5(−), CD10(−), CD103(−), and surface light chain restricted. The plasma cell component is CD138(+), CD38(bright +), CD19(+), CD56(−), and cytoplasmic light chain restricted.
- Plasma cells show frequent intranuclear pseudoinclusions (Dutcher bodies) or cytoplasmic immunoglobulin inclusions (Russell bodies).
- Amyloid or light chain deposition may be present (Figure 8-13).

DIFFERENTIAL DIAGNOSIS

- Marginal zone lymphoma with plasmacytic differentiation
- Plasmacytoma
- Chronic lymphocytic leukemia/small lymphocytic lymphoma
- Follicular lymphoma

FIGURE 8-11 This lymph node shows effaced architecture, dilated sinuses, and a monotonous neoplastic infiltrate.

FIGURE 8-12 A high-power view of the neoplastic infiltrate reveals an admixture of small lymphocytes, plasmacytoid lymphocytes, and mature plasma cells.

FIGURE 8-13 This lymph node with LPL also contains extensive immunoglobulin deposits, manifesting as amorphous eosinophilic material.

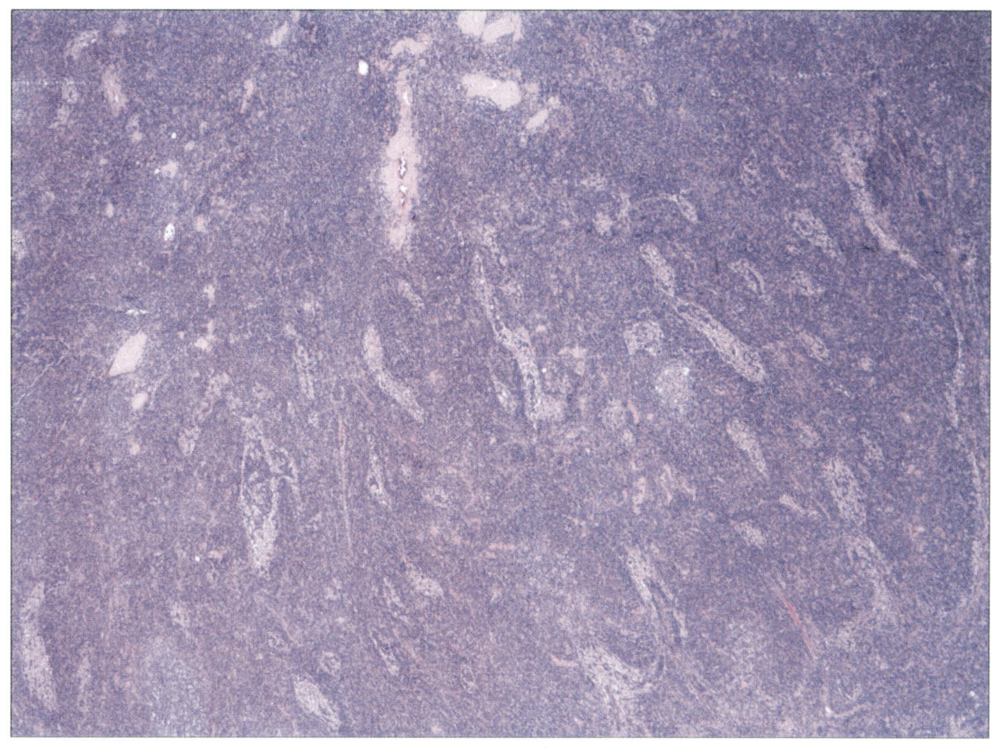

FIGURE 8-11

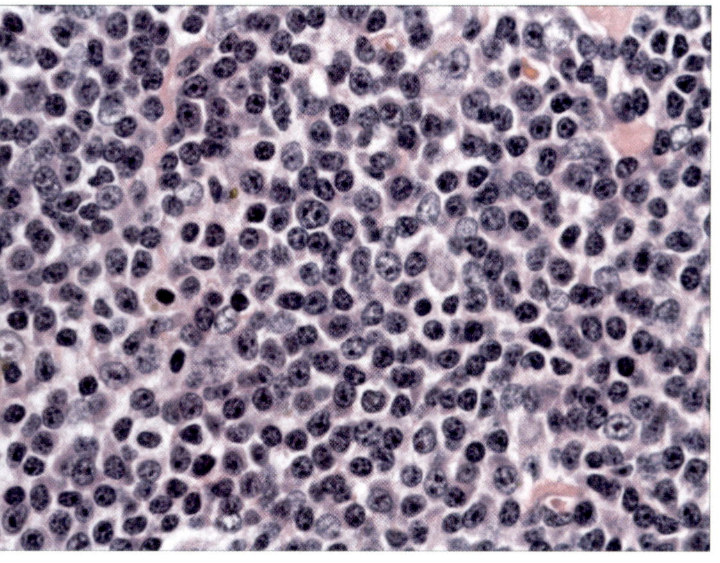

FIGURE 8-12

FIGURE 8-13

Heavy Chain Diseases (HCDs)

DEFINITION

HCDs are a set of three rare B-cell neoplasms (alpha, gamma, and mu HCD) characterized by monoclonal heavy chain production (IgA, IgG, and IgM, respectively), without accompanying light chains. Gamma HCD morphologically resembles lymphoplasmacytic lymphoma, and may involve lymph nodes. Alpha HCD is considered a variant of extranodal marginal zone lymphoma of mucosa associated lymphoid tissue (MALT lymphoma) and typically involves the small bowel. Mu HCD morphologically resembles chronic lymphocytic leukemia/small lymphocytic lymphoma and does not usually involve lymph nodes.

A. GAMMA HEAVY CHAIN DISEASE

CLINICAL FEATURES

- Gamma HCD is very rare, presenting at a median age 60 years with a slight male predominance.
- Patients present with nonspecific symptoms (weakness, weight loss).
- Autoimmune conditions, such as rheumatoid arthritis, Sjogren syndrome, systemic lupus erythematosus, are present in 25% of cases.
- Bone marrow is involved in approximately 50% of patients.

HISTOLOGIC FINDINGS

- Lymph nodes show a polymorphous infiltrate composed of small, mature lymphocytes, plasmacytoid lymphocytes, mature plasma cells, and occasional immunoblasts (Figures 8-14 and 8-15).
- Immunohistochemistry and in situ hybridization shows only gamma heavy chain expression; light chains are not demonstrable (Figure 8-16).

DIFFERENTIAL DIAGNOSIS

- Lymphoplasmacytic lymphoma
- Marginal zone lymphoma with plasmacytic differentiation

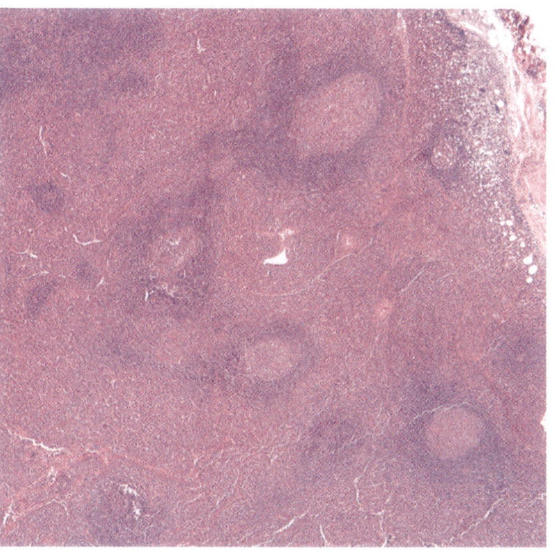

FIGURE 8-14

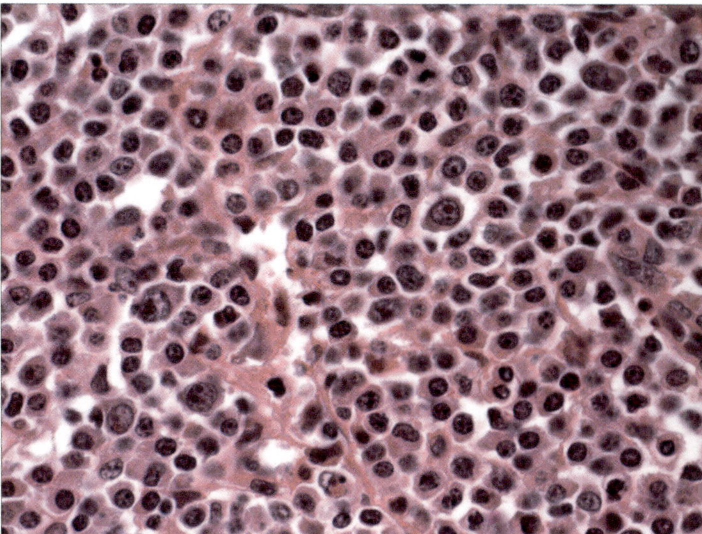

FIGURE 8-15

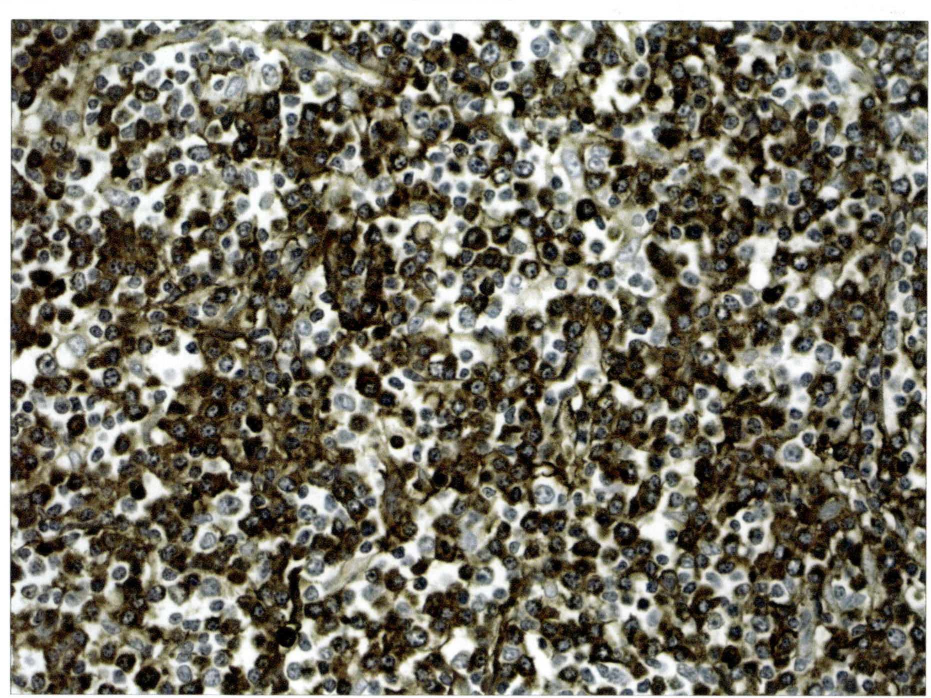

FIGURE 8-16

FIGURE 8-14 This lymph node has a partially preserved architecture with an interfollicular infiltrate between reactive follicles.

FIGURE 8-15 High-power magnification of the interfollicular infiltrate demonstrates small lymphocytes, plasmacytoid lymphocytes, plasma cells, and immunoblasts.

FIGURE 8-16 IgG immunohistochemistry demonstrates gamma heavy chain expression in the neoplastic cells.

Extraosseous Plasmacytoma

DEFINITION

Extraosseous plasmacytoma represents a collection of neoplastic plasma cells, arising in tissues other than bone.

CLINICAL FEATURES

- This is a rare plasma cell dycrasia (3–5% of plasma cell neoplasms), with a median age of 55 years and a male to female ratio of 2:1.
- Extraosseous plasmacytoma commonly occurs in the upper respiratory tract, but can also involve lymph nodes and other tissues.
- Symptoms are related to site of involvement; a monoclonal serum protein is present in 20% of cases.

HISTOLOGIC FINDINGS

- Plasmacytomas consist of sheets of plasma cells with variable morphology (Figures 8-17 and 8-18).
- Immunohistochemistry demonstrates light chain restriction in the neoplastic plasma cells.
- An immunophenotype of CD138(+), CD38(+), CD19(−), CD56(+), CD20(−) plasma cells favors a plasmacytoma over a B-cell lymphoma with plasmacytic differentiation.

DIFFERENTIAL DIAGNOSIS

- Marginal zone lymphoma with plasmacytic differentiation
- Heavy chain disease
- Plasmablastic lymphoma

FIGURE 8-17 This lymph node has an architecture that is effaced by a diffuse infiltrate of plasma cells.

FIGURE 8-18 High-power view of the neoplastic infiltrate reveals variably-sized plasma cells with eccentric nuclei, dispersed chromatin, and small nucleoli.

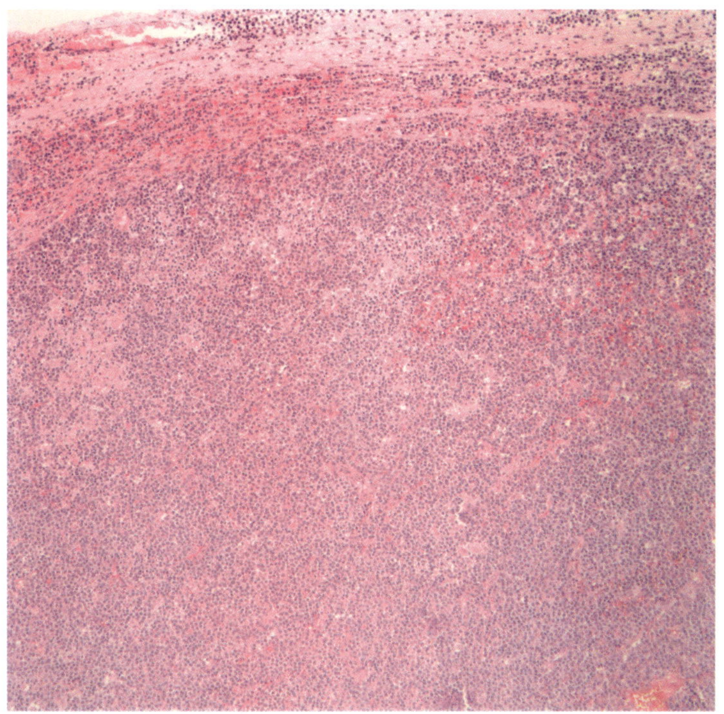

FIGURE 8-17

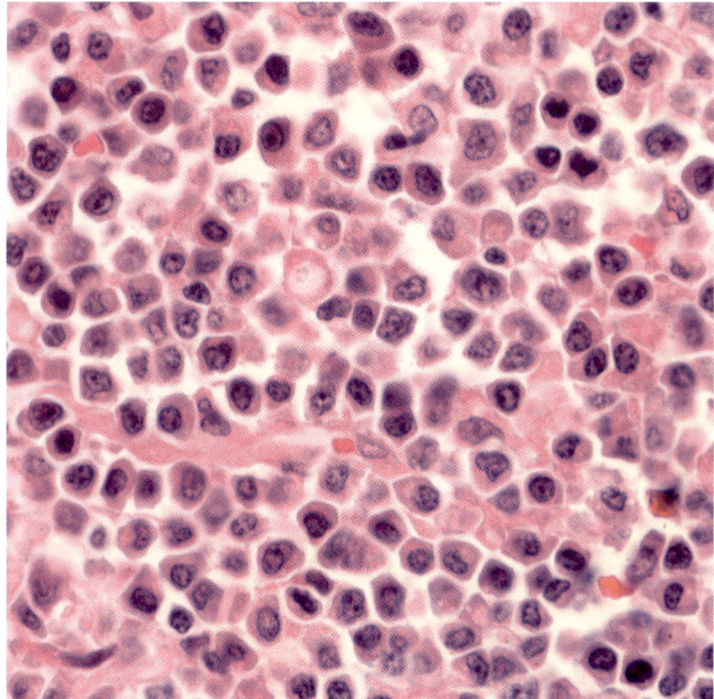

FIGURE 8-18

Nodal Marginal Zone Lymphoma (MZL)

DEFINITION

Nodal MZL is a low-grade B-cell neoplasm that involves lymph nodes, morphologically resembles lymph node involvement by MZL of splenic or extranodal origin, but lacks evidence of splenic or extranodal lymphoma.

CLINICAL FEATURES

- Nodal MZL is rare, representing 1.5–2% of lymphomas.
- It presents at a median age of 60 years, with no gender predilection.
- Patients present with localized or generalized lymphadenopathy, but are otherwise, usually asymptomatic.
- In addition to lymph nodes, bone marrow and peripheral blood are occasionally involved.

HISTOLOGIC FINDINGS

- Two main patterns are observed: cases resembling nodal involvement by extranodal MZL ("MALT type") and those resembling involvement by splenic MZL.
- In the common MALT type, the lymph node architecture is largely preserved, with neoplastic cells distributed in perisinusoidal, perivascular, and peri- or para-follicular distribution (Figure 8-19). Follicles are reactive, with intact mantles.
- In the uncommon splenic MZL-like type, the architecture is effaced by a diffuse or vaguely nodular infiltrate. Sinuses are obliterated; burnt out or naked germinal centers may be present.
- The neoplastic infiltrates consist of an admixture of centrocyte-like (marginal zone) cells, monocytoid B cells, plasma cells, and occasional transformed cells (Figure 8-20).
- Plasmacytic differentiation may be prominent, raising the differential diagnosis with lymphoplasmacytic lymphoma or plasmacytoma.
- Occasional cases may have >20% large transformed cells; however, they are usually admixed with small cells and do not represent large cell transformation.
- MZL cells are typically CD19(+), CD20(+), CD22(+), CD5(−), CD10(−), BCL2-(+), BCL-6(−), cyclin D1(−), and surface light chain restricted.
- CD43 is positive in 50% of cases and IgD is usually negative.

DIFFERENTIAL DIAGNOSIS

- Splenic MZL
- Extranodal MZL of mucosa-associated lymphoid tissue (MALT) lymphoma
- Lymphoplasmacytic lymphoma
- Chronic lymphocytic leukemia/small lymphocytic lymphoma
- Mantle cell lymphoma
- Follicular lymphoma with marginal zone differentiation

FIGURE 8-19 This lymph node contains a neoplastic infiltrate with nodules surrounded by accentuated marginal zones.

FIGURE 8-20 This high-power image demonstrates a collection of small to medium-sized cells with mild nuclear irregularities and moderately abundant pale cytoplasm.

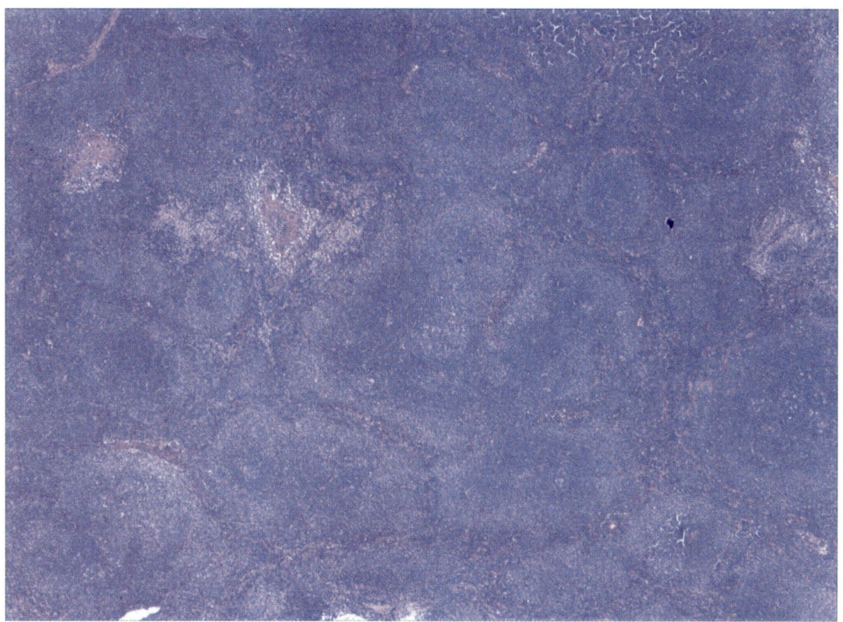

FIGURE 8-19

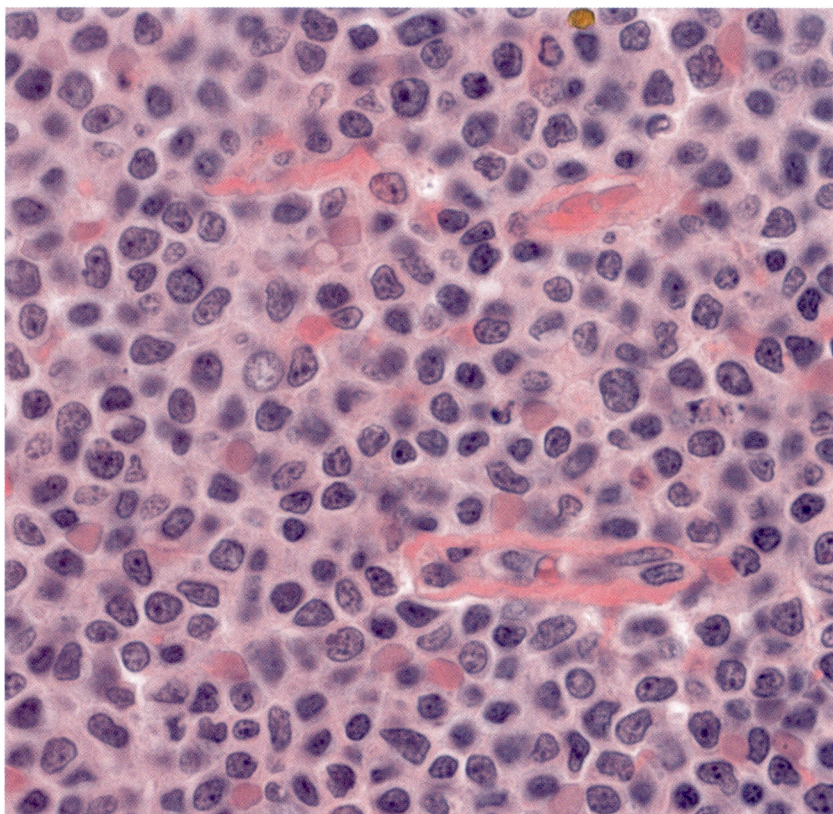

FIGURE 8-20

Follicular Lymphoma (FL)

DEFINITION

FL is a B-cell neoplasm of germinal center origin, composed of centrocytes and centroblasts, and with at least some degree of follicular pattern in the vast majority of cases.

CLINICAL FEATURES

- FL comprises 20% of lymphomas.
- It occurs at a median age of 60 years, with a male to female ratio of 1:1.7.
- FL can rarely occur in pediatric patients, usually males.
- Patients present with lymphadenopathy of varying extent, but are otherwise usually asymptomatic.
- The bone marrow is commonly involved (40–70% of cases).

HISTOLOGIC FINDINGS

- Typical cases show a follicular pattern, with back-to-back neoplastic follicles that lack polarization, tingible body macrophages, and well-defined mantle zones (Figure 8-21).
- The follicles are composed of centrocytes and a variable number of centroblasts (Figure 8-22). The number of centroblasts determines the morphologic grade: grade 1 (0–4 centroblasts/high-power field); grade 2 (5–14 centroblasts/hpf); grade 3 (≥15 centroblasts/hpf).
- Grade 3 is subdivided into 3A, if centrocytes are present, and 3B, if only centroblasts are present (Figure 8-22).
- A diffuse pattern may be present in variable proportion to the follicular pattern (Figure 8-23).
- Diffuse areas that have >15 centroblasts/hpf are reported as diffuse large B-cell lymphoma with FL.

(continued)

FIGURE 8-21 This lymph node contains a neoplastic infiltrate composed of uniform, back-to-back follicles that lack polarization, tingible body macrophages, and well-defined mantle zones.

FIGURE 8-22 Follicular lymphoma (FL), histologic grading. (A) FL grade 1, with <5 centroblasts (arrows)/hpf; (B) FL grade 2, with 5–14 centroblasts (arrows)/hpf; (C) FL grade 3A, with ≥15 centroblasts/hpf, admixed with centrocytes; (D) FL grade 3B, with follicle consisting exclusively of centroblasts.

FIGURE 8-23 This lymph node demonstrates an effaced architecture and no evidence of follicular pattern. The inset demonstrates medium-power view of the neoplastic infiltrate, composed predominantly of centrocytes.

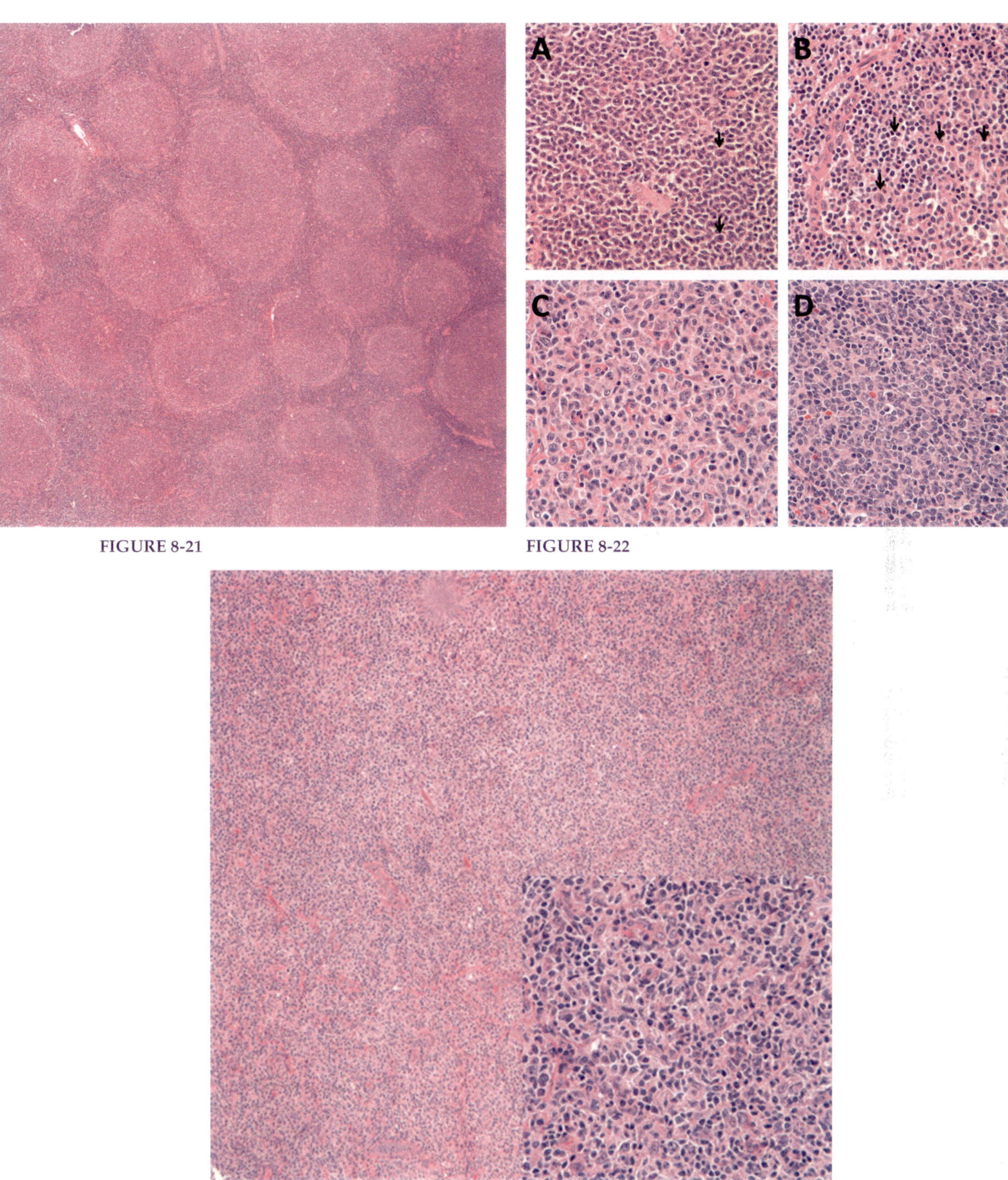

FIGURE 8-21

FIGURE 8-22

FIGURE 8-23

Follicular Lymphoma (FL) *(continued)*

- FL may have marginal zone differentiation, with follicles surrounded by a cuff of medium-sized cells with mild nuclear irregularities and abundant pale cytoplasm (Figure 8-24).
- An uncommon "floral" variant of FL may be seen, with irregularly shaped neoplastic follicles due to invagination of mantle zones into the follicles (Figure 8-25).
- The typical immunophenotype is CD19(+), CD20(+), CD5(−), CD10(+), BCL-2(+), BCL-6(+), and surface light chain restricted.
- CD10 expression may be lost, particularly in grade 3B FL or FL with marginal zone differentiation.
- BCL-2 expression may be absent, particularly in grade 3 FL.
- CD21, CD23, and CD35 highlight follicular dendritic cell meshworks corresponding to the neoplastic follicles; lack of such meshworks is helpful in confirming areas with a diffuse pattern.
- The pediatric variant of FL usually presents with localized lymphadenopathy; grade 3 morphology; and lacks BCL-2 (Figure 8-26).

DIFFERENTIAL DIAGNOSIS

- Reactive lymphadenopathy with follicular hyperplasia
- Mantle cell lymphoma
- Marginal zone lymphoma

FIGURE 8-24 In this follicular lymphoma with marginal zone differentiation, the neoplastic follicles are surrounded by a pale rim of cells with features of marginal zones cells.

FIGURE 8-25 In this floral variant of follicular lymphoma, the lymph node contains variably-sized and irregularly shaped follicles, resembling progressive transformation of germinal centers.

FIGURE 8-26 In this example of pediatric follicular lymphoma, the lymph node contains closely packed neoplastic follicles, composed almost exclusively of centroblasts (inset).

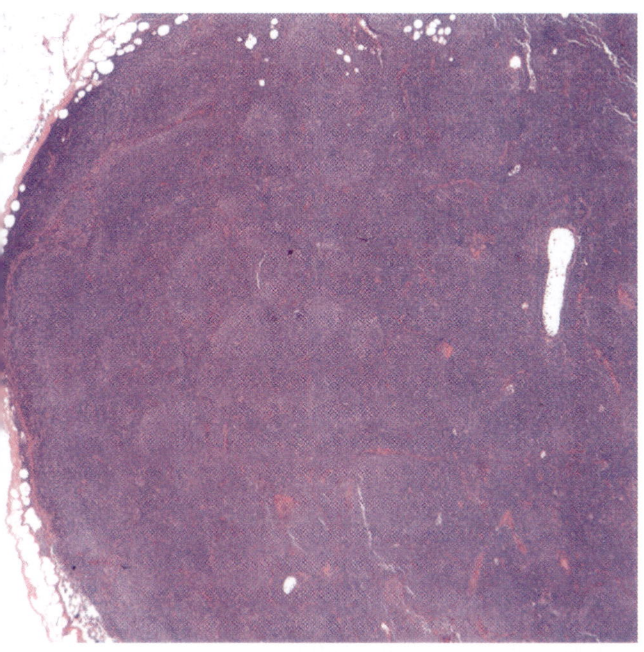

FIGURE 8-24

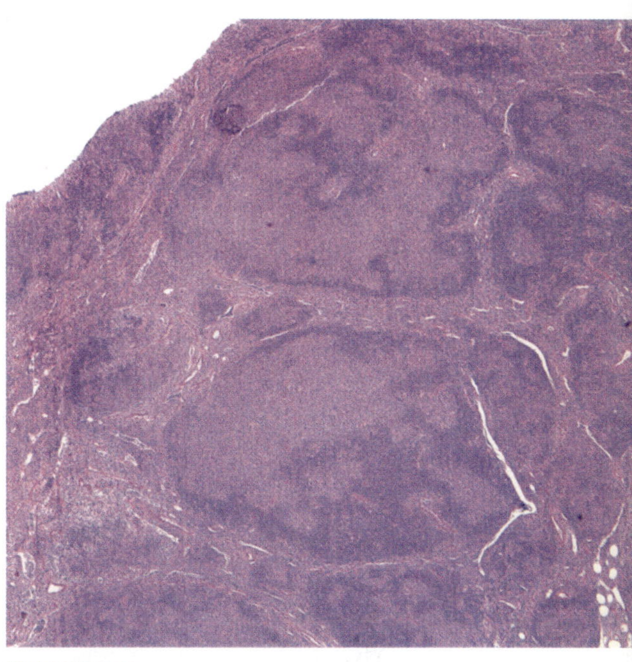

FIGURE 8-25

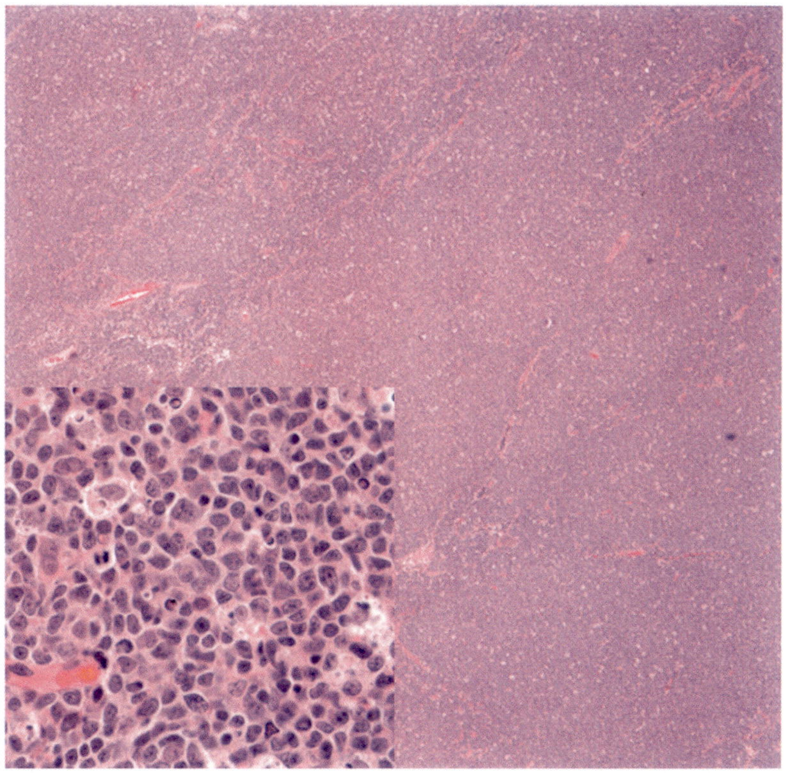

FIGURE 8-26

Mantle Cell Lymphoma (MCL)

DEFINITION

MCL is a clinically aggressive B-cell neoplasm composed of small to medium-sized cells with irregular nuclei and almost uniform cyclin D1 expression as a consequence of the t(11;14)(q13;q32) translocation.

CLINICAL FEATURES

- MCL is uncommon (3–10% of non-Hodgkin lymphomas).
- This lymphoma type occurs at a median age of 60 years, with a male to female ratio of 2:1.
- Lymph nodes are commonly involved; bone marrow and peripheral blood involvement are also present to some degree in the majority of cases.
- Gastrointestinal tract involvement is very common, and occasionally this is the presenting site of involvement (lymphomatous polyposis).
- Patients frequently present with bulky disease, with advanced clinical stage.

HISTOLOGIC FINDINGS

- MCL typically produces effaced nodal architecture with a diffuse or vaguely nodular infiltrate. Less commonly, MCL assumes distinctly nodular or mantle zone patterns.
- Classically, MCL is composed of small to medium-sized cells with variable nuclear irregularities, mature chromatin, and scanty cytoplasm (Figures 8-27 and 8-28).
- The blastoid variant of MCL consists of cells with finely dispersed chromatin and frequent mitoses (Figure 8-29).
- The pleomorphic variant of MCL shows variable cytology, with frequent large cells with occasional prominent nucleoli and abundant pale cytoplasm (Figure 8-30).
- The typical immunophenotype is CD19(+), CD20(+), CD22(+), CD5(+), CD10(−), CD23(−), FMC-7(+), BCL-6(−), BCL-2(+), SOX11(+).
- Almost all cases express cyclin D1 and have a t(11;14)(q13;q32) translocation; rare cyclin D1(−) cases are SOX11(+).

DIFFERENTIAL DIAGNOSIS

- Chronic lymphocytic leukemia/small lymphocytic lymphoma
- Marginal zone lymphoma

FIGURE 8-27 This lymph node has effaced architecture with a vaguely nodular infiltrate.

FIGURE 8-28 High-power view demonstrates that the neoplastic cells are small to medium in size, with irregular nuclear contours, condensed chromatin, and scant cytoplasm. The inset demonstrates strong cyclin D1 positivity in the lymphoma cells.

FIGURE 8-29 In this blastoid variant of mantle cell lymphoma, the malignant cells have dispersed chromatin and mildly irregular nuclei.

FIGURE 8-30 This pleomorphic variant of mantle cell lymphoma is composed of large cells with irregular nuclei, variably clumped chromatin, occasional distinct nucleoli, and eosinophilic cytoplasm.

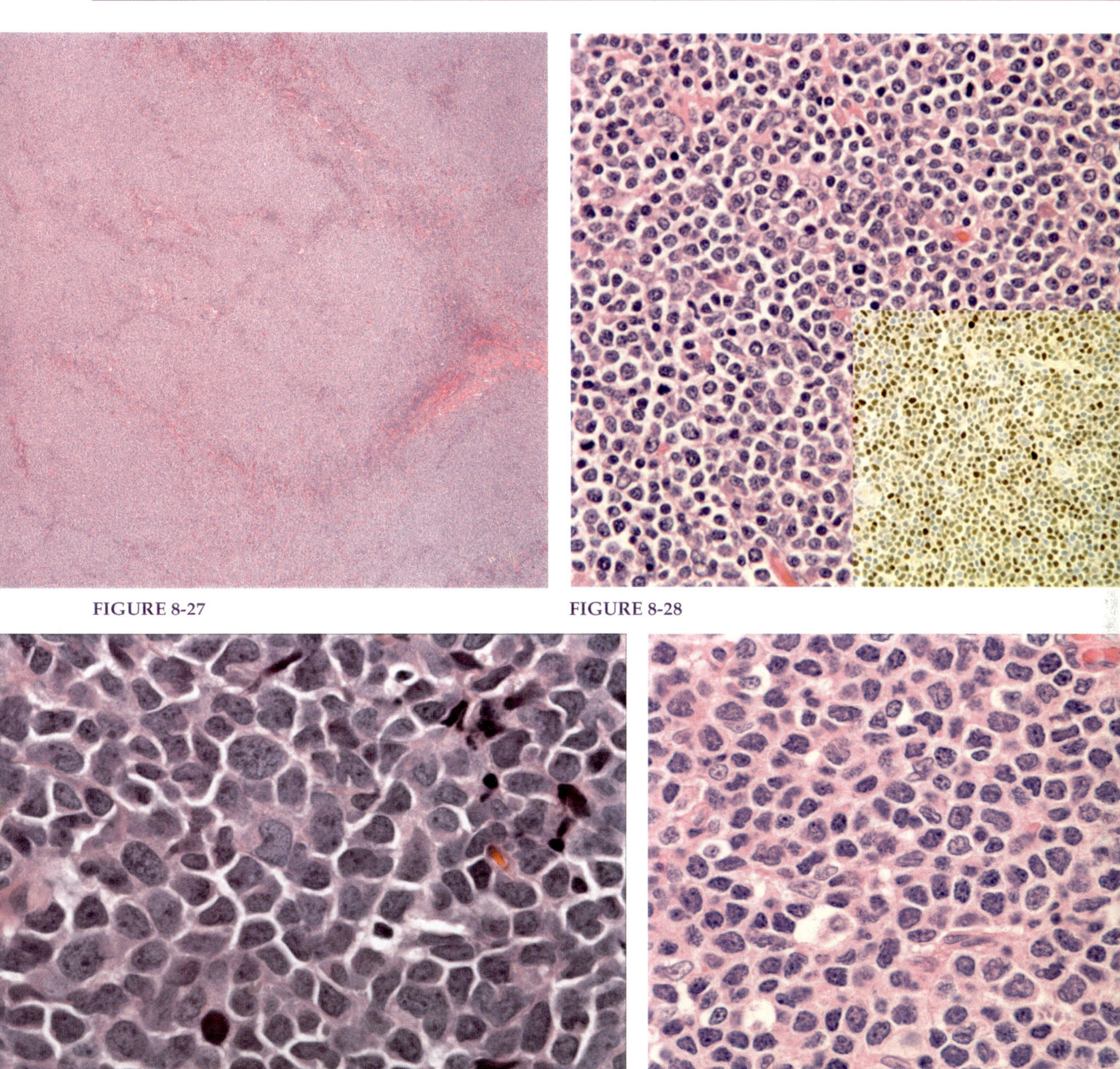

FIGURE 8-27

FIGURE 8-28

FIGURE 8-29

FIGURE 8-30

Diffuse Large B-Cell Lymphoma, Not Otherwise Specified (DLBCL, NOS)

DEFINITION

This is a heterogeneous group of lymphomas that consist of lymphocytes with a nucleus at least twice as large as the size of a normal lymphocyte, or larger than a macrophage nucleus. In addition to DLBCL, NOS, specific subtypes and entities are also recognized in the 2008 WHO classification of hematolymphoid neoplasms.

CLINICAL FEATURES

- DLBCL is common in Western countries (approximately 30% of adult non-Hodgkin lymphomas).
- It can occur at any age, but most often in older patients (median age of 70 years). There is a slight male predominance.
- DLBCL may occur de novo, or as a transformation of a prior low-grade B-cell non-Hodgkin lymphoma.
- Extranodal presentation is common (approximately 40% of cases).
- Bone marrow involvement (10–25% of cases) may have discordant (small cell) or concordant (large cell) morphology.
- Patients present with lymphadenopathy and are often otherwise asymptomatic.

HISTOLOGIC FINDINGS

- Involved lymph nodes show partial or total architectural effacement by a diffuse infiltrate composed of large neoplastic cells. Common recognized cytologic variants include centroblastic (medium to large-sized cells with regular nuclei, vesicular chromatin, several membrane bound nucleoli, and scant cytoplasm) and immunoblastic (large cells with round to oval nuclei, single, central, prominent nucleolus, and abundant amphophilic cytoplasm) (Figures 8-31 to 8-33).
- DLBCL with polylobate nuclei frequently manifests in bone or soft tissue (Figure 8-34).
- DLBCL is composed of clonal B cells that are CD19(+), CD20(+), CD22(+), and surface light chain restricted. They are commonly divided into germinal center type [CD10(+) or CD10(−), BCL6(+), IRF4/MUM1(−)] and activated B-cell type [CD10(−), IRF4/MUM1(+)]. CD5 is expressed in 5% of cases.

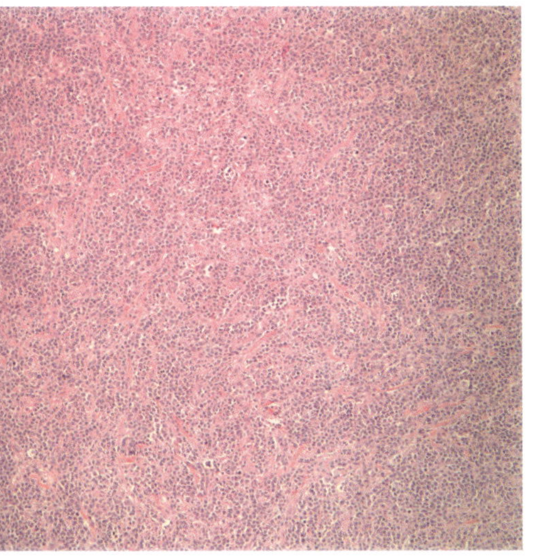

FIGURE 8-31

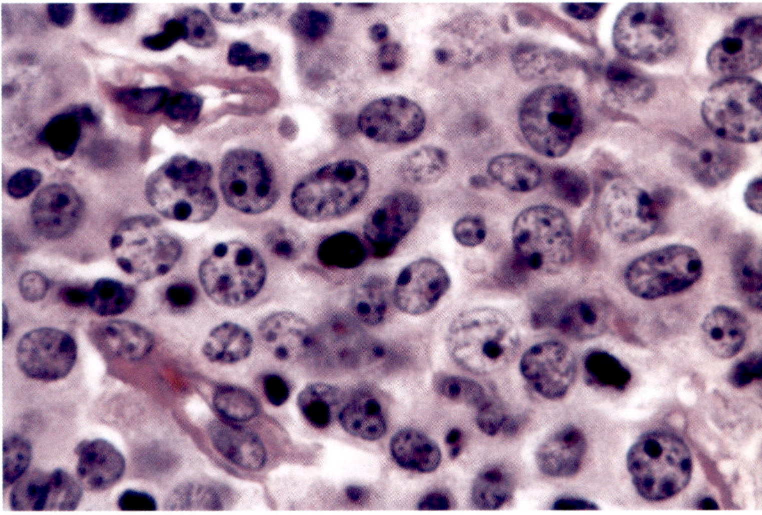

FIGURE 8-32

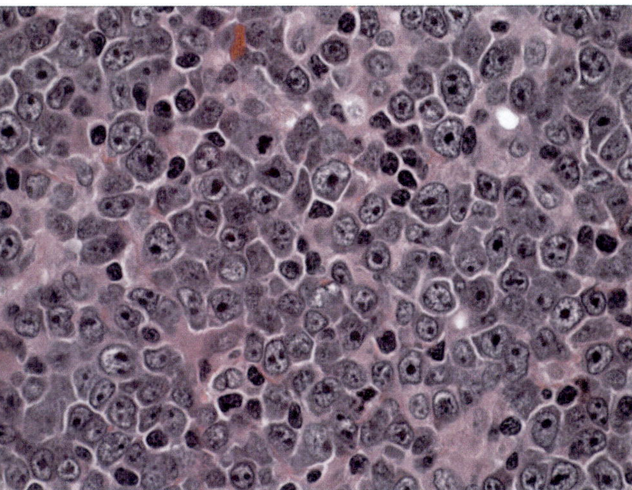

FIGURE 8-33

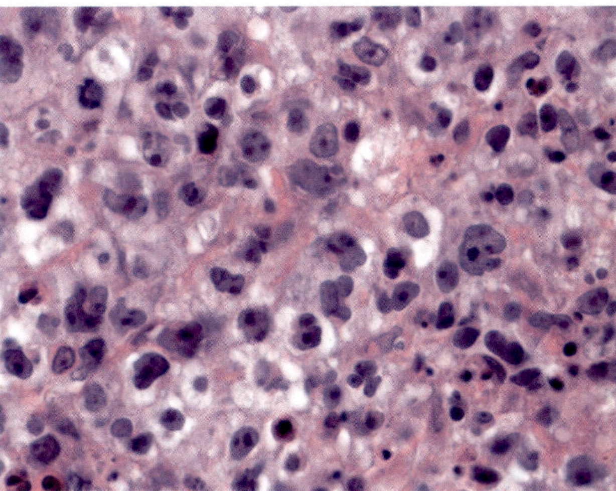

FIGURE 8-34

FIGURE 8-31 This lymph node shows effaced architecture and a diffuse infiltrate of neoplastic cells.

FIGURE 8-32 High-power view of the large cells demonstrates centroblastic morphology: regular nuclei, vesicular chromatin, and multiple, membrane-bound nucleoli.

FIGURE 8-33 This DLBCL has immunoblastic features, characterized by prominent central nucleoli and abundant amphophilic cytoplasm.

FIGURE 8-34 This example consists of large cells with polylobate nuclei.

DLBCL Subtypes

A. T CELL/HISTIOCYTE-RICH LARGE B-CELL LYMPHOMA (TCHRLBCL)

DEFINITION

This variant represents a DLBCL composed of rare large, atypical B cells, admixed with frequent T cells and histiocytes.

CLINICAL FEATURES

- TCHRLBCL comprises fewer than 10% of DLBCLs. It typically occurs in middle-aged adults.
- Patients present with systemic symptoms and lymphadenopathy or organomegaly.

HISTOLOGIC FINDINGS

- Lymph nodes demonstrate an effaced architecture and scattered atypical large B-cells in a background of numerous T cells and frequent histiocytes (Figure 8-35).

B. EBV POSITIVE DIFFUSE LARGE B-CELL LYMPHOMA OF THE ELDERLY

DEFINITION

This variant is defined as an EBV(+) large cell lymphoma occurring in individuals older than 50 years without prior history of immunodeficiency or lymphoma.

CLINICAL FEATURES

- The median age is 71 years, with a male to female ratio of 1.4:1.
- Patients commonly present with extranodal disease (70%).

HISTOLOGIC FINDINGS

- Involved lymph nodes have an effaced architecture, focal necrosis, and frequent atypical large B-cells, admixed with a variable number of small lymphocytes, plasma cells, immunoblasts, and histiocytes (Figure 8-36).
- The lymphoma cells are CD19(+), CD20(+), CD10(−), BCL-6(−), CD30(variably +), CD15(−), LMP1(+), EBNA-2(+), and EBER(+) by in situ hybridization.

DIFFERENTIAL DIAGNOSIS

- Infectious mononucleosis lymphadenitis
- Anaplastic large cell lymphoma
- Classical Hodgkin lymphoma
- Myeloid sarcoma
- Poorly differentiated carcinoma
- Melanoma

FIGURE 8-35

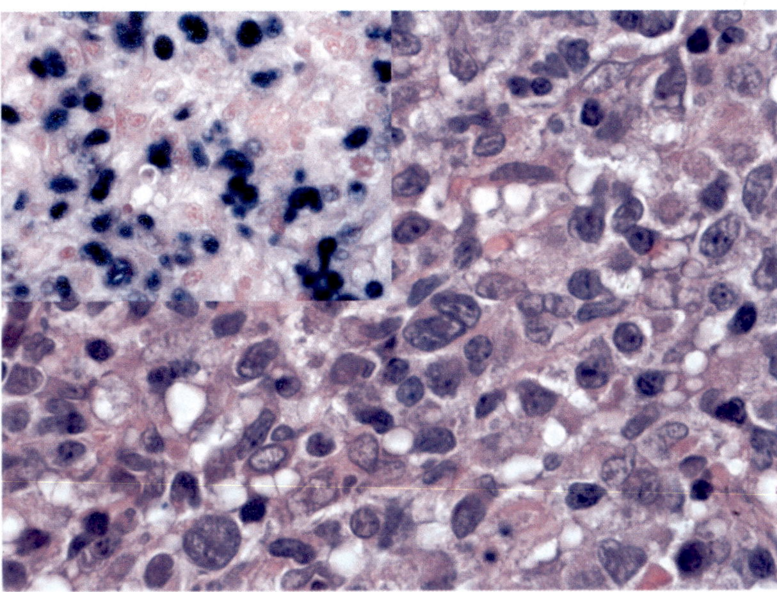

FIGURE 8-36

FIGURE 8-35 T-cell/histiocyte rich large B-cell lymphoma. A hematoxylin and eosin stained section (left) shows scattered large atypical cells, with oval nuclei, and prominent nucleoli, in a background of numerous small lymphocytes and histiocytes. CD20 immunohistochemistry (right) highlights the atypical cells, and occasional small B cells. The remaining cells are predominantly small T cells.

FIGURE 8-36 This example of EBV positive diffuse large B-cell lymphoma of the elderly consists of a polymorphous infiltrate of large cells, small lymphocytes, and histiocytes. The inset demonstrates in situ hybridization for EBER, with strong nuclear positivity in the lymphoma cells.

Primary Mediastinal Large B-Cell Lymphoma (PMLBCL)

DEFINITION

PMLBCL represents a diffuse large B-cell lymphoma of putative thymic origin, arising in the anterior mediastinum, and showing distinct clinical and pathologic features.

CLINICAL FEATURES

- This uncommon tumor (2–4% of non-Hodgkin lymphomas) occurs at a median age of 35 years with a female predominance (male:female = 1:2).
- Patients present with a bulky, anterior mediastinal mass, and lack systemic lymph node and bone marrow involvement.
- Symptoms are related to the mediastinal mass.

HISTOLOGIC FINDINGS

- The typical morphology is that of nests of lymphoma cells separated by thin bands of fibrosis (Figure 8-37).
- The lymphoma cells are medium to large in size, with regular nuclei and abundant pale cytoplasm (Figure 8-38); occasional cells with Reed-Sternberg-like morphology may be present.
- Tumor cells are typically CD19(+), CD20(+), CD22(+), CD10(−), CD15(−), BCL-2(+), BCL-6(+), IRF4/MUM1(+), and CD30(weakly+) (Figure 8-39).

DIFFERENTIAL DIAGNOSIS

- Diffuse large B-cell lymphoma, NOS
- Classical Hodgkin lymphoma
- Anaplastic large cell lymphoma
- Thymoma

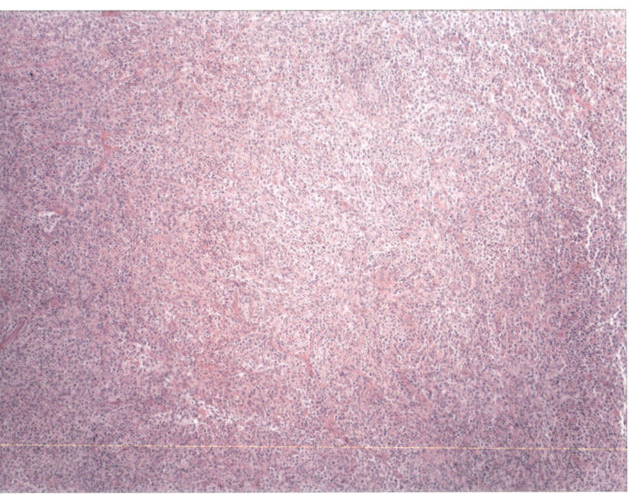

FIGURE 8-37

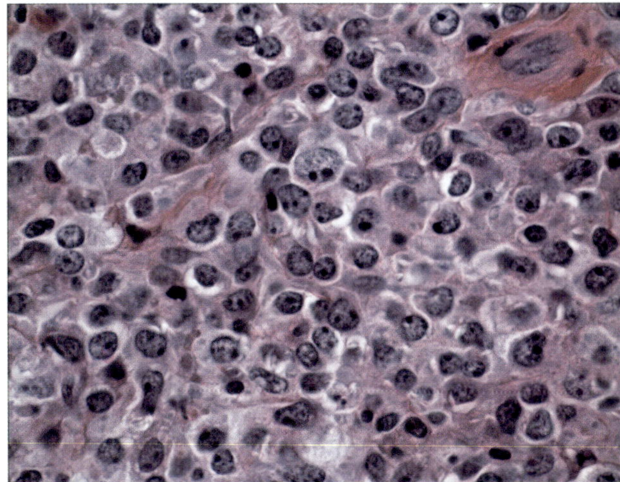

FIGURE 8-38

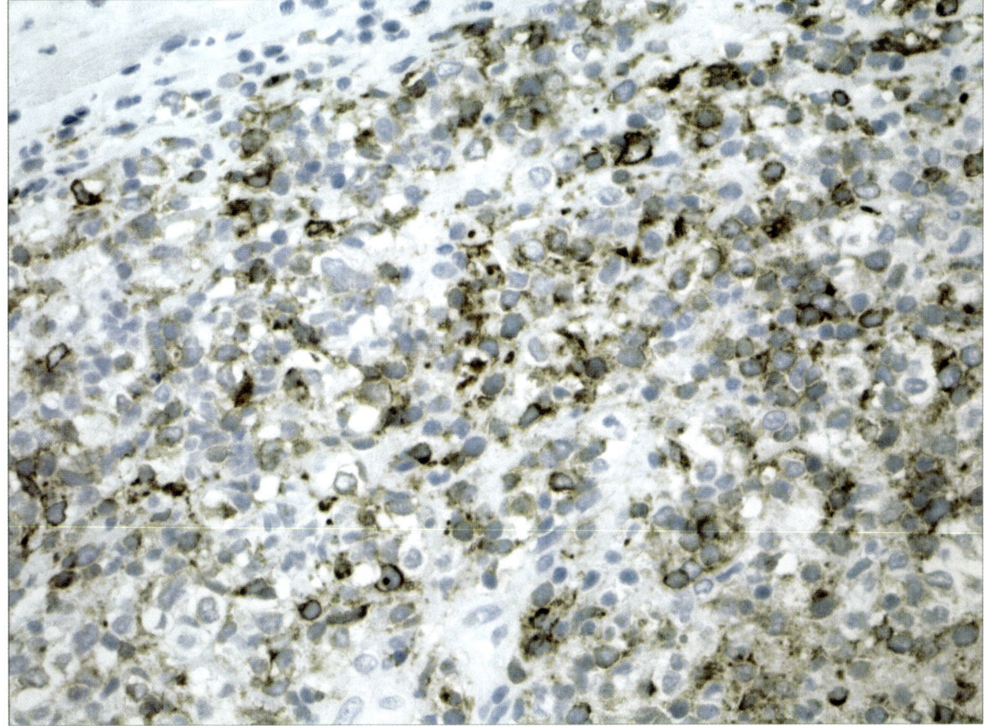

FIGURE 8-39

FIGURE 8-37 This lymph node has an effaced architecture by a neoplastic infiltrate disposes in nests separated by thin bands of fibrosis.

FIGURE 8-38 The neoplastic cells are medium to large in size with abundant pale cytoplasm, surrounded by thin collagenous strands.

FIGURE 8-39 Immunohistochemistry demonstrates variable CD30 expression in the lymphoma cells.

ALK Positive Large B-Cell Lymphoma

DEFINITION

This entity is defined as a lymphoma consisting of ALK(+) B-cells of large size with immunoblastic or plasmablastic morphology.

CLINICAL FEATURES

- This is a very rare lymphoma (<1% of diffuse large B-cell lymphomas)
- ALK(+) large B-cell lymphoma occurs at a median age of 36 years with a male predominance (male:female = 3:1).
- Patients typically present with advanced stage disease.
- Extranodal presentation is occasionally seen.

HISTOLOGIC FINDINGS

- Lymph nodes show partially or completely effaced architecture; intrasinusoidal involvement is a frequent feature. The tumor cells are monomorphic large cells with regular nuclei, prominent central nucleoli, and abundant amphophilic cytoplasm (Figure 8-40).
- The typical immunophenotype is ALK(+), CD38(+), CD138(+), EMA(+), CD3(−), CD20(−), CD30(−), CD45(−), and light chain restricted (Figure 8-41).

DIFFERENTIAL DIAGNOSIS

- Anaplastic large cell lymphoma, ALK positive
- Carcinoma

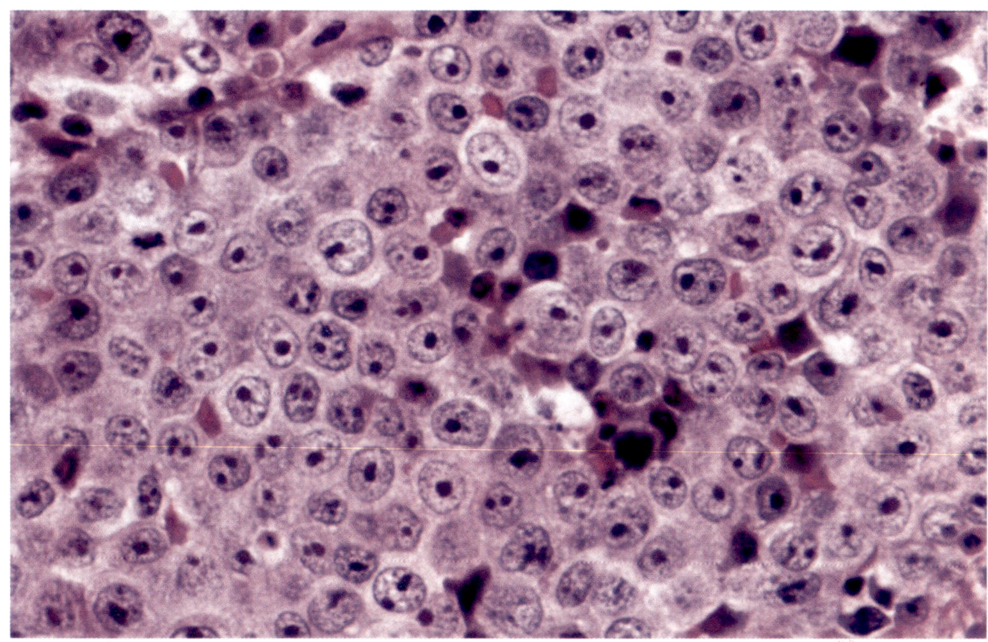

FIGURE 8-40

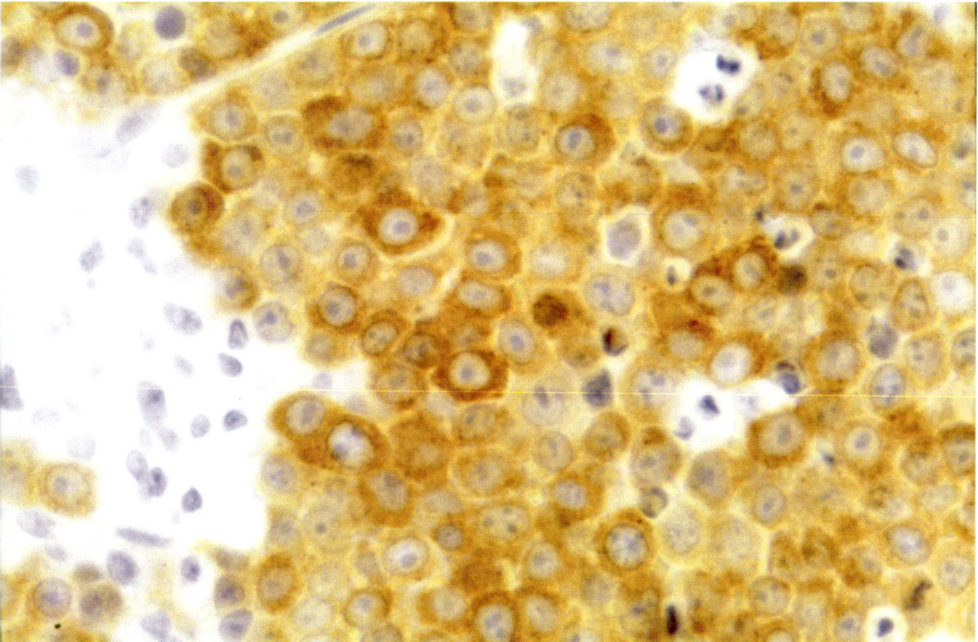

FIGURE 8-41

FIGURE 8-40 The neoplastic cells are large with regular nuclei, vesicular chromatin, and prominent central nucleoli.

FIGURE 8-41 Immunohistochemistry shows ALK positivity with a predominantly cytoplasmic pattern.

Plasmablastic Lymphoma (PBL)

DEFINITION

This is an aggressive lymphoma consisting of large cells with plasmablastic/immunoblastic morphology and plasma cell immunophenotype.

CLINICAL FEATURES

- Plasmablastic lymphoma is most often seen in HIV-infected individuals and in other immunodeficiency states.
- It occurs at a median age of 50 years.
- The typical presentation is a mass in the oral cavity, although it may also present in other extranodal sites (e.g., gastrointestinal tract).
- Nodal involvement is more common in HIV-negative patients.

HISTOLOGIC FINDINGS

- Typical morphology is that of a diffuse infiltrate of large cells with plasmablastic or immunoblastic morphology: the cells typically have regular nuclei, prominent central nucleoli, and moderately abundant, densely amphophilic cytoplasm. They may show a morphologic spectrum between immunoblasts/plasmablasts and cells with overtly plasmacytic features (Figure 8-42).
- Frequent mitoses, apoptotic debris, and tingible body macrophages (sometimes producing a starry sky appearance) are characteristic features.
- The typical immunophenotype is CD38(+), CD138(+), CD19(−), CD20(−), CD79a(variably +), PAX-5(weak +), CD45(−), CD56(variably +), and cytoplasmic light chain restricted; CD30 and EMA are frequently (+).
- EBER in situ hybridization is positive in 75% of cases (100% of cases presenting in the oral mucosa). HHV8 is negative.

DIFFERENTIAL DIAGNOSIS

- Plasmablastic myeloma
- Primary effusion lymphoma
- Diffuse large B cell lymphoma
- Anaplastic large cell lymphoma

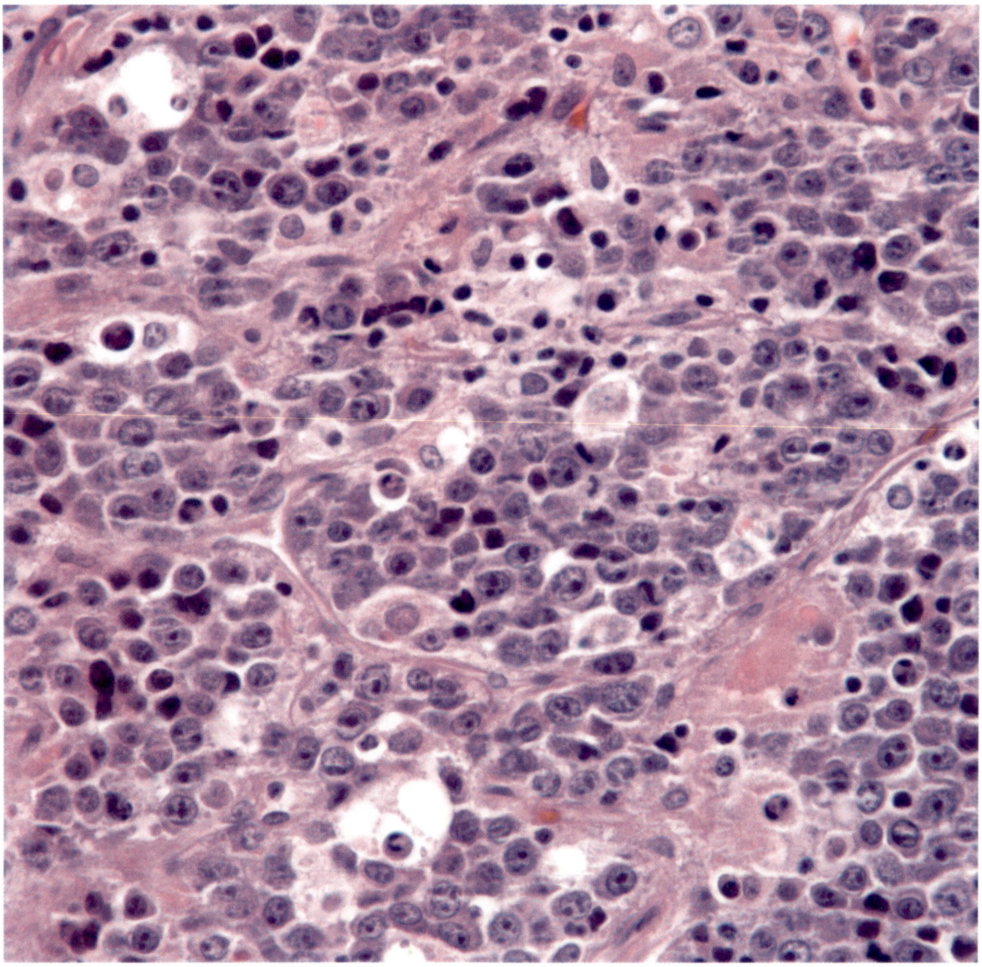

FIGURE 8-42

FIGURE 8-42 This image demonstrates an intrasinusoidal infiltrate of large cells with regular nuclei, prominent nucleoli, and basophilic cytoplasm. Frequent mitoses and apoptotic debris are also present.

Large B-Cell Lymphoma Arising in HHV8-Associated Multicentric Castleman Disease

DEFINITION

This is a distinct form of large B-cell lymphoma that occurs in the setting of HHV8(+) multicentric Castleman disease (MCD), usually in HIV-positive individuals.

CLINICAL FEATURES

- This lymphoma occurs most frequently in HIV(+) individuals who are profoundly immunosuppressed and who have developed HHV8(+) MCD.
- Lymph node and splenic involvement is typical.

HISTOLOGIC FINDINGS

- A typical lymph node with HHV8(+) MCD shows hyperplastic or regressed follicles, interfollicular infiltrates of mature plasma cells, and scattered HHV-8(+), lambda-restricted plasmablasts (large cells with eccentric nuclei, vesicular chromatin, prominent nucleoli, and dense amphophilic cytoplasm) in the follicle mantles (Figures 8-43 and 8-44).
- In some cases, HHV-8(+) plasmablasts form localized aggregates (microlymphomas) (Figure 8-45).
- When plasmablasts form confluent sheets, DLBCL arising in HHV8(+) MCD is diagnosed (Figure 8-46).
- The plasmablasts are CD20(variable +), CD138(−), and EBER in situ hybridization(−), in contrast to plasmablastic lymphoma.

DIFFERENTIAL DIAGNOSIS

- Plasmablastic lymphoma
- Primary effusion lymphoma

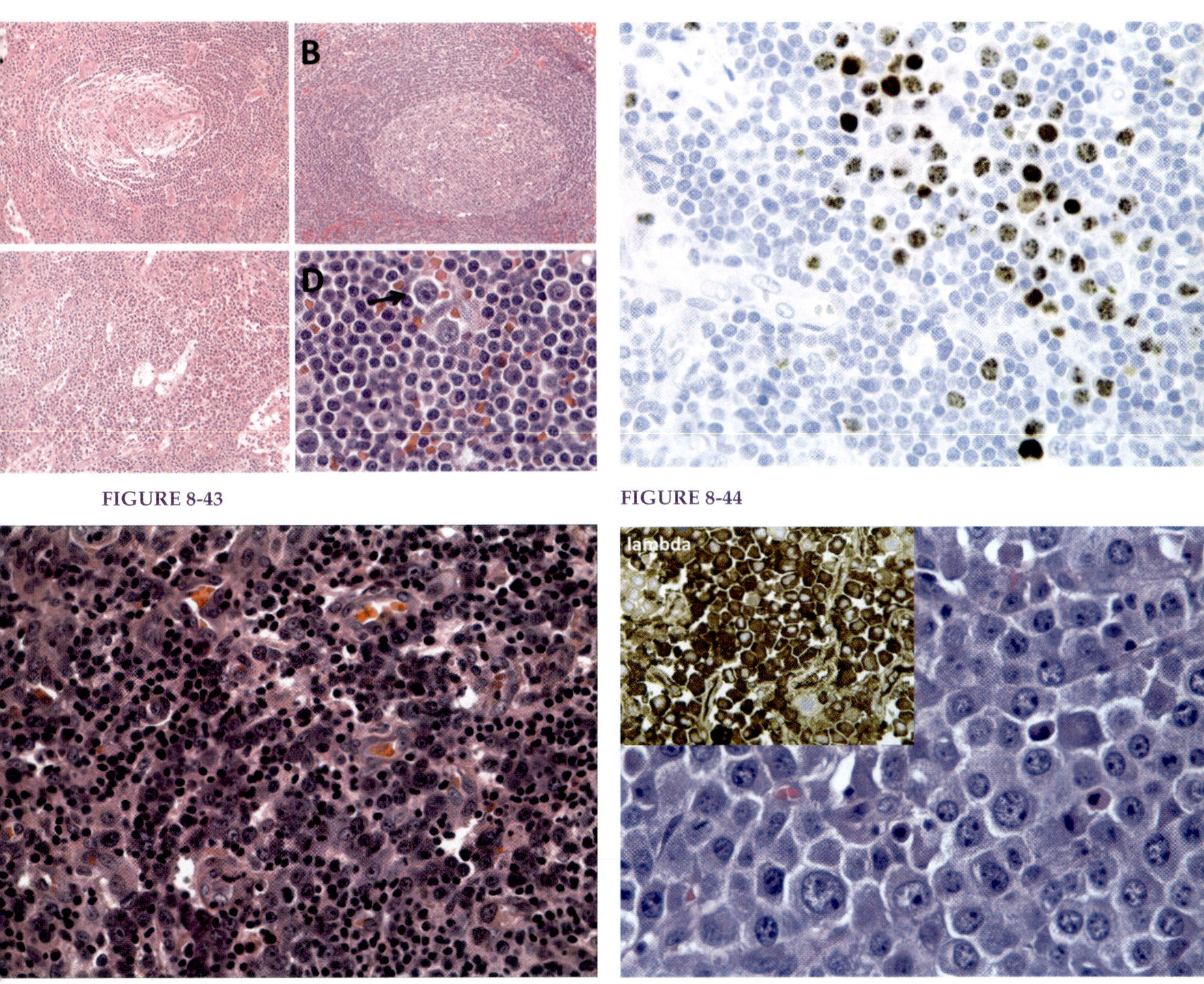

FIGURE 8-43

FIGURE 8-44

FIGURE 8-45

FIGURE 8-46

FIGURE 8-43 This composite demonstrates a lymph node with regressed follicles (**A**), follicles with expanded mantle zones (**B**), interfollicular plasma cell infiltrates (**C**), and occasional plasmablasts (**D, arrow**).

FIGURE 8-44 HHV8 immunohistochemistry highlights plasmablasts.

FIGURE 8-45 This "microlymphoma," consists of a localized aggregate of HHV8(+) plasmablasts.

FIGURE 8-46 This diffuse infiltrate of plasmablasts shows lambda light chain restriction (inset, immunohistochemistry).

Burkitt Lymphoma (BL)

DEFINITION

BL is an aggressive B-cell lymphoma composed of medium-sized cells, with rapid doubling time, and uniform association with a translocation of C-MYC with one of the immunoglobulin genes. Although it lacks a single diagnostic gold standard, the combination of typical morphology, immunophenotype, and cytogenetic features is often sufficient to make a diagnosis of BL.

CLINICAL FEATURES

- Clinical variants include endemic, sporadic and immunodeficiency-associated BL.
- Endemic BL is common in Africa, affects predominantly children (age 4–7 years) with a male predominance (male:female = 2:1), often presents as a jaw mass, and has a uniform association with EBV.
- Sporadic BL is rare (1–2% of lymphomas in Western countries), occurs at a median age of 30 years with a male predominance (male:female = 3:1), usually presents as an abdominal mass, and is only associated with EBV in 30% of cases.
- Immunodeficiency-associated BL is frequently seen in HIV-infected individuals with preserved CD4 counts, often presents with nodal involvement, and has a 30% association with EBV.
- In general, patients present with bulky disease.

HISTOLOGIC FINDINGS

- BL has typical shows a low-power "starry sky" appearance, with tingible body macrophages interrupting diffuse sheets of monotonous, medium-sized cells, with round nuclei, distinctly clumped chromatin, multiple nucleoli, and dense amphophilic, vacuolated cytoplasm (Figures 8-47 and 8-48).
- This lymphoma demonstrates brisk mitotic activity and a very high MIB-1/Ki-67 proliferation rate (>95%).
- The typical immunophenotype is CD19(+), CD20(+), CD22(+), CD10(+), BCL-2(−), BCL-6(+), CD38(bright +), and surface light chain restricted.
- A C-MYC gene translocation is present in all cases, with one of the immunoglobulin genes (heavy chain, kappa, or lambda) as a translocation partner.

DIFFERENTIAL DIAGNOSIS

- Diffuse large B-cell lymphoma with C-MYC gene translocation
- B-cell lymphoma, unclassifiable, with features intermediate between diffuse large B-cell lymphoma and Burkitt lymphoma

FIGURE 8-47 This lymph node has an architecture that is effaced by a diffuse neoplastic infiltrate demonstrating frequent tingible body macrophages ("starry sky" appearance).

FIGURE 8-48 The infiltrate consists of monomorphic medium-sized cells, with stippled chromatin, multiple small nucleoli, and amphophilic cytoplasm. The inset shows a very high proliferation rate, as demonstrated by Ki-67 immunohistochemistry.

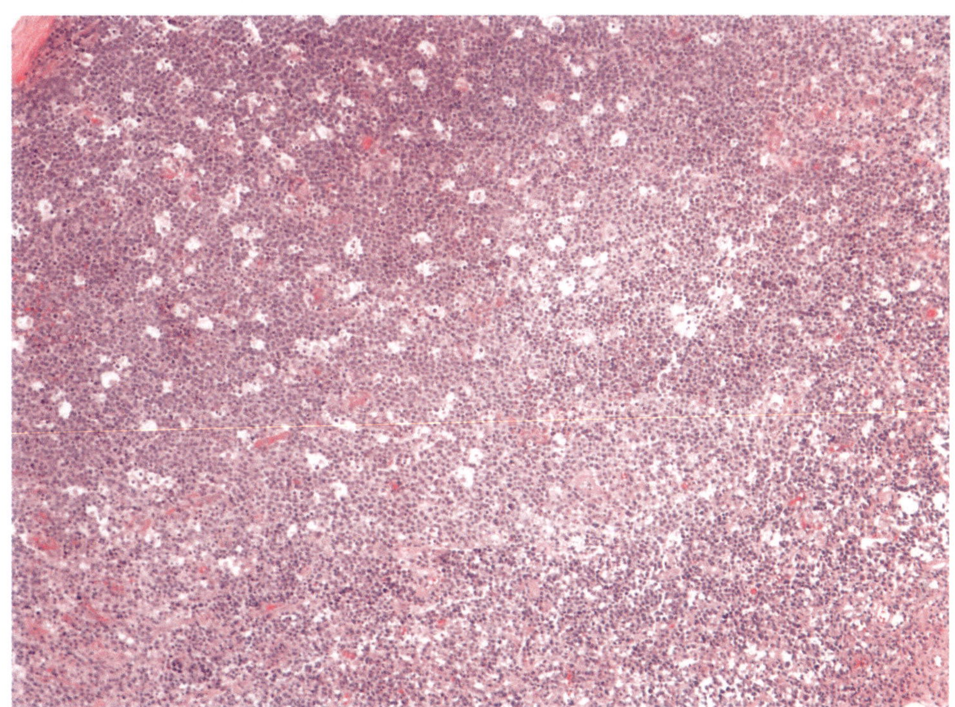

FIGURE 8-47

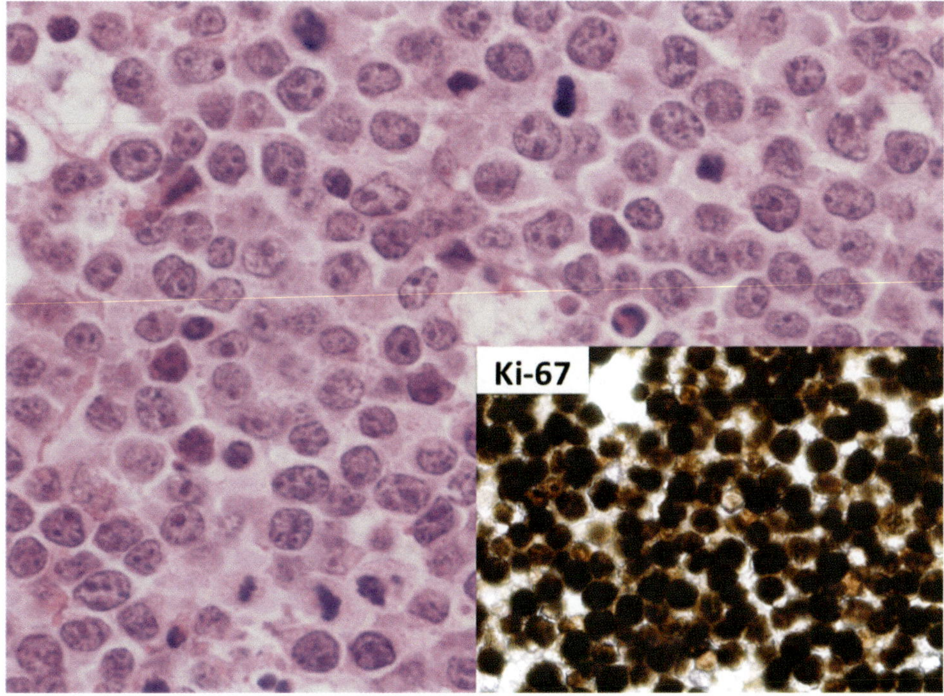

FIGURE 8-48

B-Cell Lymphoma, Unclassifiable, with Features Intermediate Between Diffuse Large B-Cell Lymphoma and Burkitt Lymphoma

DEFINITION

This represents a high-grade B-cell lymphoma with aggressive clinical course, and with overlapping morphologic and genetic features between diffuse large B-cell lymphoma (DLBCL) and Burkitt lymphoma (BL). Examples include cases with BL morphology, but unusual immunophenotype (IP) or cytogenetics; cases with BL IP and/or cytogenetics, but unusual morphology; and cases of "double-hit" lymphomas (C-MYC+BCL-2, or C-MYC+BCL-6 translocations). Cases with typical DLBCL morphology and a C-MYC gene rearrangement or a high mitotic rate (>95) do not fall in this category.

CLINICAL FEATURES

- This is a rare lymphoma, presenting mostly in adults with lymphadenopathy or organomegaly.

HISTOLOGIC FINDINGS

- This lymphoma generally consists of medium to large-sized cells, with regular to variably irregular nuclei, variable amounts of cytoplasm, and distinct nucleoli (Figures 8-49 and 8-50).
- The usual immunophenotype is CD19(+), CD20(+), CD22(+), CD79a(+), CD10(+), BCL-2(+), BCL-6(+), and light chain restricted.
- "Double hit" lymphomas are frequently CD19(dim+), CD20(dim+), CD38(bright +), and surface light chain (dim +).

DIFFERENTIAL DIAGNOSIS

- Diffuse large B-cell lymphoma
- Burkitt lymphoma

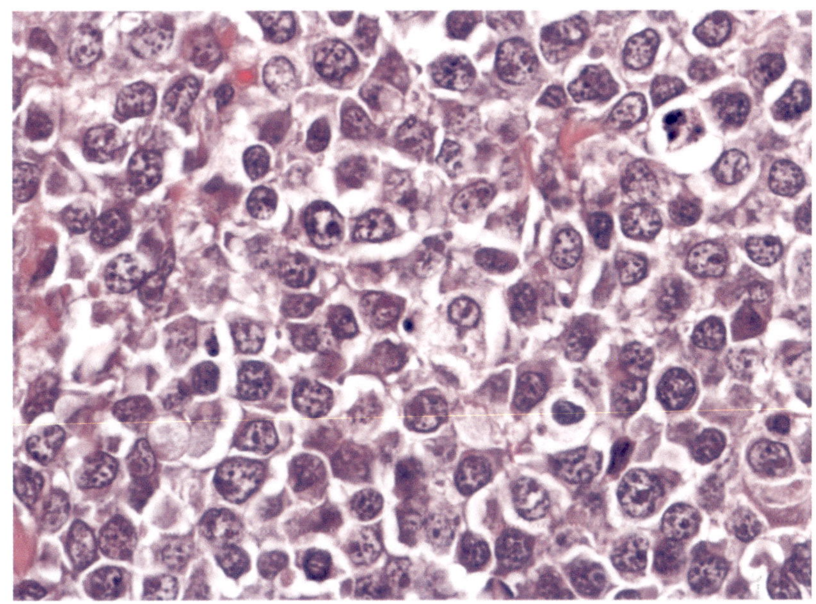

FIGURE 8-49

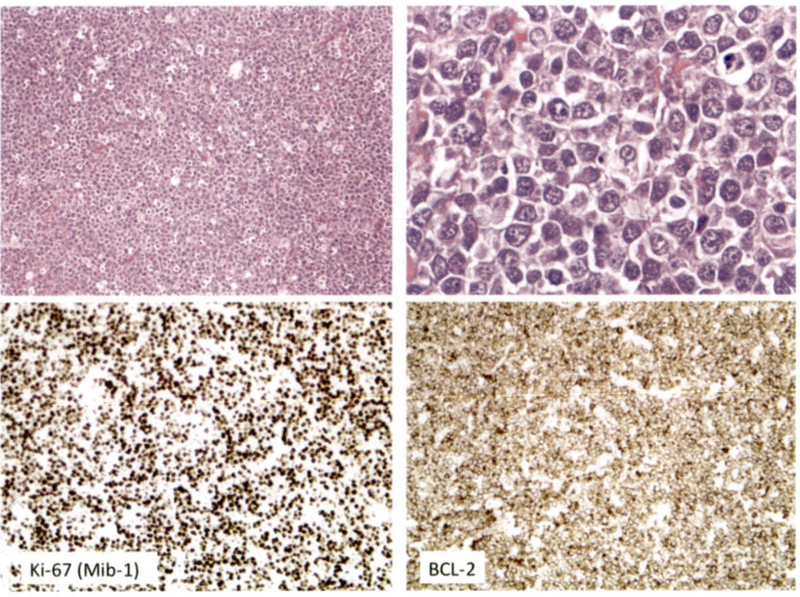

FIGURE 8-50

FIGURE 8-49 This abdominal lymph node in a patient with prior history of follicular lymphoma shows medium to large sized cells with mild nuclear irregularities, vesicular chromatin, and distinct nucleoli. Frequent apoptotic debris is present. Fluorescence in situ hybridization demonstrated both C-MYC and BCL-2 gene translocation ("double hit" lymphoma).

FIGURE 8-50 Hematoxylin and eosin stained low-power and high-power sections of the same case, demonstrating a "starry sky" appearance; immunohistochemistry showing a high (~100%) proliferation rate and strong BCL-2 positivity in the neoplastic cells.

B-Cell Lymphoma, Unclassifiable, with Features Intermediate Between Diffuse Large B-Cell Lymphoma and Classical Hodgkin Lymphoma

DEFINITION

This is defined as a B-cell lymphoma with aggressive clinical course and overlapping morphologic and genetic features between diffuse large B-cell lymphoma (DLBCL) and Hodgkin lymphoma (cHL). Examples include cases with DLBCL morphology and CD30(+)/CD15(+) lymphoma cells; or cases with cHL morphology, strong CD20 expression, and numerous neoplastic cells.

CLINICAL FEATURES

- This uncommon tumor often presents with a mediastinal mass in young men (age, 20–40 years).

HISTOLOGIC FINDINGS

- This entity consists of pleomorphic, large lymphoma cells with a variable number of cells with Reed-Sternberg morphology, embedded in a fibrotic stroma (Figures 8-51 and 8-52).
- The immunophenotype is usually CD45(+), CD30(+), CD15(+), CD20(+), CD79a(+), PAX-5(+), CD10(−), ALK(−).

DIFFERENTIAL DIAGNOSIS

- Primary mediastinal large B-cell lymphoma
- Diffuse large B-cell lymphoma
- Classical Hodgkin lymphoma
- Anaplastic large cell lymphoma

FIGURE 8-51 This image demonstrates a dense infiltrate of atypical, variably-sized cells, with oval nuclei, vesicular chromatin, prominent nucleoli, and abundant cytoplasm. Admixed are plasma cells, eosinophils, and frequent apoptotic debris.

FIGURE 8-52 This high-power view demonstrates large, atypical pleomorphic cells, some with Reed-Sternberg morphology, surrounded by fibrotic stroma.

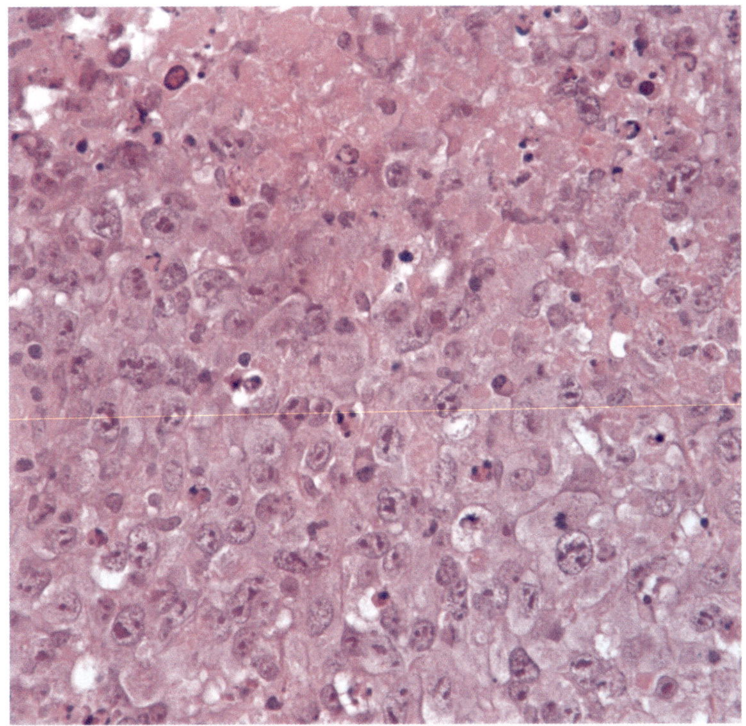

FIGURE 8-51

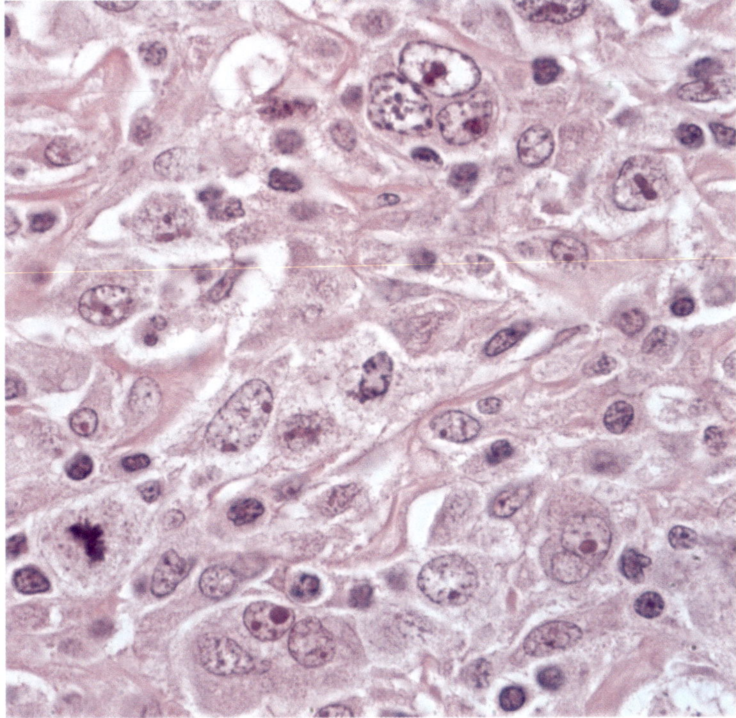

FIGURE 8-52

9

Mature T- and NK-Cell Neoplasms

T-CELL PROLYMPHOCYTIC LEUKEMIA

AGGRESSIVE NK-CELL LEUKEMIA/LYMPHOMA

ADULT T-CELL LEUKEMIA/LYMPHOMA

SEZARY SYNDROME/MYCOSIS FUNGOIDES

PERIPHERAL T-CELL LYMPHOMA, NOT OTHERWISE SPECIFIED

ANGIOIMMUNOBLASTIC T-CELL LYMPHOMA

ANAPLASTIC LARGE CELL LYMPHOMA, ALK POSITIVE

ANAPLASTIC LARGE CELL LYMPHOMA, ALK NEGATIVE

T-Cell Prolymphocytic Leukemia

DEFINITION

T-cell prolymphocytic leukemia (T-PLL) is a rare lymphoproliferative disorder overall, though it is the most common mature T-cell lymphoproliferative disorder.

CLINICAL FEATURES

- T-PLL is predominantly a disease of the middle aged and elderly; the median age is 65 years.
- Most patients present with marked leukocytosis and extensive bone marrow involvement.
- Lymphadenopathy is observed in approximately 25–60% of cases. Hepatosplenomegaly is common. Skin rashes may be observed in 20–50% of cases.
- The disease pursues an aggressive course in the majority of cases, though up to 25% have an indolent course. This neoplasm appears to be exquisitely sensitive to alemtuzumab therapy (anti-CD52 antibody).

HISTOLOGIC FINDINGS

- Lymph nodes show an effaced, diffuse architecture and increased vascularity (Figure 9-1).
- Neoplastic lymphocytes expand the paracortical area and most commonly consist of a monotonous, small to medium-sized cellular infiltrate (Figure 9-2). The cytology can be quite variable from case to case, with nuclei ranging from round and regular (mimicking CLL/SLL) to mildly or moderately irregular to frankly convoluted, Sezary-like morphology. Nucleoli are frequently observed in a proportion of tumor cells in involved tissues. Most cases show mature, condensed chromatin.
- Tumor cells show the following immunophenotype: CD4(+)/CD8(-) in 60% of cases, CD4(+)/CD8(+) in 25% of cases, and CD4(-)/CD8(+) in 15% of cases. Co-expression of CD4 and CD8, though present in only a quarter of cases, is nearly unique to T-PLL amongst mature T-cell neoplasms. Most cases are positive for CD2, CD3, CD5, CD7, and CD45RO.
- TCL-1 overexpression by immunohistochemistry is observed in the majority of cases but is neither a sensitive nor specific marker of T-PLL. 80% of cases show an inversion 14(q11;q32).

DIFFERENTIAL DIAGNOSIS

- Peripheral T-cell lymphoma, NOS
- Sezary syndrome/Mycosis fungoides
- T- lymphoblastic leukemia/lymphoma
- Chronic lymphocytic leukemia/small lymphocytic lymphoma

FIGURE 9-1 The neoplastic infiltrate shows effacement of the lymph node architecture in a diffuse pattern.

FIGURE 9-2 The neoplastic infiltrate expands the paracortex and is associated with increased vascularity and congestion of some sinuses (left). High-power magnification of the neoplastic infiltrate reveals slightly enlarged lymphocytes with mature chromatin and mild nuclear irregularity.

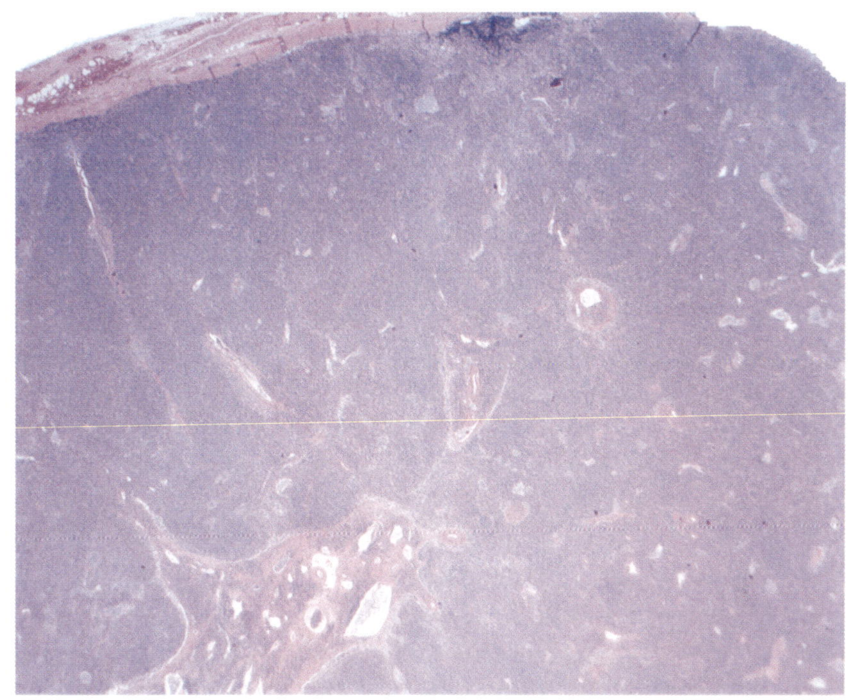

FIGURE 9-1

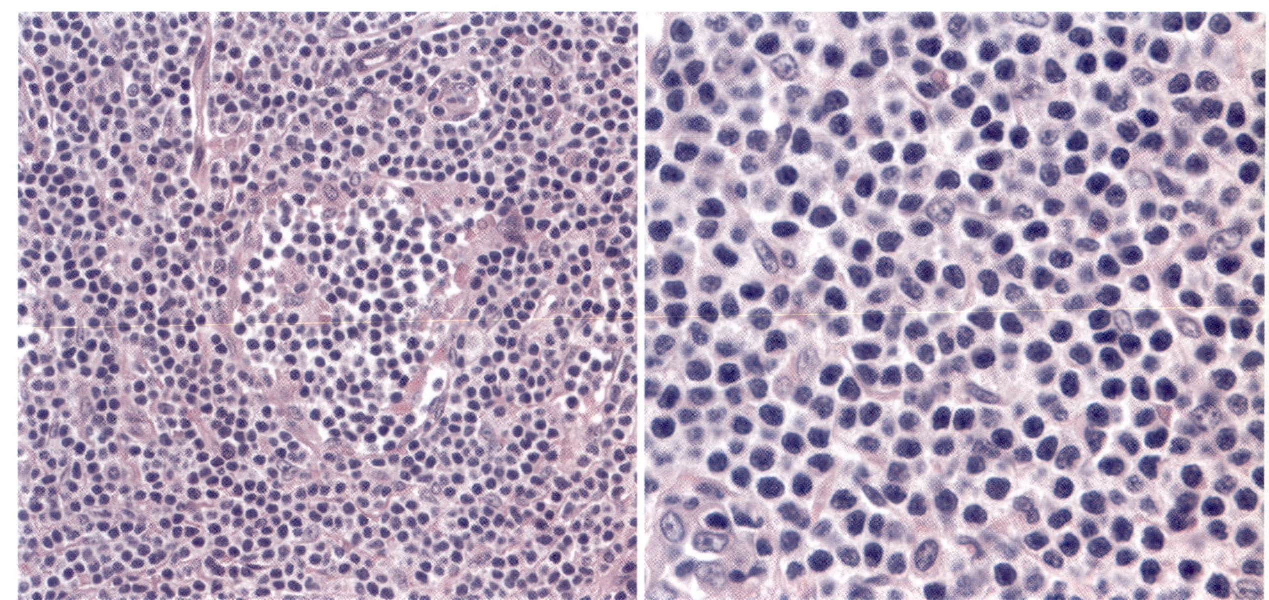

FIGURE 9-2

Aggressive NK-Cell Leukemia/Lymphoma

DEFINITION

Aggressive NK-cell leukemia is a rare leukemia that is most prevalent in Asia and has a fulminant clinical course. Reports on tissue involvement are rare, as this diagnosis is most frequently made on blood and/or bone marrow evaluation. Morphologically, aggressive NK-cell leukemia/lymphoma may exist on a continuum with extranodal NK/T-cell lymphoma, nasal type.

CLINICAL FEATURES

- This lymphoma affects young adults, with median age ranges of 30–41 years, in small case series. The prevalence is highest in Asians.
- Most patients present with fever, hepatosplenomegaly, cytopenias, and occasionally lymphadenopathy. Peripheral blood and bone marrow involvement are frequent.
- Associated hemophagocytic syndrome occurs in many cases.
- The disease has an aggressive course, with <2 months median survival.

HISTOLOGIC FINDINGS

- Involved lymph nodes show effaced architecture with prominent intrasinusoidal infiltration by the neoplastic cells.
- Neoplastic cells are medium to large in size and have variable nuclear features, ranging from round and regular with condensed chromatin to irregular and pleomorphic (Figure 9-3). Areas of necrosis and apoptosis and mitotic figures are frequent.
- The tumor cells stain positive for CD2, CD3ε, CD56, granzyme B, and TIA-1.
- Most cases are positive for EBER in situ hybridization studies.

DIFFERENTIAL DIAGNOSIS

- Extranodal NK/T-cell lymphoma, nasal type
- Peripheral T-cell lymphoma, not otherwise specified

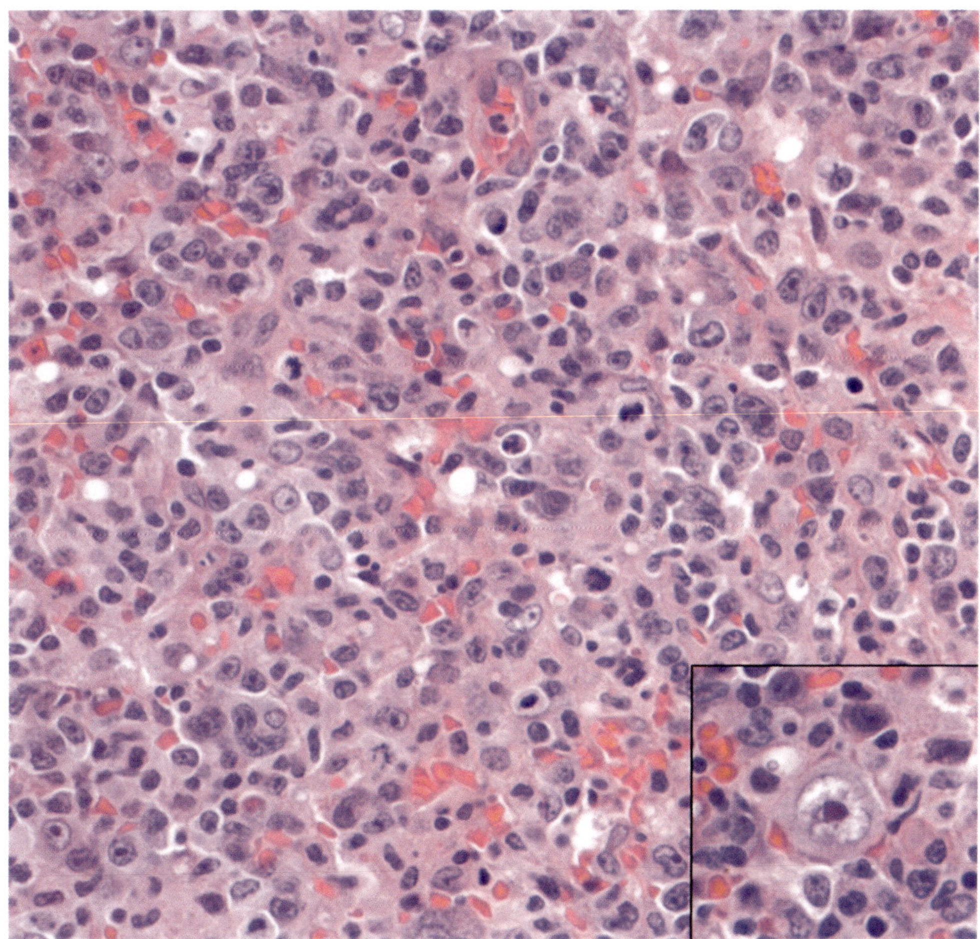

FIGURE 9-3

FIGURE 9-3 The neoplastic infiltrate in this inguinal lymph node shows large cell size and pleomorphism, with frequent mitotic figures and apoptotic debris. Frequent Reed-Sternberg-like cells were observed (inset).

Adult T-Cell Leukemia/Lymphoma

DEFINITION

Adult T-cell leukemia/lymphoma (ATLL) is a mature T-cell neoplasm associated with human T-cell leukemia virus (HTLV-1) that is characterized by a variable clinical presentation and course. This malignancy occurs decades following HTLV-1 exposure; endemic regions include: Japan, Caribbean, and Africa.

CLINICAL FEATURES

- ATLL is a disease of adults, with an average age of onset of 59 years old.
- Several clinical subtypes of ATLL exist: acute, lymphomatous, chronic, and smoldering. The acute subtype is the most common and consists of leukemic involvement by highly atypical lymphocytes termed "flower cells," lymphadenopathy, hepatosplenomegaly, hypercalcemia, and skin rash. The lymphomatous variant consists of lymphadenopathy in the absence of leukemic involvement. Additionally, the chronic form may have lymphadenopathy.
- The acute and lymphomatous variants have the poorest prognoses, with <1 year overall survivals.
- ATLL patients are frequently immunosuppressed and therefore subject to infectious complications.

HISTOLOGIC FINDINGS

- Several different patterns have been described in the ATLL lymph node, including: Hodgkin's-like, pleomorphic small cell, pleomorphic (medium and large cell), anaplastic, and angioimmunoblastic T-cell lymphoma-like (AILT-like) ATLL.
- The neoplastic cells are CD4(+) and CD25(+), representing regulatory T-cells. Characteristically, the tumor cells lack CD7 expression.
- The majority of cases show diffuse effacement by pleomorphic, medium to large-sized lymphoma cells with marked nuclear irregularity and mature chromatin (pleomorphic medium and large cell type) (Figures 9-4 and 9-5). Reed-Sternberg-like cells may be observed. The anaplastic variant consists of neoplastic cells that are larger in size and show marked pleomorphism with prominent nucleoli. Both of these ATLL types have the poorest prognoses.
- The Hodgkin's-like ATLL type shows preservation of the lymph node architecture with paracortical expansion by a small to medium-sized lymphocyte population and interspersed Reed-Sternberg-like cells. The RS-like cells stain like conventional RS cells.
- The small cell ATLL type shows a predominance of small to medium-sized lymphocytes with mild nuclear atypia.
- The AILT-like variant shows increased vascularity and clusters of atypical, enlarged lymphocytes with clear to lightly eosinophilic cytoplasm in a background of a variable mixed inflammatory cell infiltrate.
- HTLV-1 DNA is present in the lymphoma cells in all cases of ATLL.

DIFFERENTIAL DIAGNOSIS

- Peripheral T-cell lymphoma, not otherwise specified
- Anaplastic large cell lymphoma
- Classical Hodgkin lymphoma
- HTLV-1-associated lymphadenitis

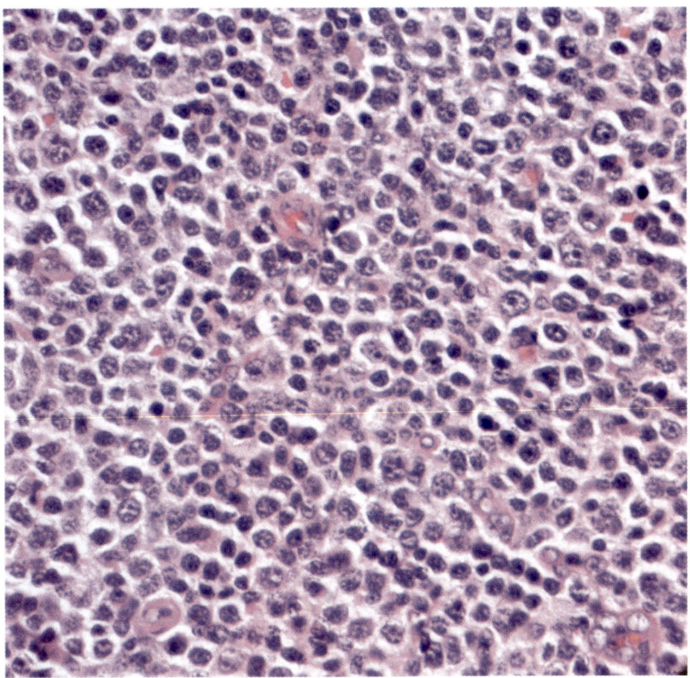

FIGURE 9-4

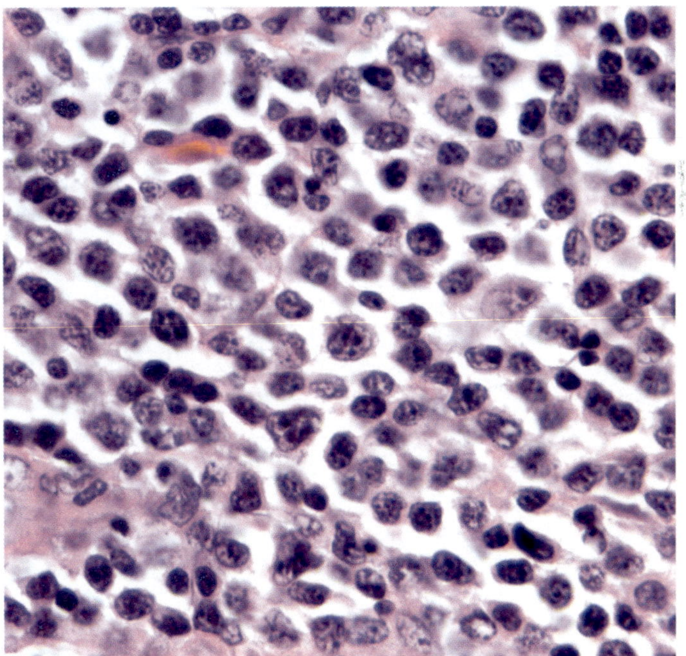

FIGURE 9-5

FIGURE 9-4 Intermediate magnification reveals a densely cellular tumor composed of medium to large lymphocytes with variable nuclear irregularity and coarse chromatin.

FIGURE 9-5 Higher power image of the case illustrated in Figure 9-4.

Sezary Syndrome/Mycosis Fungoides

DEFINITION

Sezary syndrome (SS) is characterized by the triad of erythroderma, generalized adenopathy, and neoplastic, cerebriform lymphocytes in the blood. Mycosis fungoides (MF) is characterized by skin involvement by these neoplastic lymphocytes and may secondarily involve lymph nodes during advanced stages of the disease.

CLINICAL FEATURES

- SS patients have erythroderma with mild, generalized peripheral lymphadenopathy. MF patients have disease confined to the skin initially, which may be in the patch, plaque, or tumor stage. Abnormal lymph nodes in SS/MF patients are defined clinically as peripheral nodes >1.5 cm in greatest dimension and/or palpable on physical examination.
- SS is a disease of adults, often presenting after the 5th decade of life. There is a male predominance.
- Large cell transformation may occur in SS/MF patients and should be suspected when a rapidly enlarging lymph node is detected.

HISTOLOGIC FINDINGS

- Dermatopathic lymphadenopathy is a frequent finding in SS/MF patients, whether or not the lymph nodes are involved by neoplastic lymphocytes. It is characterized by a paracortical expansion of dendritic cells, mostly Langerhans cells, and histiocytes containing variable melanin pigment (Figure 9-6) (see Chapter 2).
- Involved nodes may show intact or partially or completely disrupted architecture.
- Variable numbers of atypical lymphocytes infiltrate the lymph node, ranging from subtle involvement to architectural effacement. Neoplastic lymphocytes can be variable in size, though they uniformly have convoluted, cerebriform nuclei (Figure 9-7).
- The International Society for Cutaneous Lymphomas and the cutaneous lymphoma task force of the European Organization of Research and Treatment of Cancer (ISCL/EORTC) have proposed the following histologic staging system: N1- no involvement; N2- early involvement with preservation of architecture; and N3- partial or complete effacement with neoplastic lymphocytes.
- Large cell transformation is characterized by architectural effacement and >25% large lymphoid cells (Figure 9-8).

DIFFERENTIAL DIAGNOSIS

- Dermatopathic lymphadenopathy
- Adult T-cell leukemia
- Peripheral T-cell lymphoma, not otherwise specified

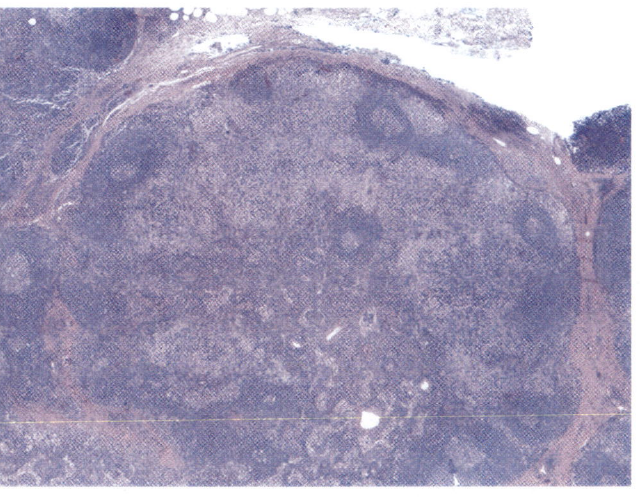

FIGURE 9-6

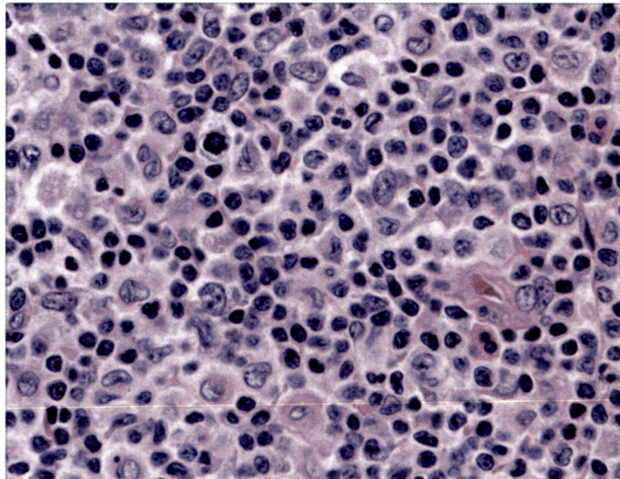

FIGURE 9-7

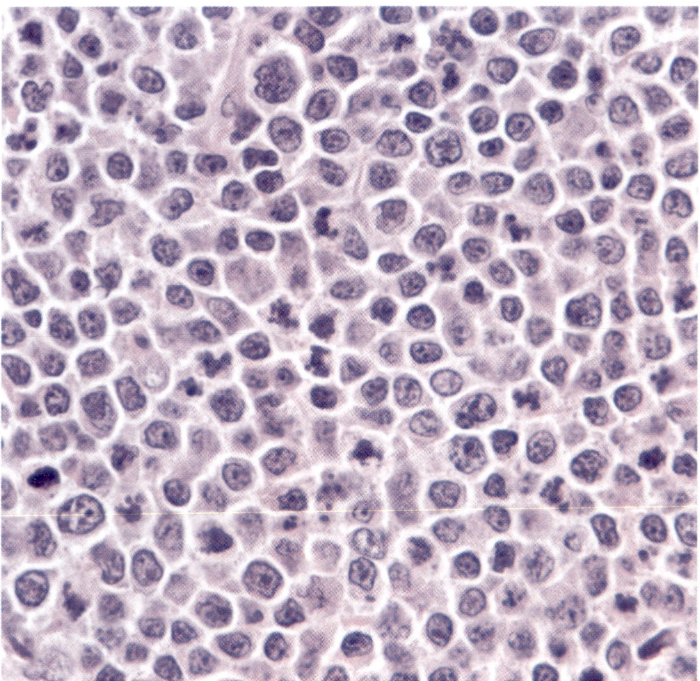

FIGURE 9-8

FIGURE 9-6 This low-power image of a lymph node involved by mycosis fungoides demonstrates the characteristic pale, cortical infiltrates of dermatopathic lymphadenopathy.

FIGURE 9-7 High-power of a dermatopathic area demonstrates small lymphocytes with irregular, hyperchromatic nuclei, and a few larger atypical lymphocytes with distinct nucleoli.

FIGURE 9-8 Large cell transformation of previously diagnosed Sezary syndrome. Sheets of large lymphocytes with irregular nuclei and multiple distinct nucleoli are present in this massively enlarged lymph node from a Sezary patient.

Peripheral T-Cell Lymphoma, Not Otherwise Specified

DEFINITION

Peripheral T-cell lymphoma, not otherwise specified (PTCL, NOS), is a heterogeneous group of mature T-cell neoplasms. All mature T-cell lymphomas that do not meet WHO criteria for a specific T-cell malignancy are classified in this diagnostic category.

CLINICAL FEATURES

- The median age is 60 years. There is a 2:1 male predominance.
- Peripheral lymph nodes are most commonly affected; extranodal disease is present in >60% of cases. Most patients present with advanced stage disease.
- Blood involvement is uncommon.
- The disease has an aggressive course with a 5-year overall survival of approximately 30%. CD30 positivity in >80% of tumor cells predicts an even worse overall survival in PCTL, NOS.

HISTOLOGIC FINDINGS

- Involved lymph nodes most often show architectural effacement, though few cases may show paracortical expansion with retention of normal architecture.
- PTCL, NOS has a wide morphological spectrum (Figures 9-9 to 9-13). Cytologically, the neoplastic lymphocytes have mature chromatin patterns and range from small to medium-sized cells with mild to moderate nuclear irregularity to large cells with pleomorphic nuclei. Tumor cells commonly have more abundant cytoplasm than normal lymphocytes. There is often a background inflammatory cell infiltrate, composed of variable numbers of eosinophils, plasma cells, and histiocytes (Figure 9-10). Reed-Sternberg-like cells are present in some cases.

(continued)

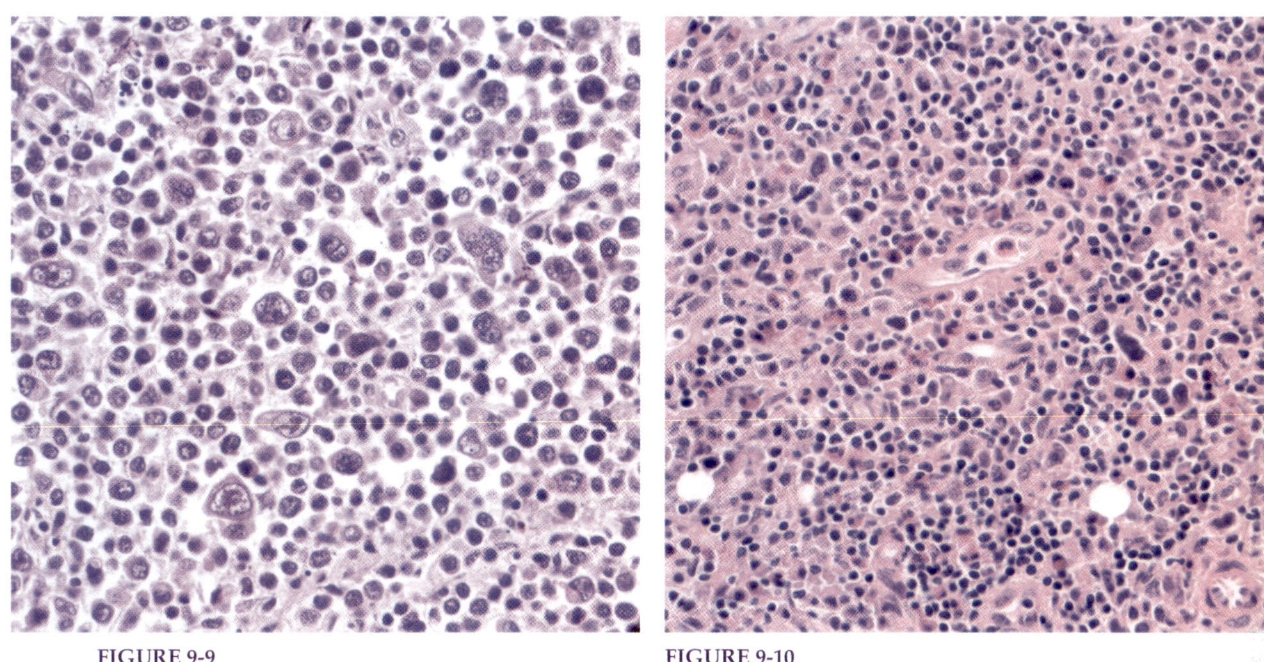

FIGURE 9-9 FIGURE 9-10

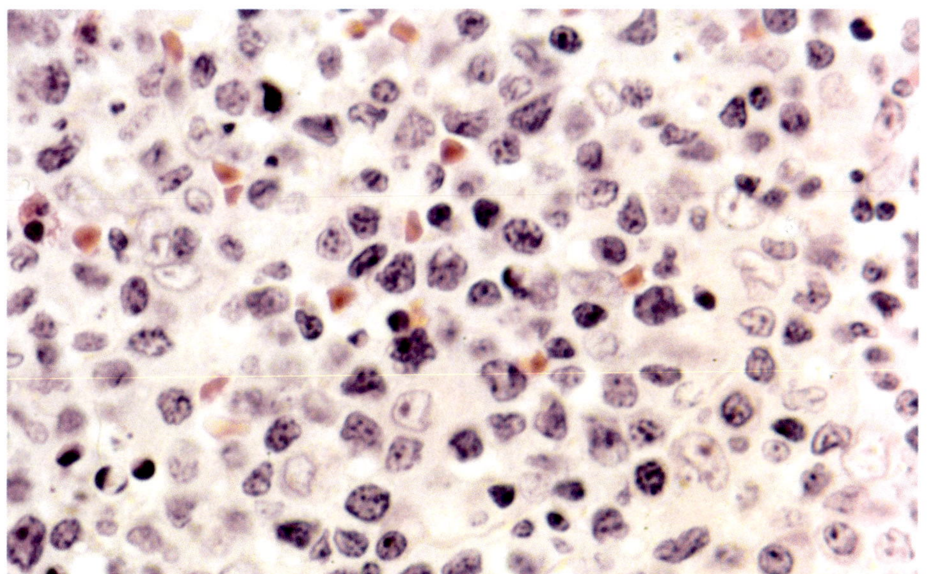

FIGURE 9-11

FIGURE 9-9 Tumor cells show marked atypia and variation in cell size with occasional forms resembling Reed-Sternberg cells.

FIGURE 9-10 The neoplastic cells show pleomorphism and are embedded in an inflammatory milieu, containing eosinophils, histiocytes, and neutrophils.

FIGURE 9-11 In this example, tumor cells are small to medium in size with prominent nuclear irregularity and pale cytoplasm.

Peripheral T-Cell Lymphoma, Not Otherwise Specified *(continued)*

- Several defined histologic variants of PTCL, NOS exist, including the lymphoepitheliod, follicular, and T-zone variants. The lymphoepitheliod variant consist of a monotonous population of fairly bland, small to medium-sized lymphocytes admixed with epithelioid histiocytes, and can be difficult to differentiate from reactive conditions without ancillary studies (Figure 9-13). The T-zone variant has similar bland cytology and involves the perifollicular areas. The follicular variant demonstrates atypical T-lymphocytes with clear cytoplasm within follicles; it is likely related to and may be difficult to distinguish from angioimmunoblastic T-cell lymphoma.
- PTCLs show variable expression of T-cell antigens. Aberrant expression of CD3, CD5, and CD7 are most common. The majority of cases are CD4(+).

DIFFERENTIAL DIAGNOSIS

- Diffuse large B-cell lymphoma
- Anaplastic large cell lymphoma
- Classical Hodgkin lymphoma
- T-cell prolymphocytic leukemia
- Adult T-cell leukemia/lymphoma
- Extranodal NK/T-cell lymphoma
- Paracortical hyperplasia (Lymphoepitheliod and T-zone variants)

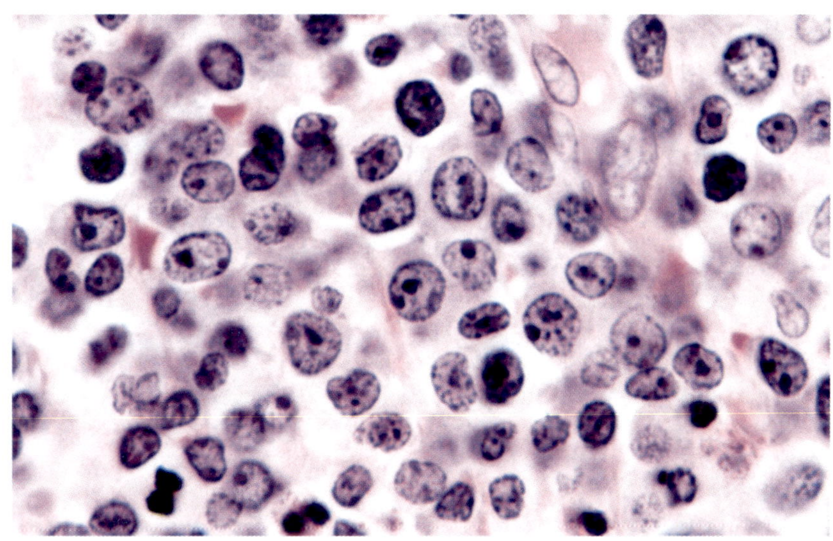

FIGURE 9-12

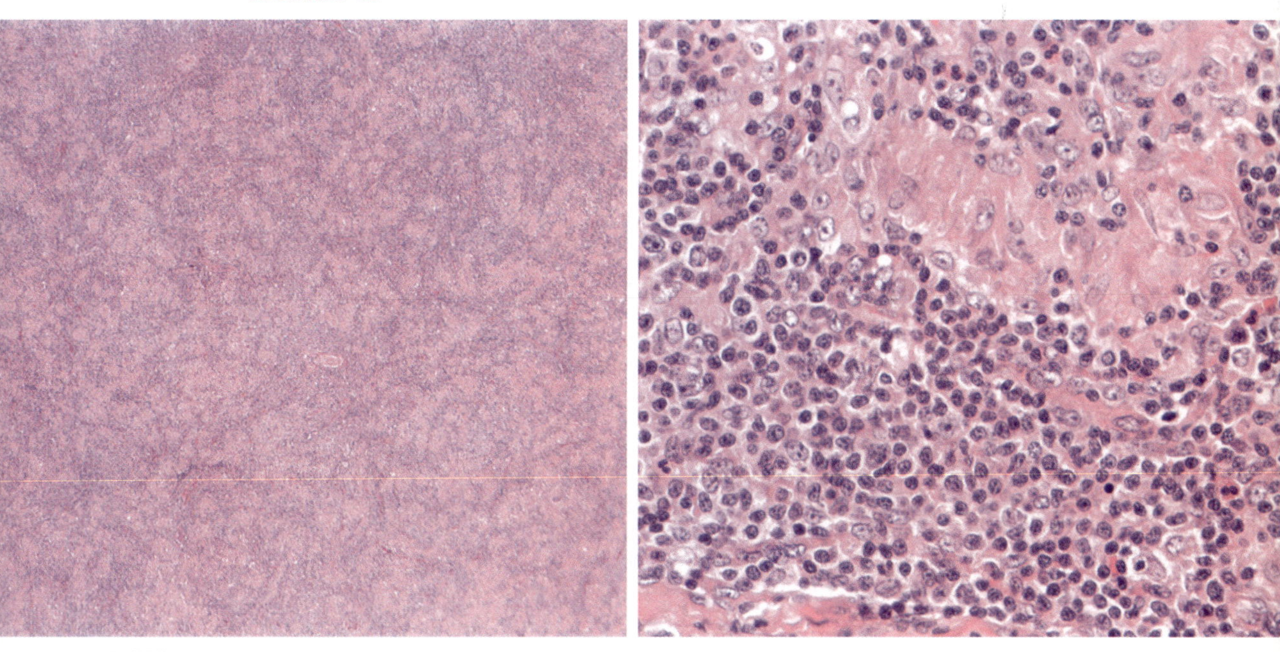

FIGURE 9-13

FIGURE 9-12 This example closely resembles a diffuse large B-cell lymphoma, with regular nuclei, vesicular chromatin, and prominent nucleoli.

FIGURE 9-13 Peripheral T-cell lymphoma, not otherwise specified, lymphoepithelioid variant. This lymph node shows effaced architecture with a diffuse granulomatous infiltrate (left). On higher power, the infiltrate is bland and consists of small to medium-sized lymphocytes that lack atypia, in a background of non-necrotizing granulomata (right). An aberrant T-cell population was identified by flow cytometry.

Angioimmunoblastic T-Cell Lymphoma

DEFINITION

Angioimmunoblastic T-cell lymphoma (AITL) is a mature T-cell neoplasm that appears to be derived from CD4(+) follicular helper T cells. It is one of the more common subtypes of T-cell lymphomas, accounting for 15–20% of T-cell lymphomas. Historically, it was postulated to represent a reactive condition and has been called several entities in the literature, including angioimmunoblastic lymphadenopathy with dysproteinemia and immunoblastic lymphadenopathy.

CLINICAL FEATURES

- AITL is a disease of adults, with cases reported between 37 and 84 years of age.
- Patients present with generalized lymphadenopathy, fever, hepatosplenomegaly, rash, and anemia. Extranodal disease is common, with frequent lung, spleen, skin, and bone marrow involvement.
- Patients are often immunosuppressed.
- AITL has a generally poor prognosis; the median overall survival is <3 years.
- Diffuse large B-cell lymphoma may arise in AITLs, presumably as clonal outgrowths of the B-immunoblast component.

HISTOLOGIC FINDINGS

- Three histologic patterns (Patterns I–III) have been described in AITL (Figure 9-14), which vary in architectural effacement and follicular dendritic cell (FDC) expansions.
- Pattern I represents AITL with hyperplastic follicles; this type is most often confused with a reactive adenopathy. The lymph node architecture is partially intact with an expanded paracortex surrounded by hyperplastic follicles.
- Pattern II shows loss of the normal nodal architecture with few, scattered attenuated follicles. FDC meshworks are prominent and expanded.
- Pattern III is the most common histologic pattern and shows complete effacement of the nodal architecture. FDC meshworks are prominent and expanded.
- In all patterns, the paracortex is expanded by a heterogeneous infiltrate, composed of variable numbers of atypical lymphocytes, histiocytes, eosinophils, plasma cells, and immunoblasts. Lymphocytes have a range of morphology, showing essentially no atypia to mild or moderate atypia. Collections of lymphocytes with clear cytoplasm and variable nuclear irregularity can frequently be found in a perivascular distribution (Figures 9-15 and 9-16).

(*continued*)

FIGURE 9-14 Low-power images of two AITL lymph nodes showing architectural pattern II (left) with regressed follicles (arrows) and pattern III (right) with complete architectural effacement.

FIGURE 9-15 This intermediate power view shows increased vascularity and perivascular collections of lymphocytes with clear cytoplasm.

FIGURE 9-16 A mixed inflammatory infiltrate composed of lymphocytes, eosinophils, plasma cells, and immunoblasts is characteristic of AITL.

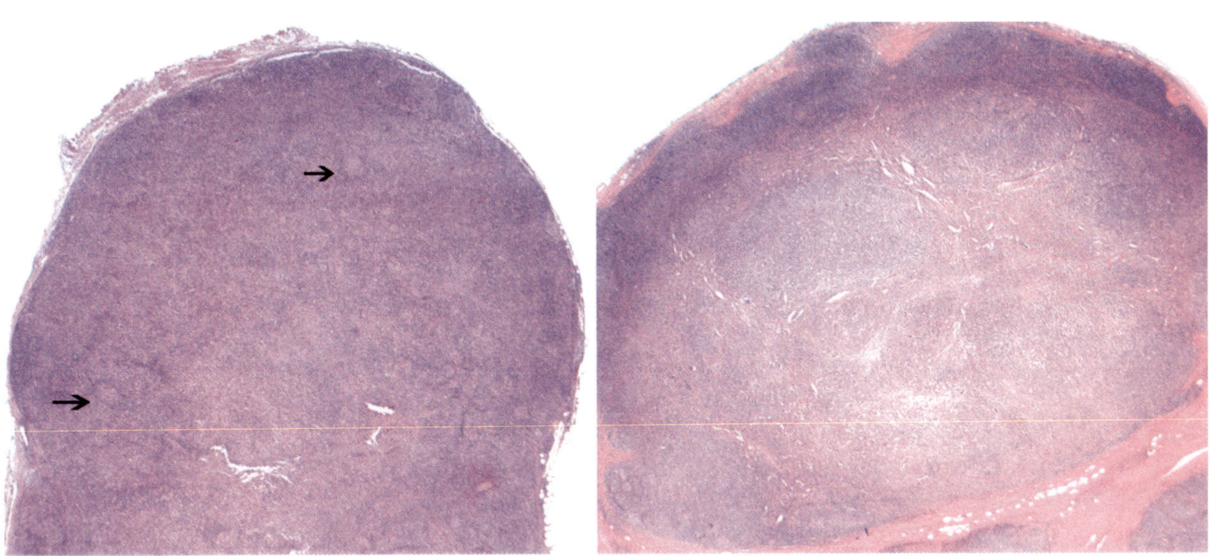

FIGURE 9-14

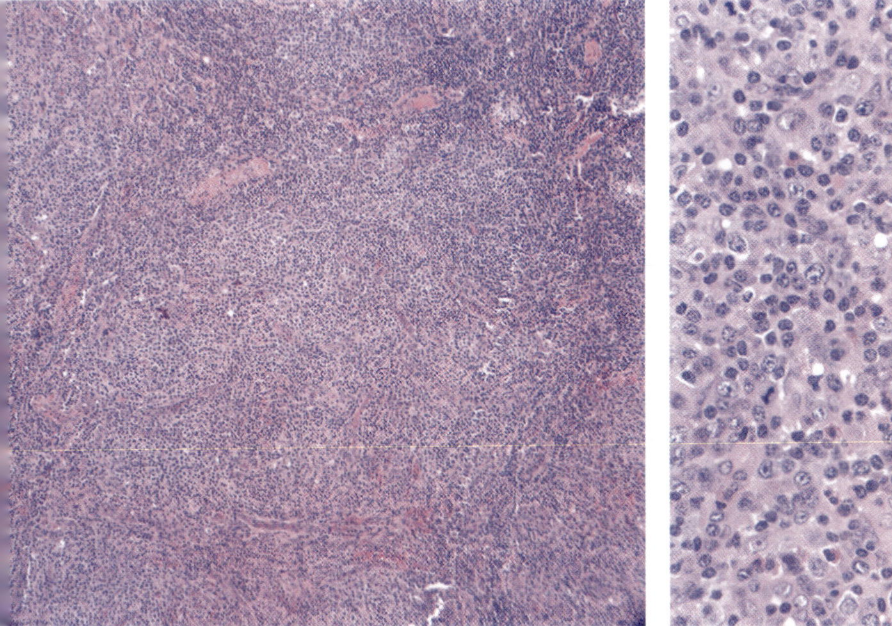

FIGURE 9-15

FIGURE 9-16

Angioimmunoblastic T-Cell Lymphoma *(continued)*

- Vascularity is uniformly increased in the paracortex.
- Most cases, including histologic pattern I cases, show immunophenotypic aberrancy of the neoplastic cells by flow cytometry. Underexpression of CD3 is the most frequent aberrancy.
- Reactive EBV(+) B-immunoblasts are present in variable numbers in the majority of AITLs (Figure 9-17). Occasionally these immunoblasts can resemble and immunophenotype as Reed-Sternberg cells (Figure 9-18). These EBV(+) B cells are part of the reactive milieu.
- The neoplastic lymphocytes are CD4(+) T cells and are usually positive for CD10. Increased CD10 expression in lymphocytes outside of the germinal centers, in the paracortex, is highly suggestive of AITL in the appropriate histologic and clinical context.
- The expanded follicular dendritic meshworks characteristic of AITL can be demonstrated with stains for follicular dendritic cells (CD21 or CD35)(Figure 9-19).

DIFFERENTIAL DIAGNOSIS

- Peripheral T-cell lymphoma, not otherwise specified
- Infectious mononucleosis
- Paracortical hyperplasia
- T-cell/histiocyte-rich large B-cell lymphoma
- Classical Hodgkin lymphoma

FIGURE 9-17 High-power magnification reveals an atypical small to medium-sized lymphocyte population with moderate nuclear irregularity and abundant pale cytoplasm admixed with scattered immunoblasts.

FIGURE 9-18 Reed-Sternberg-like cells (arrowed) were observed in this AITL.

FIGURE 9-19 The CD21 stain reveals expanded FDC meshworks. An EBER stain reveals scattered positive immunoblasts. A CD10 stain highlights increased numbers of CD10(+) lymphocytes outside of germinal centers.

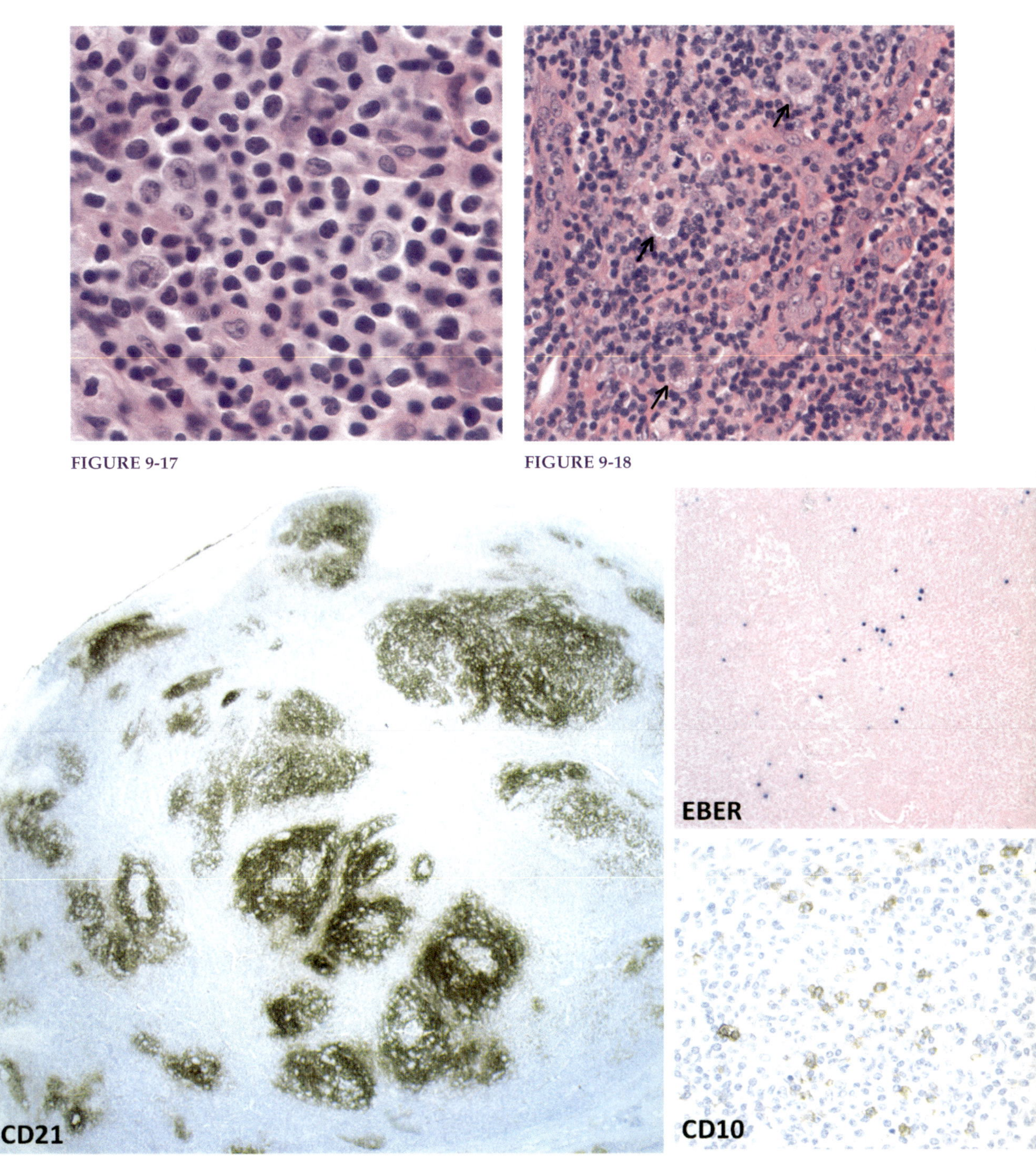

FIGURE 9-17

FIGURE 9-18

FIGURE 9-19

Anaplastic Large Cell Lymphoma, ALK Positive

DEFINITION

ALK$^+$ anaplastic large cell lymphoma (ALCL) is a mature T-cell neoplasm characterized by strong CD30 expression, hallmark cells, and translocations t(2;5) or t(2;v) involving the ALK gene, resulting in over-expression of novel chimeric ALK proteins. It accounts for approximately 3% of non-Hodgkin lymphomas.

CLINICAL FEATURES

- The majority of cases occur in the first 3 decades, with an increased incidence in the pediatric population. ALCLs account for 30% of pediatric lymphomas.
- The median age for adults is 34 years. There is a male predilection.
- Most patients present with advanced stage disease.
- Peripheral and abdominal lymph nodes are most commonly involved. Extranodal involvement is observed in 60% of cases, with skin, bone, and soft tissues most frequently involved.
- ALK$^+$ ALCLs have a better prognosis than their ALK$^-$ counterpart, though a recent study suggests that this prognostic difference is negated when patients are age-matched.

HISTOLOGIC FINDINGS

- Lymph nodes have partially or completely effaced architecture, with neoplastic cells frequently showing at least a partial intrasinusoidal pattern of involvement.
- Lymphoma cells are predominantly large in size, heterogeneous in morphology, and arranged frequently in cohesive clusters (Figures 9-20 and 9-21). Variable numbers of hallmark cells, characterized by eccentric, reniform or C-shaped nuclei, paranuclear clear to eosinophilic hofs, multiple distinct nucleoli, and abundant eosinophilic cytoplasm, are present. Imprints of these cells show prominent cytoplasmic vacuolization.

(*continued*)

FIGURE 9-20 High-power magnification reveals large tumor cells with frequent reniform nuclei, mature chromatin, abundant cytoplasm, and multiple prominent small nucleoli, representing hallmark cells.

FIGURE 9-21 Several hallmark cells are observed at this high-power magnification.

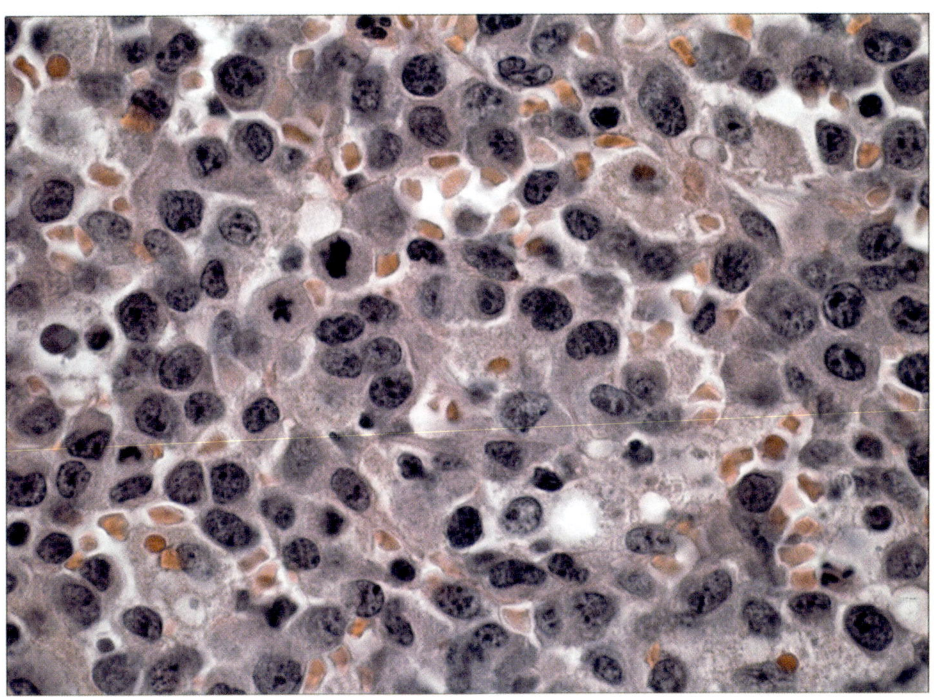

FIGURE 9-20

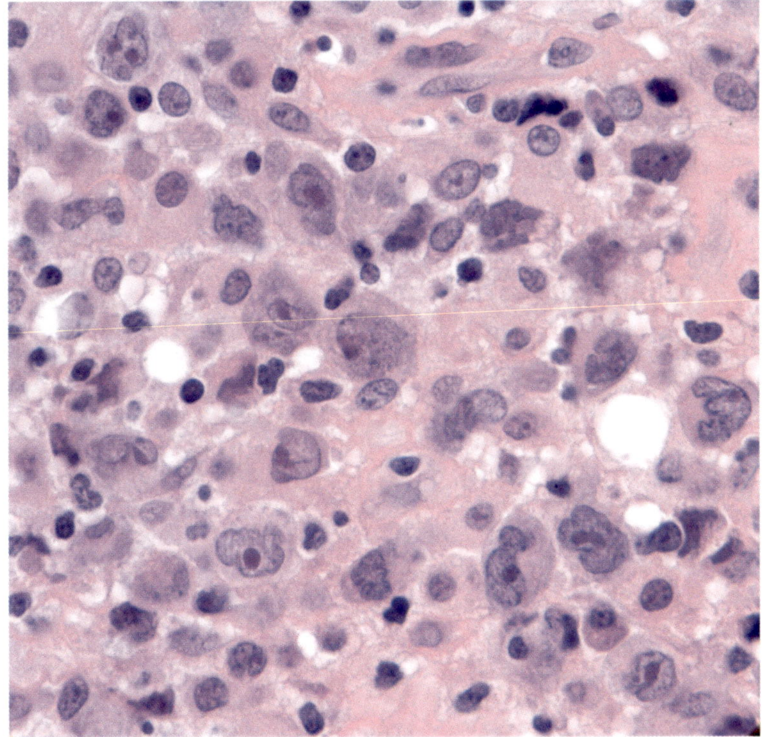

FIGURE 9-21

Anaplastic Large Cell Lymphoma, ALK Positive *(continued)*

- Several variants are described, including the lymphohistiocytic and small cell variants. The lymphohistiocytic variant accounts for 5–10% of ALCLs and is composed of neoplastic cells admixed with numerous histiocytes (Figure 9-22). The small cell variant accounts for a similar percentage of ALCLs and consists of a predominance of small to medium-sized neoplastic cells with hyperchromatic, irregular nuclei and small numbers of more typical large cells, including hallmark cells, typically in a perivascular distribution (Figure 9-23). The small tumor cells show variable CD30 expression, in contrast to the strong CD30(+) large cells.

(continued)

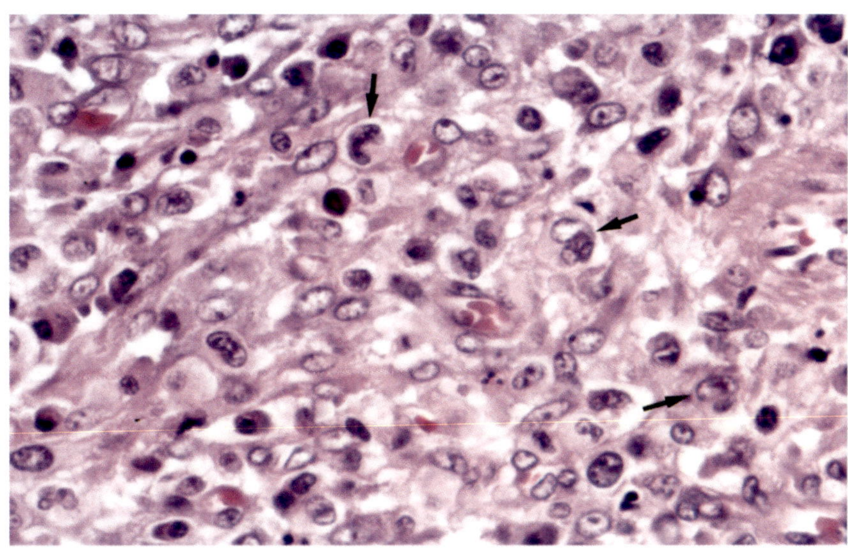

FIGURE 9-22

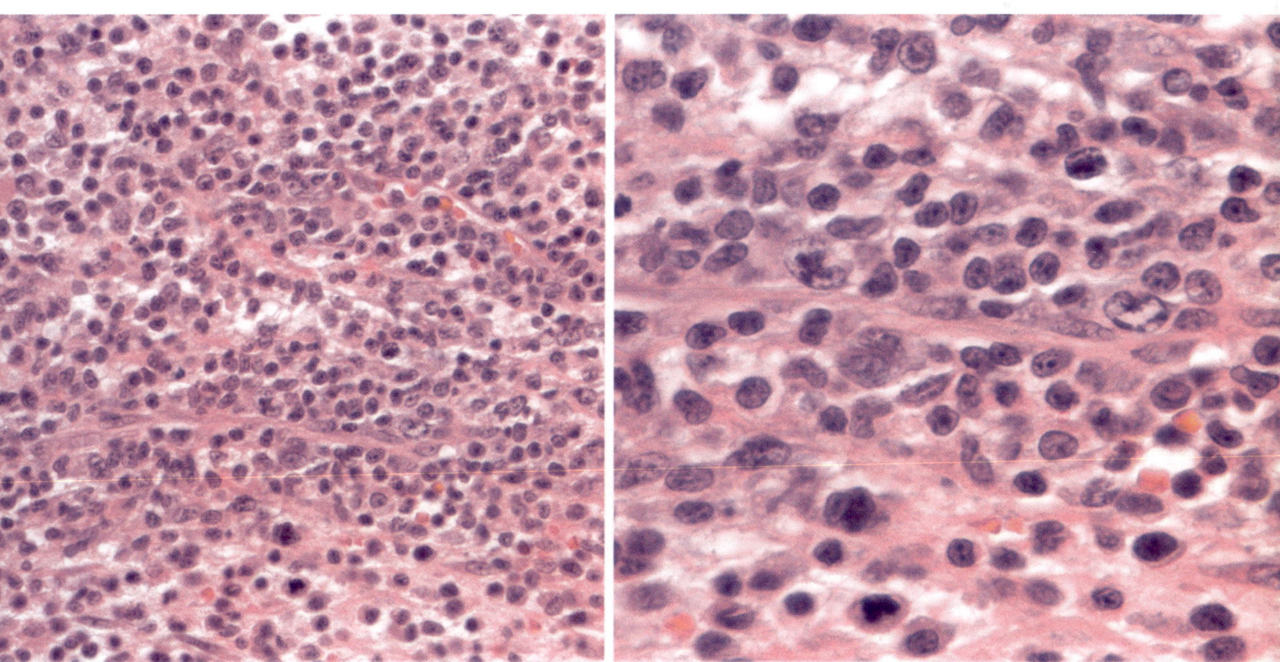

FIGURE 9-23

FIGURE 9-22 Lymphohistiocytic variant of anaplastic large cell lymphoma, ALK$^+$. The majority of cells in the infiltrate are benign histiocytes. Neoplastic cells (arrows) may be inconspicuous, obscured by the histiocytic infiltrate.

FIGURE 9-23 Small cell variant of anaplastic large cell lymphoma, ALK$^+$. The neoplastic cells are predominantly small to medium in size. Scattered hallmark cells are observed on higher magnification (right). An ALK stain was positive.

Anaplastic Large Cell Lymphoma, ALK Positive *(continued)*

- By definition, with the exception of the small cell variant, the neoplastic cells stain uniformly strong positive for CD30 (Figure 9-24). ALCLs express variable T cell antigens, though notably up to 75% of cases are CD3(-). CD4 expression is more common than CD8 expression. Null cell cases are occasionally encountered.

DIFFERENTIAL DIAGNOSIS

- Classical Hodgkin lymphoma
- ALK^+ large B-cell lymphoma
- Anaplastic large cell lymphoma, ALK^-
- Peripheral T-cell lymphoma, not otherwise specified
- Metastatic carcinoma, including embryonal carcinoma

FIGURE 9-24 Neoplastic cells show strong uniform CD30 expression with Golgi accentuation (Top) and nuclear and cytoplasmic expression of ALK-1 protein (bottom). This pattern of ALK expression is observed in cases with the conventional translocation, t(2;5).

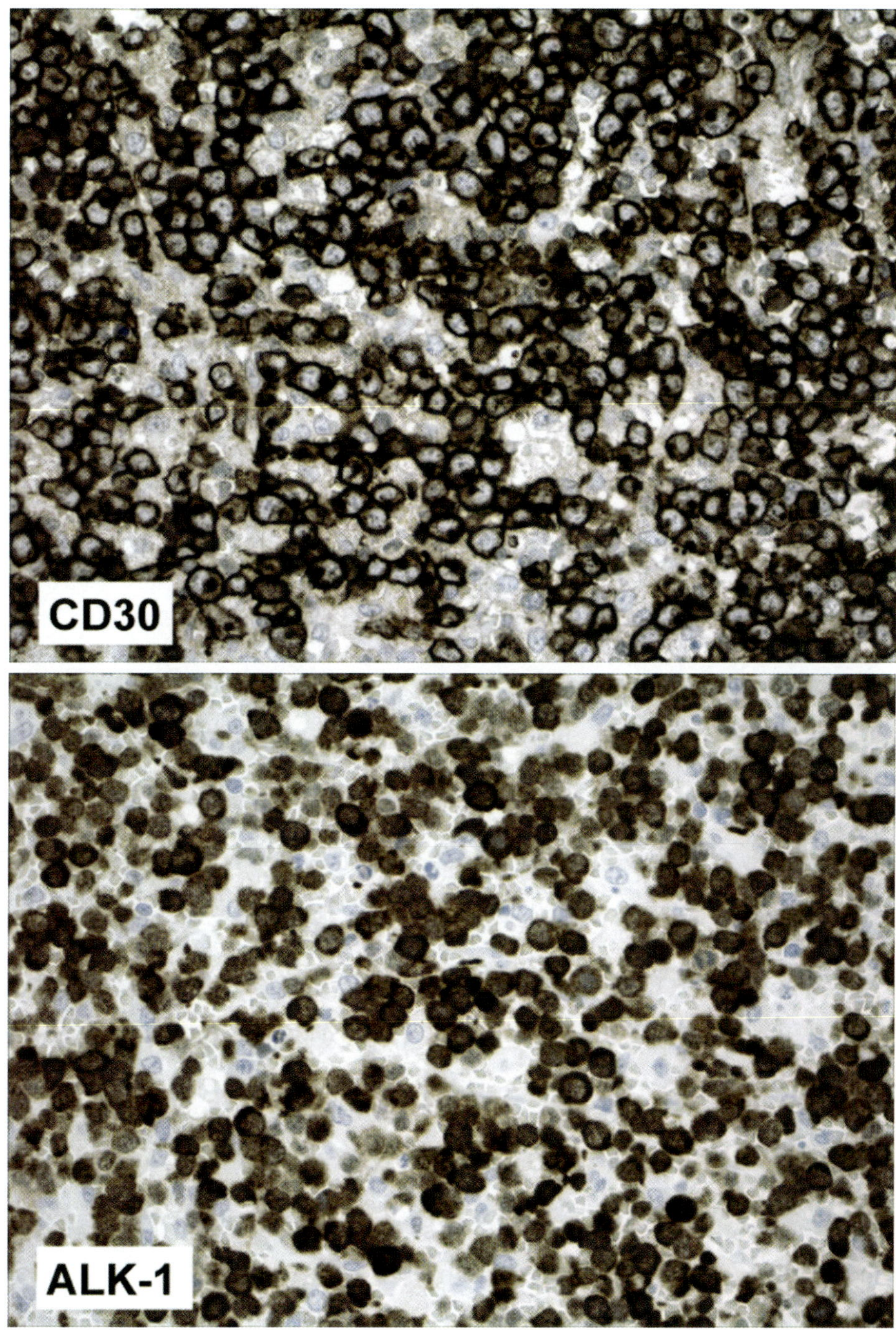

FIGURE 9-24

Anaplastic Large Cell Lymphoma, ALK Negative

DEFINITION

ALK⁻ anaplastic large cell lymphoma (ALCL) is a mature T-cell neoplasm that is morphologically and immunophenotypically similar to ALK⁺ ALCL, but that differs in that it lacks ALK gene rearrangements and ALK protein expression. It is a provisional entity in the 2008 WHO classification, though some argue it represents a variant of peripheral T-cell lymphoma, not otherwise specified (PTCL, NOS).

CLINICAL FEATURES

- The majority of cases occur in adults, in contrast to ALK⁺ ALCL, with a median age of 58 years. There is a male predilection (1.5:1).
- Most patients present with advanced stage disease. Approximately 50% of cases are limited to nodal involvement at diagnosis. Extranodal disease is observed most commonly in the skin, liver, and lung.
- The prognosis is worse in ALK⁻ ALCL than in ALK⁺ cases, though when age-adjustments are made, this outcome difference may be negated. Better overall survivals are obtained in ALK⁻ ALCLs than in PTCL, NOS.

HISTOLOGIC FINDINGS

- Involved lymph nodes display partially or completely effaced architecture, with neoplastic cells frequently showing an intrasinusoidal pattern of involvement (Figure 9-25).
- Lymphoma cells are predominantly large in size, heterogeneous in morphology, and frequently arranged in cohesive clusters (Figure 9-26). Variable numbers of hallmark cells are present, characterized by eccentric, reniform or C-shaped nuclei, paranuclear clear to eosinophilic hofs, multiple distinct nucleoli, and abundant eosinophilic cytoplasm.
- By definition, the neoplastic cells stain uniformly strong positive for CD30. ALCLs express variable T-cell antigens, though approximately 50% of cases are CD3(–). CD4 expression is more common than CD8 expression. EMA is expressed in only 40% of cases, compared to 80% of ALK⁺ ALCLs.

DIFFERENTIAL DIAGNOSIS

- Classical Hodgkin lymphoma
- Diffuse large B-cell lymphoma
- Anaplastic large cell lymphoma, ALK⁺
- Peripheral T-cell lymphoma, not otherwise specified
- Metastatic carcinoma, including embryonal carcinoma

FIGURE 9-25 This low-power image of an ALK(-) ALCL demonstrates striking intrasinusoidal infiltration highlighted by a CD30 stain.

FIGURE 9-26 This high-power image reveals large neoplastic cells that show frequent hallmark morphology. The tumor cells stained weakly positive for CD3 and were ALK(-). The histology of this case is virtually identical to an ALK⁺ case.

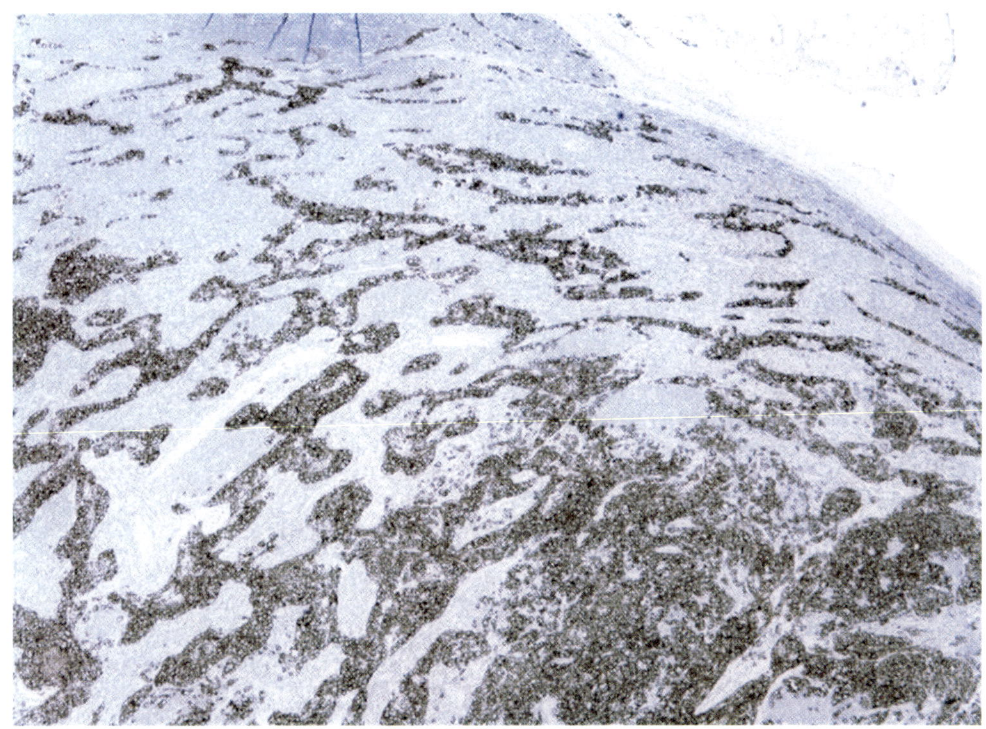
FIGURE 9-25

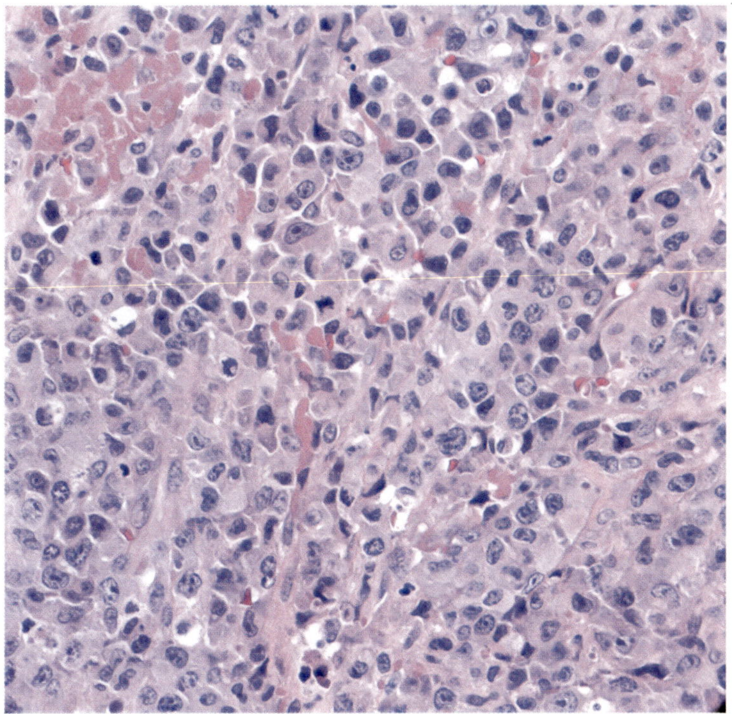
FIGURE 9-26

10

Hodgkin Lymphoma

NODULAR LYMPHOCYTE PREDOMINANT HODGKIN LYMPHOMA

NODULAR SCLEROSIS CLASSICAL HODGKIN LYMPHOMA

MIXED CELLULARITY CLASSICAL HODGKIN

LYMPHOCYTE RICH CLASSICAL HODGKIN LYMPHOMA

LYMPHOCYTE-DEPLETED CLASSICAL HODGKIN LYMPHOMA

Nodular Lymphocyte Predominant Hodgkin Lymphoma

DEFINITION

Nodular lymphocyte predominant Hodgkin lymphoma (NLPHL) is an uncommon form of Hodgkin lymphoma, accounting for non-classical cases. It is an indolent disease with a good prognosis, although there is a propensity for late recurrences.

CLINICAL FEATURES

- Most affected patients are between the ages of 30–50 years. There is a male predominance (3:1).
- Cervical lymph nodes are most commonly affected, and the majority of patients present with limited stage disease. Mediastinal involvement is not observed. Extranodal disease, including marrow involvement, is rare.
- Most patients present without B symptoms.
- NLPHL has an indolent clinical behavior and a good prognosis, though late stage recurrences (10–20 years from presentation) are common.
- Approximately 5% of cases may transform to diffuse large B-cell lymphoma.

HISTOLOGIC FINDINGS

- The lymph node has a nodular architecture. Nodules appear "moth-eaten" and are contain expanded follicular dendritic meshworks (Figure 10-1). Diffuse areas may be present, but any nodularity, given the appropriate neoplastic cell immunophenotype, requires classification as NLPHL, according to the 2008 WHO classification.
- "LP" or "popcorn" cells are the neoplastic cells within the nodules (Figure 10-2). These are large cells with frequently irregular, multilobated, and convoluted nuclei and multiple small basophilic nucleoli. Occasional LP cells may have large, eosinophilic nucleoli, similar to classic Reed-Sternberg cells. LP cells are admixed with small, mature lymphocytes lacking atypia and histiocytes.
- The LP cells stain positive for CD20, PAX-5, BCL-6, and CD45 and are negative for CD15 and CD30. CD57(+) T cells are enriched within the nodules and often encircle the LP cells.
- Progressive transformation of germinal centers (PTGC) may be observed in some cases of NLPHL. PTGCs has also been reported to precede the diagnosis of NLPHL in few cases, though the vast majority of PTGC are not related to NLPHL.

DIFFERENTIAL DIAGNOSIS

- Classical Hodgkin lymphoma
- T cell/histiocyte-rich large B cell lymphoma
- Progressive transformation of germinal centers
- Angioimmunoblastic T-cell lymphoma
- Reactive follicular and/or paracortical hyperplasia

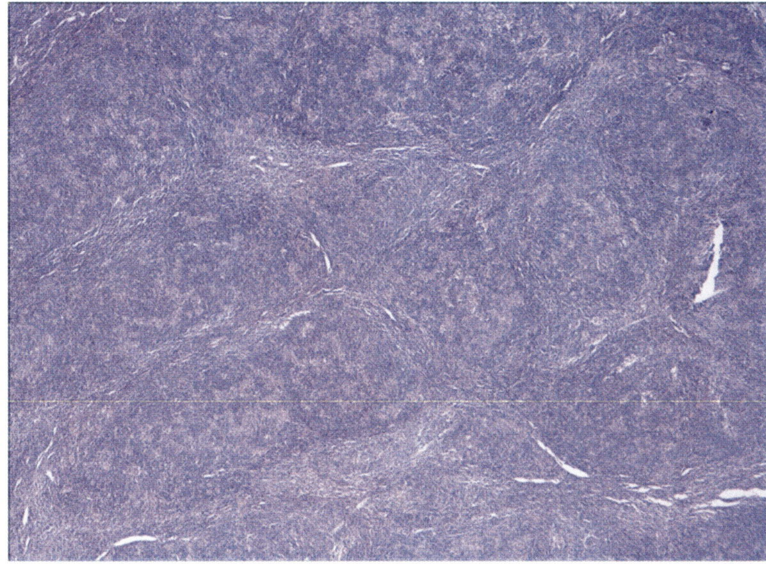

FIGURE 10-1

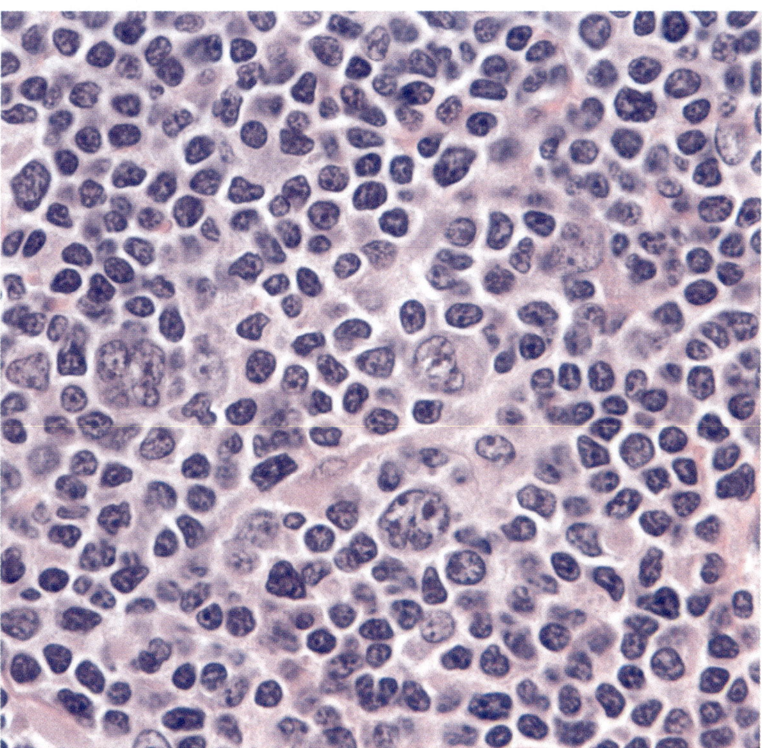

FIGURE 10-2

FIGURE 10-1 The lymph node shows an effaced architecture with multiple nodules showing a moth-eaten appearance.

FIGURE 10-2 High-power examination of the nodular areas reveals multilobated LH cells surrounded by small lymphocytes that lack atypia.

Nodular Sclerosis Classical Hodgkin Lymphoma

DEFINITION

Nodular sclerosis classical Hodgkin lymphoma (NSCHL) is the most common subtype of Hodgkin lymphoma, accounting for approximately 20% of lymphomas in the U.S. and Europe. It is characterized by dense sclerotic bands separating the infiltrate into nodules within the lymph node; this nodularity is often observable on gross examination.

CLINICAL FEATURES

- The peak incidence is between ages 15-34 years, with no gender predilection.
- 80% of patients present with mediastinal involvement. Cervical and axillary lymph nodes are also commonly involved. Bulky disease is observed in 50% of cases.
- Extranodal disease, including marrow involvement, is uncommon.
- Poor prognostic factors include bulky disease for early stage lymphoma and ≥ 5 of the following for advanced disease: age ≥45 years, stage IV, male sex, white blood cell count ≥15,000/µL, lymphopenia (<600/µL), albumin <4g/dL, and hemoglobin <10.5g/dL.

HISTOLOGIC FINDINGS

- The lymph node capsule is frequently thickened. Variably thick bands of sclerosis extend from the capsule into the parenchyma and divide the lymph node into nodules (Figure 10-3).
- Nodules are composed of Reed-Sternberg cells embedded in an inflammatory cell milieu, consisting of small B and T lymphocytes, eosinophils, neutrophils, histiocytes, and plasma cells (Figure 10-4). Neutrophilic and/or eosinophilic microabscesses may be observed.
- The RS cells often have "lacunar" morphology due to retraction artifact caused by formalin fixation. RS cells are large in size and have frequently multilobated nuclei, variably prominent eosinophilic nucleoli (usually smaller than in classical RS cells), and abundant cytoplasm. When the RS cells are arranged in cohesive clusters, the "syncytial variant" designation may be applied, though there is no clinical/prognostic significance to this variant.
- Large areas of geographic necrosis occur in some cases, particularly in syncytial areas (Figure 10-5).

(*continued*)

FIGURE 10-3 The lymph node shows a markedly thickened fibrous capsule and thick, hypocellular fibrous bands organizing the parenchyma into nodules.

FIGURE 10-4 Intermediate magnification of a nodule reveals many RS cells admixed with lymphocytes, eosinophils, neutrophils, and histiocytes.

FIGURE 10-5 Extensive areas of necrosis were present in this case.

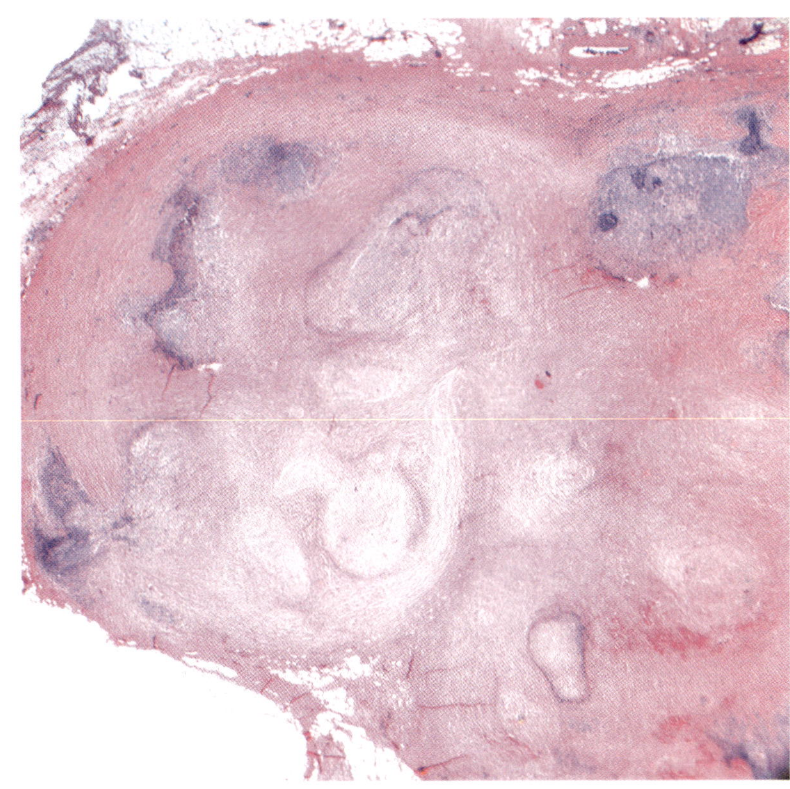

FIGURE 10-3

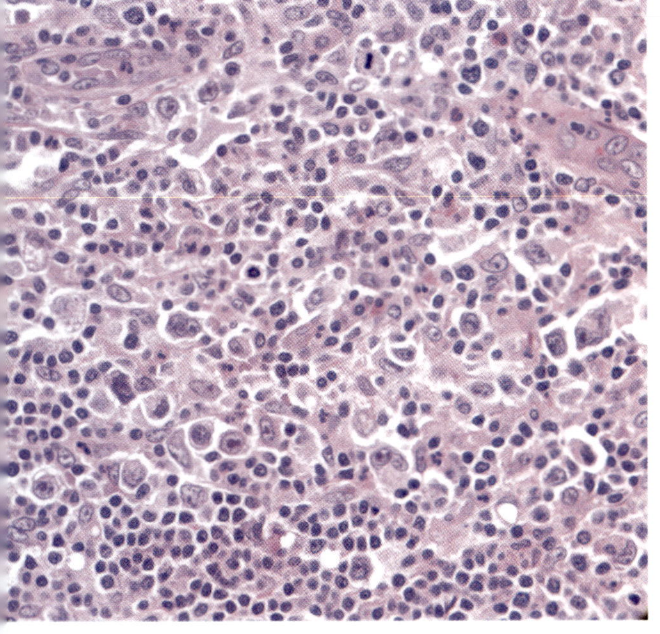

FIGURE 10-4

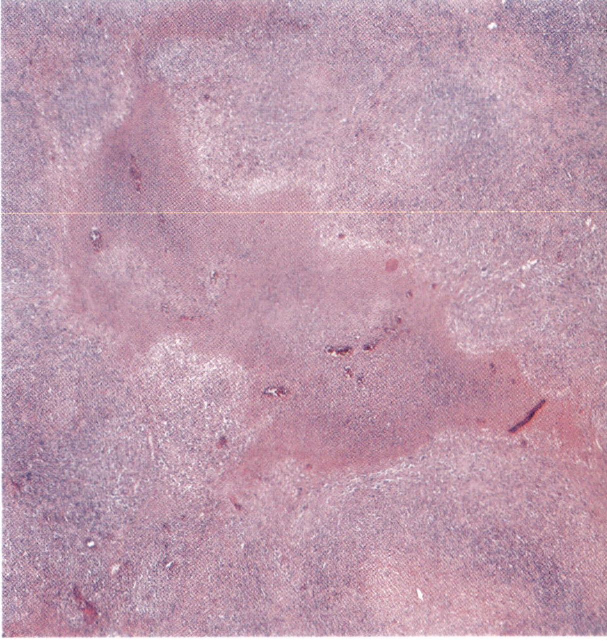

FIGURE 10-5

Nodular Sclerosis Classical Hodgkin Lymphoma *(continued)*

- Classical RS cells are positive for CD15, CD30, and PAX-5 and are negative for CD45 (Figure 10-6). RS cells express CD20 in approximately 20–30% of cases; when present, it is typically weak and expressed in only a subset of RS cells.

DIFFERENTIAL DIAGNOSIS

- Primary mediastinal (thymic) large B-cell lymphoma
- B-cell lymphoma, unclassifiable, with features intermediate between DLBCL and classical Hodgkin lymphoma
- Nodular lymphocyte predominant Hodgkin lymphoma
- Peripheral T-cell lymphoma, NOS
- Anaplastic large cell lymphoma

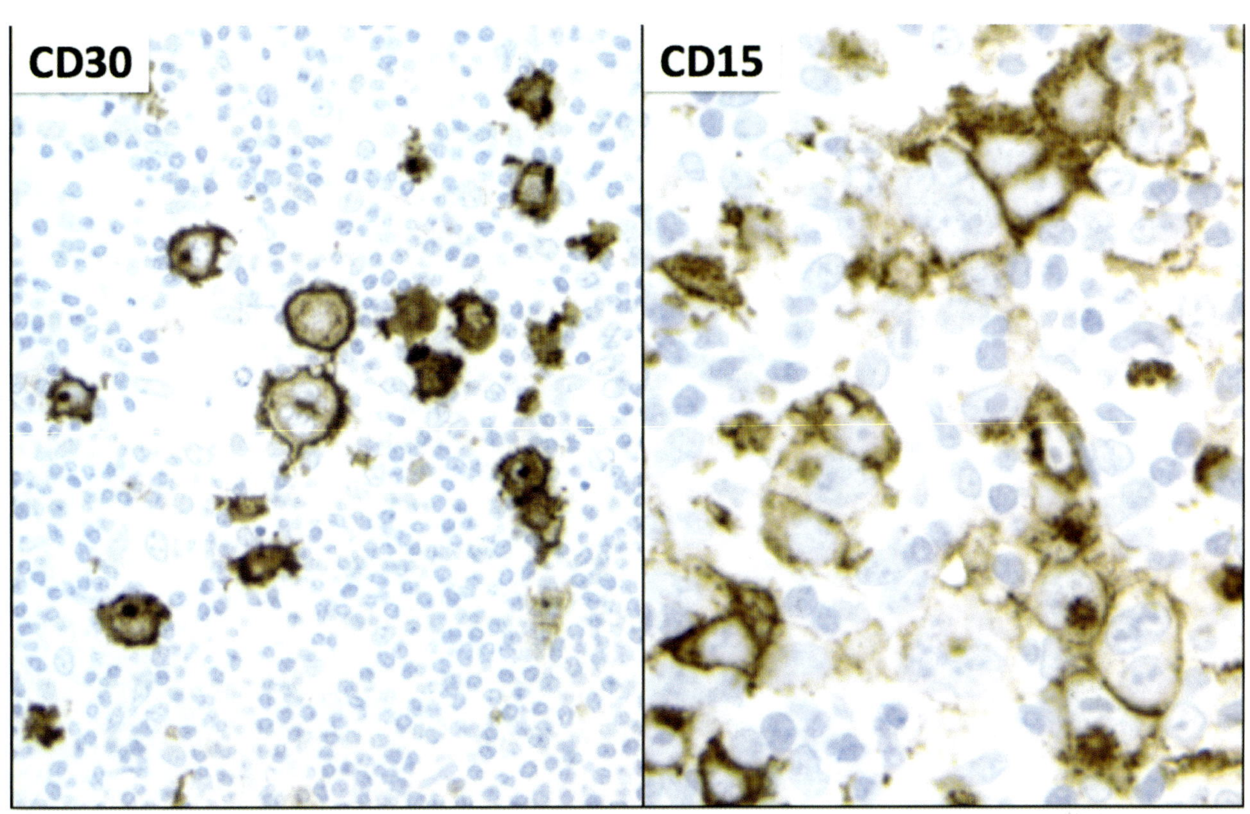

FIGURE 10-6

FIGURE 10-6 The RS cells are positive for CD30 and CD15 by immunohistochemistry.

Mixed Cellularity Classical Hodgkin

DEFINITION

Mixed cellularity classical Hodgkin lymphoma (MCCHL) is the second most common Hodgkin lymphoma subtype in the U.S. and Europe and is characterized by classic Reed-Sternberg cells embedded in a mixed inflammatory cell infiltrate.

CLINICAL FEATURES

- The median age of presentation is 38 years old, though there is a bimodal age incidence including pediatric and elderly patients. The majority of cases occur in males (70%).
- Peripheral lymph nodes, including cervical and axillary sites, are most commonly involved; generalized involvement is more common in this subtype than other subtypes (with the exception of lymphocyte-depleted). The mediastinum is uncommonly involved.
- Mixed cellularity classical Hodgkin lymphoma is more commonly associated with a poor prognosis, when comparing all Hodgkin lymphomas.

HISTOLOGIC FINDINGS

- The lymph node architecture is effaced by a diffuse infiltrate (Figure 10-7), with occasional cases showing vaguely nodular or interfollicular involvement.
- Organized fibrosis is not present.
- Classic RS cells are embedded within an inflammatory cell milieu, consisting of variable numbers of small lymphocytes lacking atypia, eosinophils, neutrophils, plasma cells, and histiocytes (Figure 10-8).
- The RS cells are large in size and may show multilobated nuclei or multinucleation. Nucleoli are large and eosinophilic. Classical RS cells are positive for CD15, CD30, and PAX-5 and are negative for CD45. RS cells express CD20 in approximately 20–30% of cases; when present, it is typically weak and expressed in only a subset of RS cells.
- EBV positivity is most commonly observed in MCCHL, compared to other subtypes. Approximately 75% of cases show EBV positivity in the RS cells.

DIFFERENTIAL DIAGNOSIS

- Nodular sclerosis classical Hodgkin lymphoma
- Peripheral T-cell lymphoma, NOS
- T-cell/histiocyte rich large B-cell lymphoma

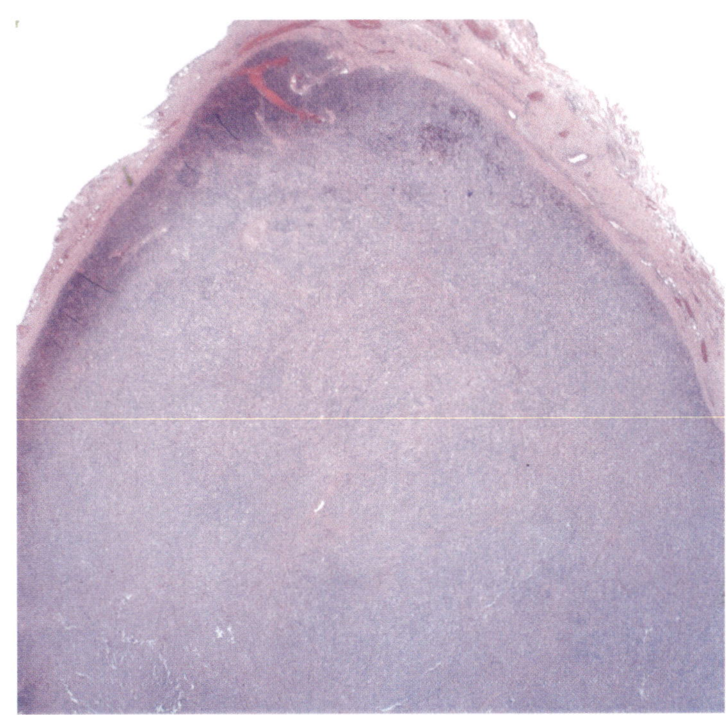

FIGURE 10-7

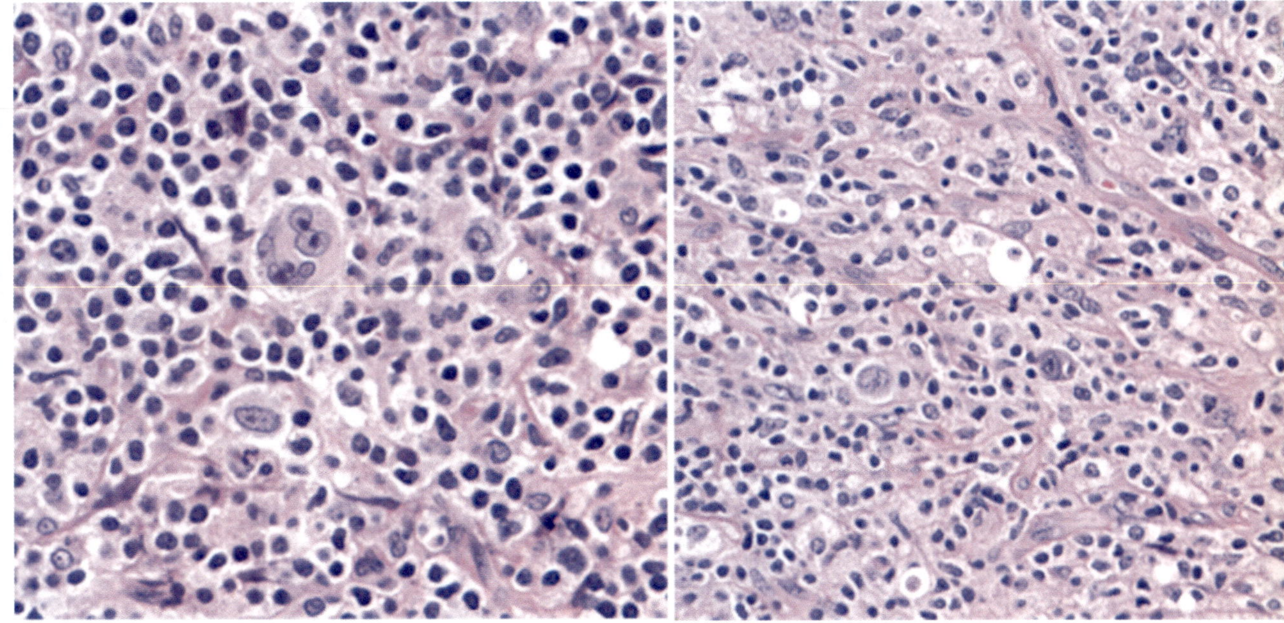

FIGURE 10-8

FIGURE 10-7 The lymph node shows an effaced architecture.
FIGURE 10-8 RS cells are observed in both lymphocyte-rich (left) and histiocyte-rich (right) areas within the same lymph node.

Lymphocyte Rich Classical Hodgkin Lymphoma

DEFINITION

Lymphocyte rich classical Hodgkin lymphoma (LRCHL) accounts for 5% of all classical Hodgkin lymphomas and is defined by a predominance of small lymphocytes, male predilection, and excellent prognosis.

CLINICAL FEATURES

- The median age is 38-43 years old, comparable to nodular lymphocyte predominant Hodgkin lymphoma (NLPHL) and older than other classical Hodgkin subtypes. There is a male predilection.
- Peripheral adenopathy is most commonly observed, with most cases presenting in low clinical stage (I-II). Mediastinal involvement is uncommon. B symptoms are infrequent.
- LRCHL has an excellent prognosis.
- Late relapses are observed, but not as commonly as in NLPHL.

HISTOLOGIC FINDINGS

- The majority of cases have a nodular architecture, though rare cases may have a diffuse growth pattern (Figure 10-9).
- The nodules are composed of small mature lymphocytes, which show immunophenotypic features of mantle zone cells. Germinal centers may be found within these nodules, and are usually small and attenuated. Importantly, the predominant lymphocyte population does not show atypia.
- The RS cells are few in number and are typically located at the periphery of these nodules, outside of the germinal centers (Figures 10-10 and 10-11). The RS cells may show classic morphology or intermediate features between classic RS cells and LP cells; therefore, immunophenotyping is essential.
- Classic RS cells stain positive for CD15, CD30, and PAX-5 and are negative for CD45. RS cells express CD20 in approximately 20–30% of cases; when present, it is typically weak and expressed in only a subset of RS cells.

DIFFERENTIAL DIAGNOSIS

- Nodular lymphocyte predominant Hodgkin lymphoma
- Mixed cellularity classical Hodgkin lymphoma
- Nodular sclerosis classical Hodgkin lymphoma
- Progressive transformation of germinal centers

FIGURE 10-9

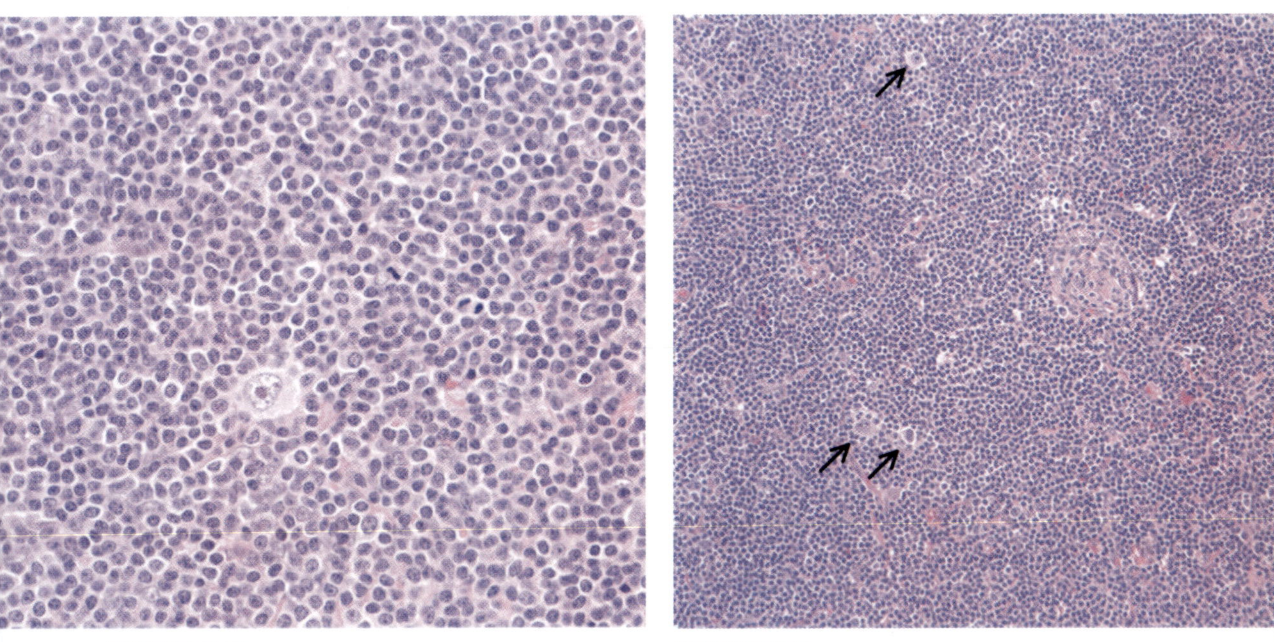

FIGURE 10-10

FIGURE 10-11

FIGURE 10-9 The lymph node shows an effaced, vaguely nodular architecture.

FIGURE 10-10 A single Reed-Sternberg cell is present in a background of numerous, histologically unremarkable small lymphocytes.

FIGURE 10-11 An atrophic germinal center is rimmed by mantle zone lymphocytes with occasional admixed Reed-Sternberg cells (arrowed).

Lymphocyte-Depleted Classical Hodgkin Lymphoma

DEFINITION

Lymphocyte-depleted classical Hodgkin lymphoma (LDCHL) is a rare subtype of classical Hodgkin lymphoma (CHL), with an incidence of <1% of all Hodgkin lymphoma. It is more commonly encountered in developing countries and is often associated with HIV infection.

CLINICAL FEATURES

- Presentation is most common in the 2nd and 3rd decades (median 30 years old). There is a male predilection.
- Approximately 75% of patients present with advanced stage, including extranodal disease, extensive lymphadenopathy, large mediastinal masses, and bone marrow and liver involvement. B symptoms are frequent.
- LDCHL has the worst prognosis of the HL subtypes, with 5 year overall survivals of 83% compared to 92% for all other CHLs, though limited data suggests that this prognostic difference has been eliminated with modern intensive chemotherapy regimens.
- Relapsed disease is common.

HISTOLOGIC FINDINGS

- The lymph node has an effaced, distorted architecture (Figure 10-12).
- RS cells predominate and are embedded in a variably fibrotic background (Figures 10-13 and 10-14). Background inflammatory cells are sparse and consist mostly of few small, mature lymphocytes. RS cells may be pleomorphic.
- RS cells have the classic immunophenotype: CD15(+), CD20(-), CD30(+), PAX-5(+), and CD45(-).

DIFFERENTIAL DIAGNOSIS

- Diffuse large B-cell lymphoma
- Anaplastic large cell lymphoma
- High grade pleomorphic sarcoma

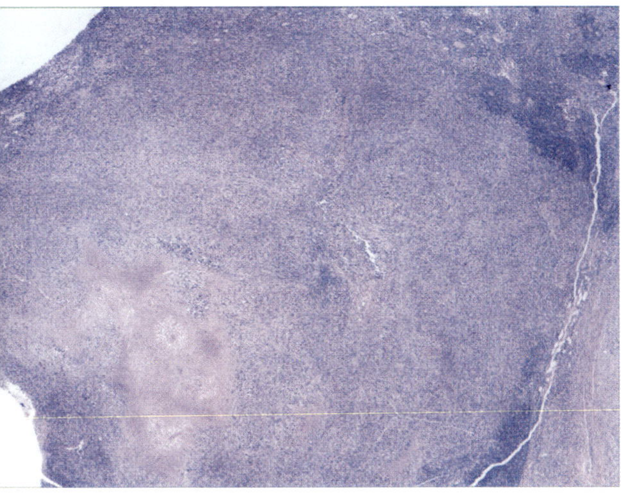

FIGURE 10-12

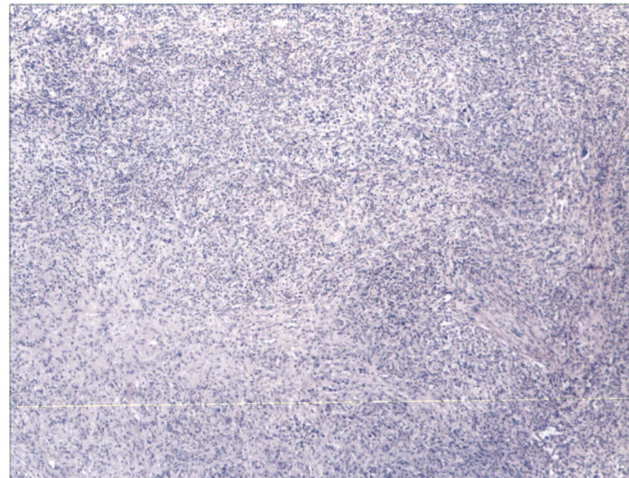

FIGURE 10-13

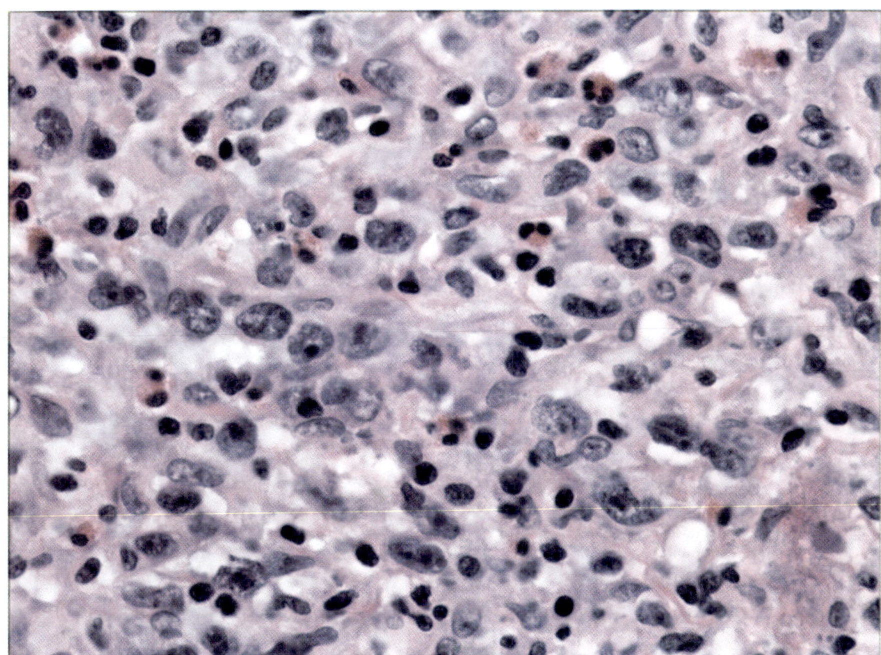

FIGURE 10-14

FIGURE 10-12 The lymph node shows an effaced architecture with areas of geographic necrosis.

FIGURE 10-13 Intermediate power of the same case as Figure 10-12 demonstrates a vague storiform pattern, mimicking a sarcoma.

FIGURE 10-14 High-power of the same case shows frequent large, atypical cells, eosinophils, and histiocytes, but few lymphocytes.

11

Immunodeficiency-Associated Lymphoproliferative Disorders

LYMPHOMAS ASSOCIATED WITH HIV INFECTION

POST-TRANSPLANT LYMPHOPROLIFERATIVE DISORDERS (PTLD)

Early Lesions: Plasmacytic Hyperplasia and Infectious Mononucleosis (IM)-Like PTLD

Polymorphic PTLD

Monomorphic PTLD

Classical Hodgkin Lymphoma Type PTLD

OTHER IATROGENIC IMMUNODEFICIENCY-ASSOCIATED LYMPHOPROLIFERATIVE DISORDERS

Lymphomas Associated With HIV Infection

DEFINITION

Lymphomas in HIV are a heterogeneous group of lymphomas that develop in HIV-positive individuals. Common lymphomas included in this category and discussed in this chapter are: Burkitt lymphoma (BL), diffuse large B-cell lymphoma (DLBCL), and Hodgkin lymphoma (HL). Primary effusion lymphoma (PEL), plasmablastic lymphoma (PBL), and large B-cell lymphoma arising in HHV8-associated multicentric Castleman disease morphology will be discussed separately.

CLINICAL FEATURES

- The incidence of non-Hodgkin lymphomas (NHLs) is 60–200 times higher than in the general population.
- The introduction of highly active antiretroviral therapy (HAART) has contributed to decreased incidence of AIDS-associated NHL, but also to increased incidence of HL.
- Extranodal presentation is common.
- Frequently, patients present with bulky disease, with advanced clinical stage and elevated LDH.
- DLBCL tends to occur in severely immunosuppressed patients, while BL presents in individuals with less severe immunosuppression.
- These lymphomas, with the exception of HL, are considered AIDS-defining conditions, and may constitute the initial presentation of AIDS.

HISTOLOGIC FINDINGS

- AIDS-associated BL demonstrate some typical BL morphologic features, including a low-power "starry sky" appearance and a diffuse infiltrate of medium-sized cells with distinctly clumped chromatin and dense, amphophilic cytoplasm containing vacuoles. However, compared to BL in non-immunosuppressed patients, AIDS-associated BL often has atypical features, including variability in nuclear size and shape, single, central nucleoli, and plasmacyoid differentation (Figures 11-1 and 11-2).
- DLBCL can show either centroblastic or immunoblastic morphology; some cases demonstrate a polymorphic appearance, similar to post-transplant lymphoproliferative disorders, and consist of an admixture of cells, ranging from small lymphocytes to immunoblasts and plasmacytoid cells.
- Classical HL is frequently of the mixed cellularity or lymphocyte depleted subtype (Figures 11-3 and 11-4).
- HL in AIDS shows essentially a 100% association with Epstein-Barr virus; DLBCL and BL are EBV(+) in 30–50% of cases.

DIFFERENTIAL DIAGNOSIS

- For DLBCL: BL; follicular lymphoma grade 3b; anaplastic large cell lymphoma; myeloid sarcoma; carcinoma; melanoma
- For BL: DLBCL; lymphoblastic lymphoma; small cell carcinoma

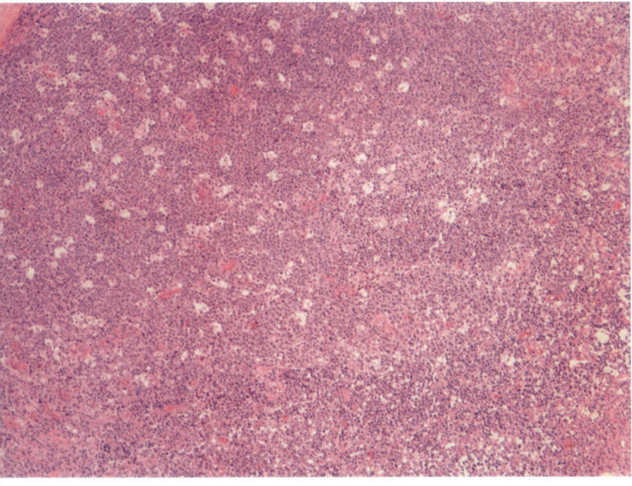

FIGURE 11-1

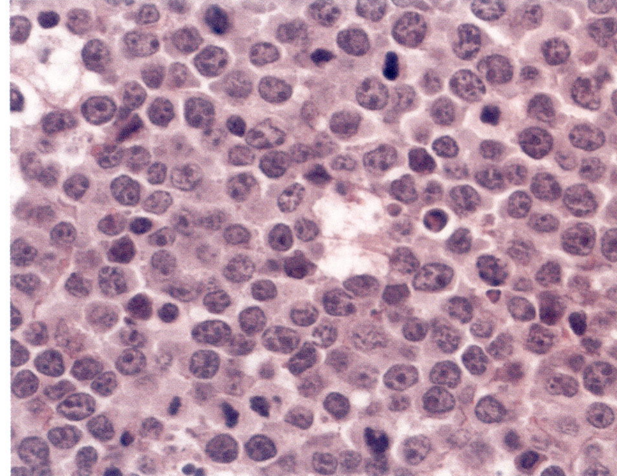

FIGURE 11-2

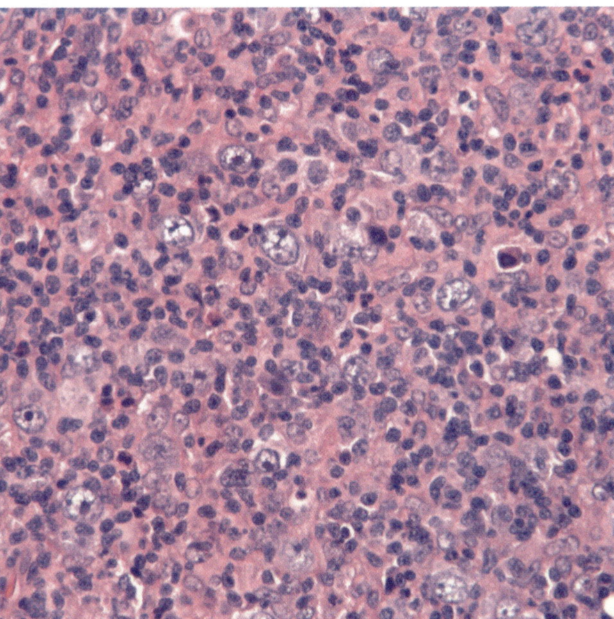

FIGURE 11-3

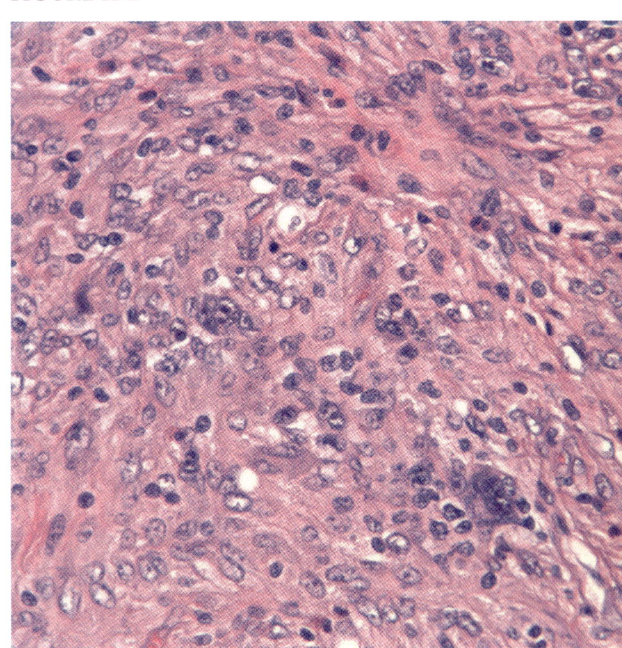

FIGURE 11-4

FIGURE 11-1 This Burkitt lymphoma associated with HIV infection manifests as a lymph node with effaced architecture and "starry sky" low-power appearance.

FIGURE 11-2 This Burkitt lymphoma associated with HIV infection consists of the tumor consists of medium-sized cells with distinctly clumped chromatin and distinct nucleoli. Frequent mitoses are also present.

FIGURE 11-3 This mixed cellularity classical Hodgkin lymphoma associated with HIV infection is characterized by frequent mononuclear Reed-Sternberg cells seen in a background of frequent lymphocytes, eosinophils, and occasional neutrophils.

FIGURE 11-4 This lymphocyte-depleted classical Hodgkin lymphoma associated with HIV infection is characterized by few Reed-Sternberg cells in a background of frequent histiocytes and occasional eosinophils and lymphocytes.

Post-Transplant Lymphoproliferative Disorders (PTLD)

DEFINITION

These lymphoid or plasmacytic proliferations arise as a consequence of immunosuppression in recipients of solid organ or stem cell/bone marrow transplants.

CLASSIFICATION

This is a heterogeneous group of disorders, divided in the following categories by the 2008 WHO classification of hematolymphoid neoplasms:

1. Early lesions
   a. Plasmacytic hyperplasia
   b. Infectious mononucleosis-like lesion
2. Polymorphic PTLD
3. Monomorphic PTLD
   a. B-cell neoplasms
      i. Diffuse large B-cell lymphoma
      ii. Burkitt lymphoma
      iii. Plasma cell myeloma
      iv. Plasmacytoma-like lesion
      v. Other (excludes indolent small B-cell lymphomas)
   b. T-cell neoplasms
      i. Peripheral T-cell lymphoma, NOS
      ii. Hepatosplenic T-cell lymphoma
      iii. Other
4. Classical Hodgkin lymphoma-type PTLD

Post-Transplant Lymphoproliferative Disorders (PTLD)

CLINICAL FEATURES

- The frequency of these disorders depends on the type of transplant (more common in solid organ vs. stem cell/bone marrow) and age (more common in children vs. adults).
- PTLDs are usually of host origin in solid organ recipients, and of donor origin in bone marrow recipients.
- Lymph nodes (LNs), gastrointestinal tract, liver and lungs are commonly involved.
- EBV(+) PTLDs present often in the first year after transplantation in BM and solid organ recipients treated with calcineurin inhibitors; EBV(−) PTLDs tend to present later (4–5 years after transplantation).

Early Lesions: Plasmacytic Hyperplasia and Infectious Mononucleosis (IM)-Like PTLD

DEFINITION

Early lesion PTLDs are characterized by non-destructive growth pattern and reactive-appearing cytologic features. They usually present as mass lesions in adenoids, tonsils or lymph nodes of allograft recipients.

CLINICAL FEATURES

- PTLD early lesions are common in children/young adults without prior EBV infection.
- These may regress, either spontaneously or upon reduction of immunosuppression.

HISTOLOGIC FINDINGS

- The involved organ usually has a maintained architecture, patent sinuses or preserved tonsillar crypts, and various degrees of follicular hyperplasia (Figure 11-5).
- Plasmacytic hyperplasia is composed of frequent mature plasma cells, admixed with small lymphocytes and rare immunoblasts (Figure 11-6).
- IM-like PTLD resembles typical IM, with paracortical hyperplasia including numerous immunoblasts, in a background of frequent plasma cells and small T lymphocytes (Figures 11-7 and 11-8).
- Plasma cells and B lymphocytes are polytypic; EBV is positive in the majority of cases (particularly the IM-like early lesions).

DIFFERENTIAL DIAGNOSIS

- Reactive lymphadenopathy or tonsillar hyperplasia

FIGURE 11-5 This example of plasmacytic hyperplasia PTLD demonstrates a lymph node with partially effaced architecture and expanded interfollicular areas.

FIGURE 11-6 This high-power view reveals interfollicular collections of plasma cells. The plasma cells are mature, and lack cytologic atypia.

FIGURE 11-7 This infectious mononucleosis-like PTLD manifests as paracortical and follicular hyperplasia.

FIGURE 11-8 High-power view of area of paracortical expansion shows frequent immunoblasts, plasma cells, and small lymphocytes.

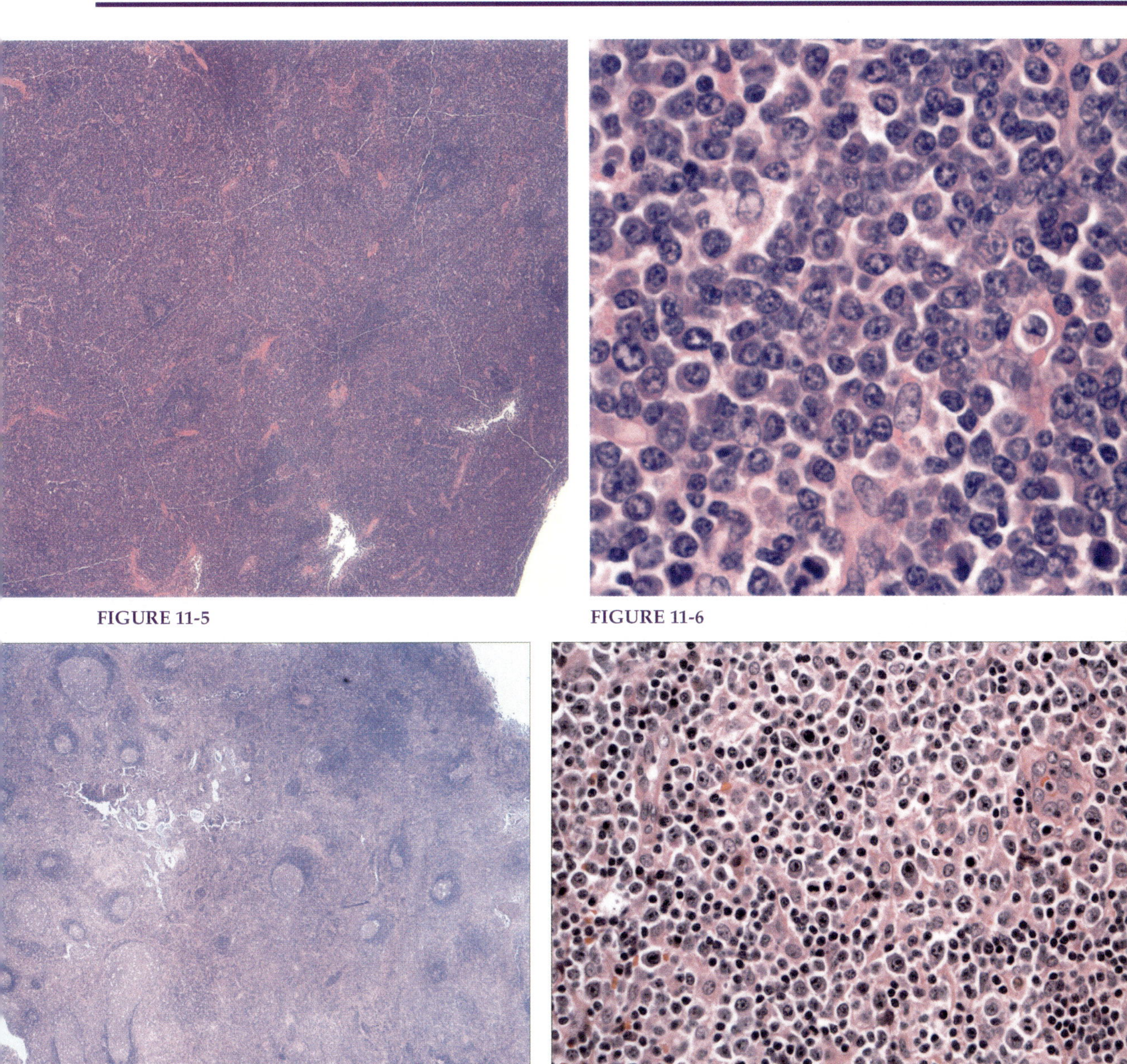

FIGURE 11-5

FIGURE 11-6

FIGURE 11-7

FIGURE 11-8

Polymorphic PTLD

DEFINITION

Polymorphic PTLDs efface normal tissue architecture or form extranodal masses, and consist of a polymorphic cell admixture that includes immunoblasts, plasma cells, and variably-sized lymphocytes.

CLINICAL FEATURES

- This is the most common PTLD in children.
- Polymorphic PTLDs may in some cases regress after reduction of immunosuppression.

HISTOLOGIC FINDINGS

- This form of PTLD demonstrates effacement of lymph node architecture with areas of geographic necrosis and a neoplastic infiltrate showing a morphologic continuum between small lymphocytes, medium-sized cells, immunoblasts, plasma cells, and occasional atypical, Reed-Sternberg-like cells (Figure 11-9).
- B cells may be polytypic or light chain restricted.
- Reed-Sternberg-like cells are CD30(+), CD20(+), CD15(−).
- EBER in situ hybridization is positive in most cases.

DIFFERENTIAL DIAGNOSIS

- Monomorphic PTLD
- IM-like PTLD

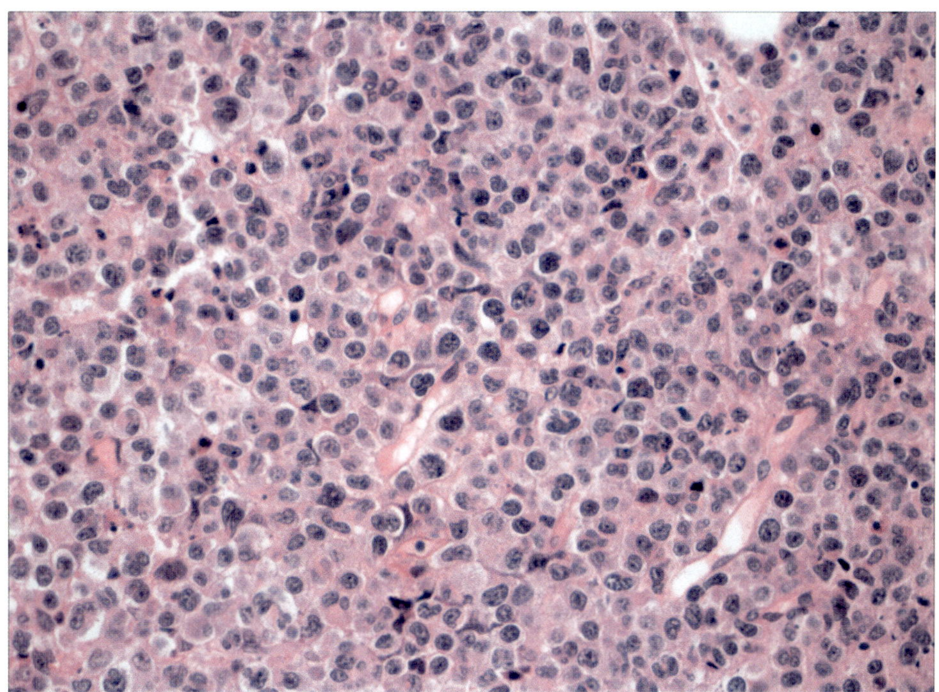

FIGURE 11-9

FIGURE 11-9 This polymorphic post-transplant lymphoproliferative disorder consists of a heterogeneous infiltrate composed of small lymphocytes, immunoblasts, lymphoplasmacytoid cells, and plasma cells.

Monomorphic PTLD

DEFINITION
This is a group of PTLDs that fulfill the morphologic criteria of specific B or NK/T-cell neoplasms encountered in the immunocompetent host. Small B-cell lymphomas, such as follicular lymphoma, marginal zone lymphoma, and mantle cell lymphoma, are excluded from this category.

A. MONOMORPHIC B-CELL PTLD

DEFINITION
Monomorphic PTLDs morphologically resemble diffuse large B-cell lymphoma (DLBCL), Burkitt lymphoma (BL) or plasma cell myeloma (PCM)/plasmacytoma.

CLINICAL FEATURES
- These present in a similar manner as comparable tumors in immunocompetent patients.

HISTOLOGIC FINDINGS
- Morphologic features of DLBCL, BL or PCM are present (Figures 11-10–11-13).
- Although some pleomorphism, including cell size variation and the presence of Reed-Sternberg-like cells, may be appreciated, the full morphologic spectrum of B-cell maturation, characteristic of polymorphic PTLDs, is missing.
- EBV expression in the neoplastic cells is variable.

DIFFERENTIAL DIAGNOSIS
- Polymorphic PTLD

(*continued*)

FIGURE 11-10 In this example of monomorphic B-cell post-transplant lymphoproliferative disorder, diffuse large B-cell lymphoma, the lymph node has effaced architecture and large area of geographic necrosis.

FIGURE 11-11 This Monomorphic post-transplant lymphoproliferative disorder represents a diffuse large B-cell lymphoma with immunoblastic morphology.

FIGURE 11-12 This high-power view of a monomorphic post-transplant lymphoproliferative disorder, Burkitt lymphoma, reveals a monotonous infiltrate of medium-sized cells with stippled chromatin and small nucleoli.

FIGURE 11-13 This high-power view of monomorphic post-transplant lymphoproliferative disorder, diffuse large B-cell lymphoma, shows a lymphoma with plasmacytic/plasmablastic morphology.

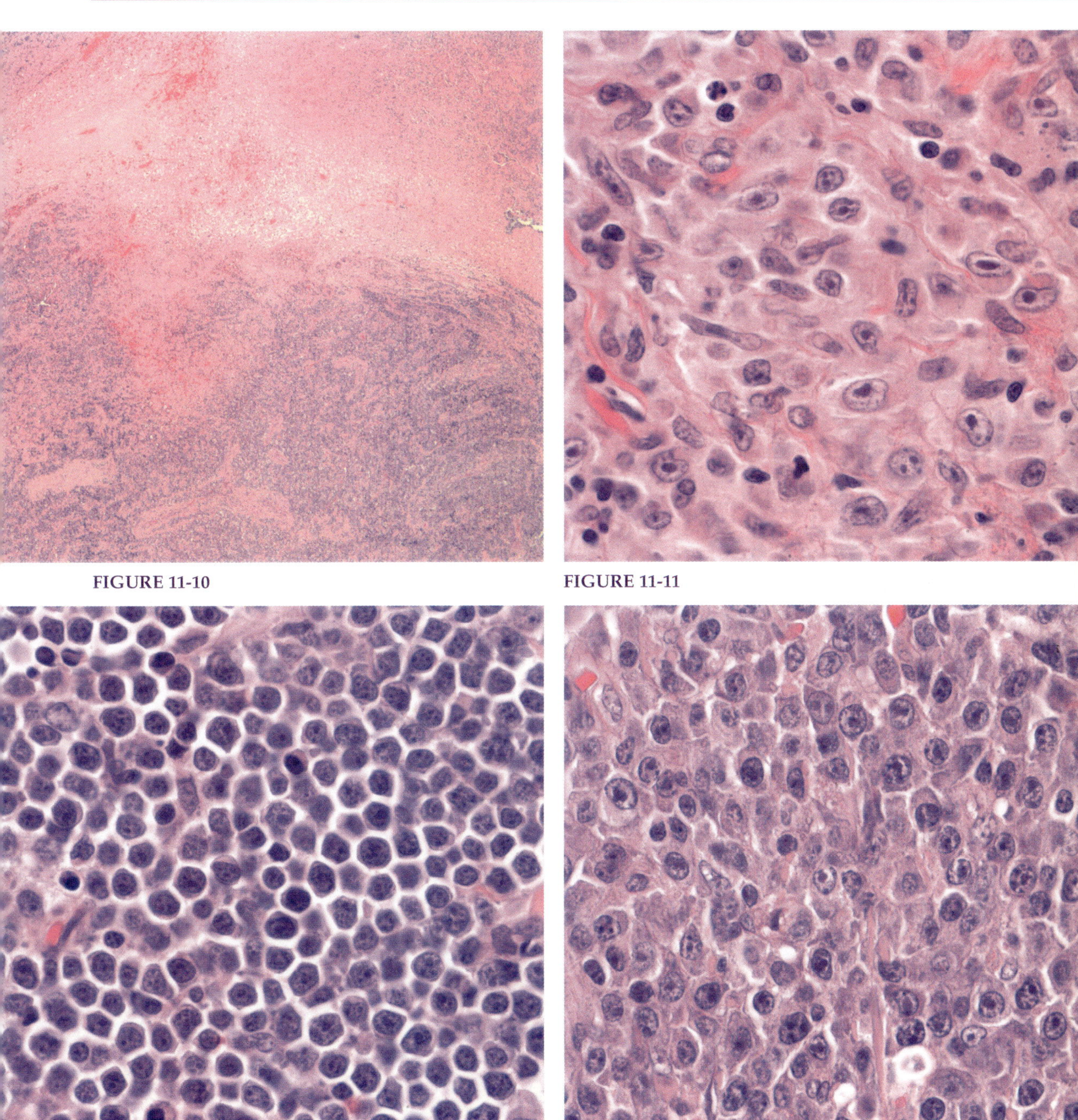

FIGURE 11-10

FIGURE 11-11

FIGURE 11-12

FIGURE 11-13

Monomorphic PTLD *(continued)*

B. MONOMORPHIC T/NK-CELL PTLD

DEFINITION

These PTLDs morphologically resemble any of the T- or NK-cell lymphomas, such as peripheral T-cell lymphomas (PTCL), NOS; hepatosplenic T-cell lymphoma; T-cell large granular lymphocyte leukemia; adult T-cell leukemia/lymphoma; extranodal NK/T-cell lymphoma, nasal type; mycosis fungoides/Sezary syndrome; and anaplastic large cell lymphoma.

CLINICAL FEATURES

- These present in a similar manner as comparable tumors in immunocompetent patients.

HISTOLOGIC FINDINGS

- The morphologic features of the corresponding entities in immunocompetent individuals are present (Figure 11-14).
- Of note, all types of T/NK-cell PTLDs are considered monomorphic, unlike B-cell PTLDs.
- EBV expression is present in 31% of cases.

DIFFERENTIAL DIAGNOSIS

- Polymorphic PTLD

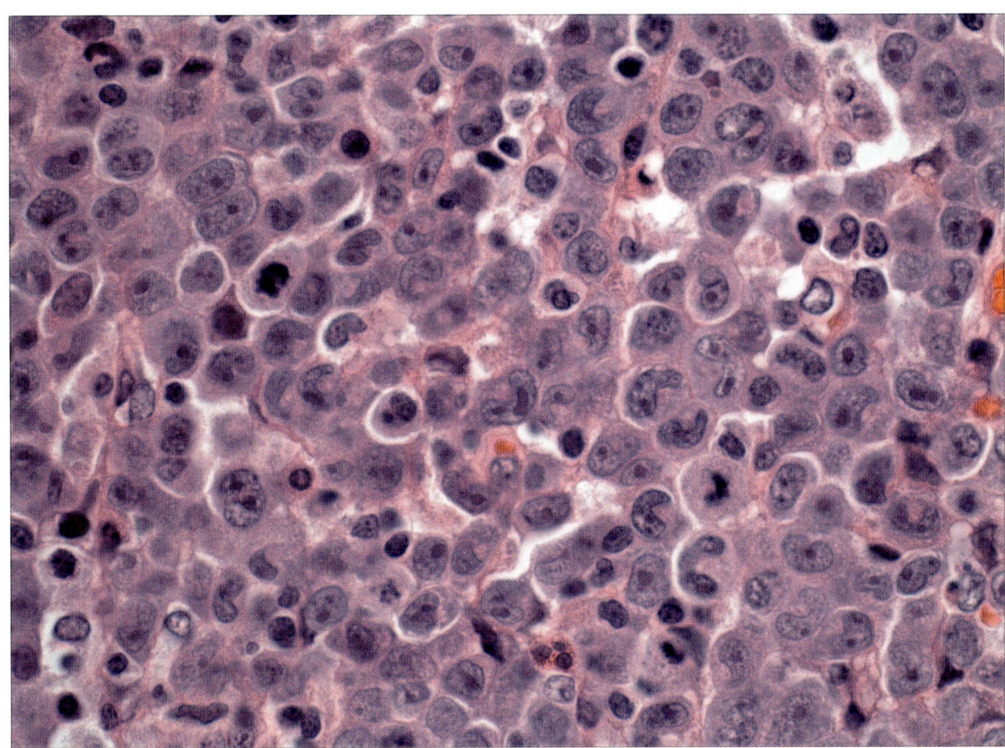

FIGURE 11-14

FIGURE 11-14 This monomorphic post-transplant lymphoproliferative disorder arising after solid organ transplant manifested as a CD30(+)/ALK(−) large T-cell lymphoma. It would be classified as an ALK(−) anaplastic large cell lymphoma in an immunocompetent individual.

Classical Hodgkn Lymphoma Type PTLD

DEFINITION

This is a PTLD with classical Hodgkin lymphoma (cHL) morphology and immunophenotype.

CLINICAL FEATURES

- This entity most commonly occurs post-renal transplant.

HISTOLOGIC FINDINGS

- The lymph node shows typical cHL morphology and immunophenotype, including CD30(+), CD15(+), CD45(−) Reed-Sternberg cells (Figures 11-15 and 11-16).
- EBV is almost always positive in the neoplastic cells.

DIFFERENTIAL DIAGNOSIS

- Polymorphic (Hodgkin-like) PTLD
- Monomorphic PTLD

FIGURE 11-15 Frequent Reed-Sternberg cells are present with irregular nuclei, vesicular chromatin, and prominent nucleoli.

FIGURE 11-16 Immunohistochemistry shows strong CD30 expression in the Reed-Sternberg cells.

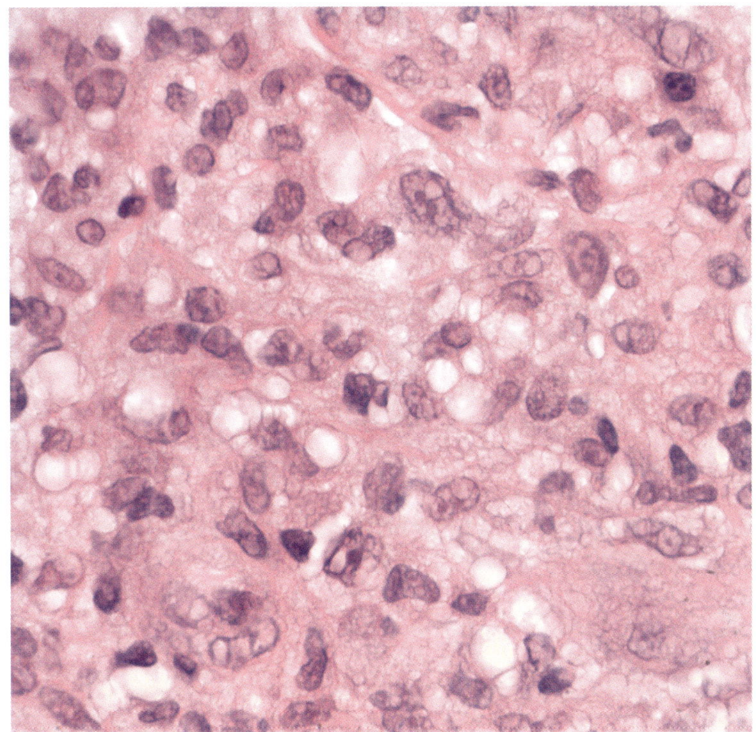

FIGURE 11-15

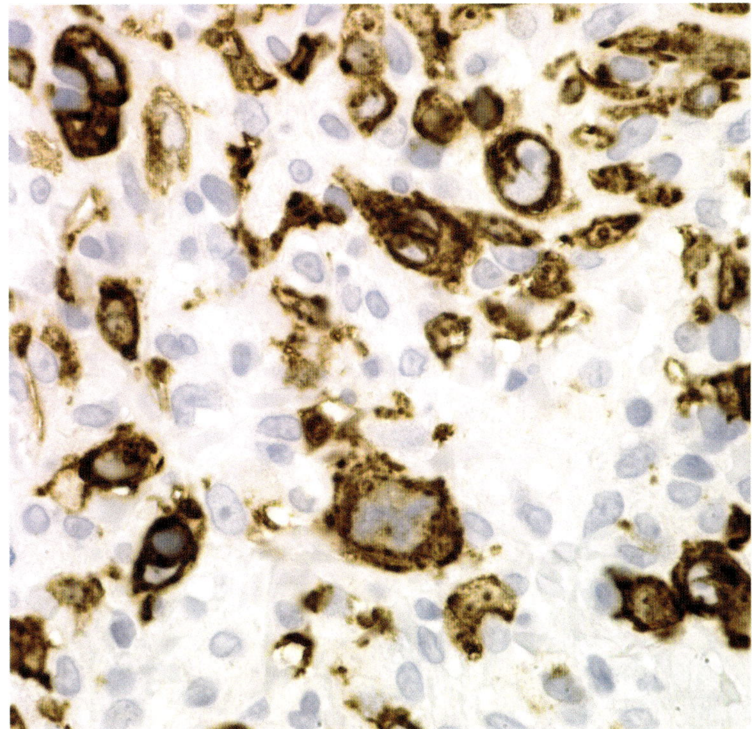

FIGURE 11-16

Other Iatrogenic Immunodeficiency-Associated Lymphoproliferative Disorders

DEFINITION

Lymphoproliferative disorders (LPDs) arise in patients treated with immunosuppressive drugs for autoimmune conditions.

CLINICAL FEATURES

- These lesions are most commonly seen in patients with rheumatoid arthritis treated with methotrexate, or in patients with Crohn's disease, treated with TNF alpha inhibitors, such as infliximab.
- Up to 50% of cases present with extranodal disease.

HISTOLOGIC FINDINGS

- The morphology is variable, ranging from polymorphic post-transplant lymphoproliferative disorder to diffuse large B-cell lymphoma, classical Hodgkin lymphoma, or hepatosplenic T-cell lymphoma (Figure 11-17).
- EBV is positive in approximately 40% of cases (Figure 11-18).

DIFFERENTIAL DIAGNOSIS

- Similar to the corresponding entities occurring in immunocompetent patients

FIGURE 11-17 This lymph node from a 69-year-old woman with history of rheumatoid arthritis treated with methotrexate shows a polymorphic lymphoid infiltrate. The atypical cells were B cells.

FIGURE 11-18 EBER in situ hybridization of the same case demonstrates EBV positivity in the neoplastic cells.

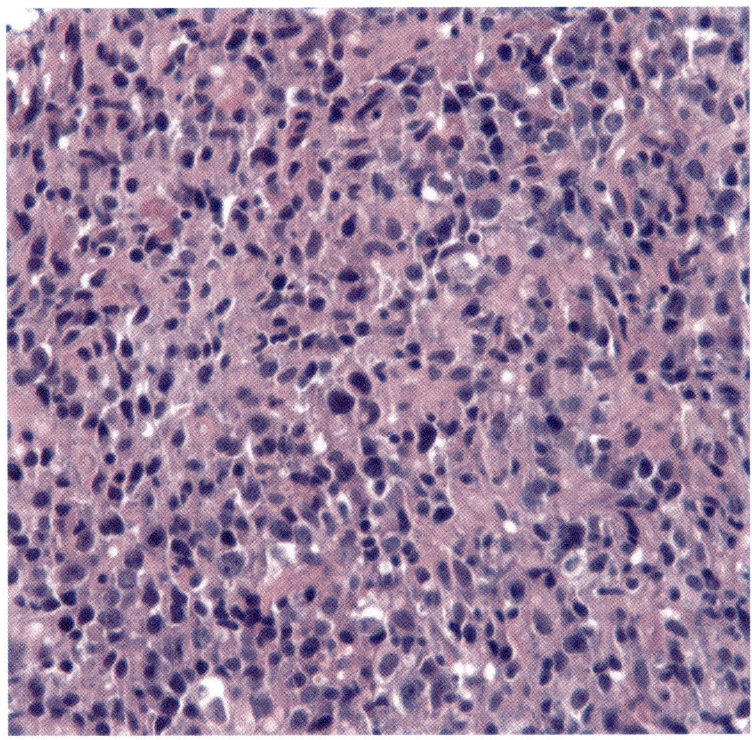

FIGURE 11-17

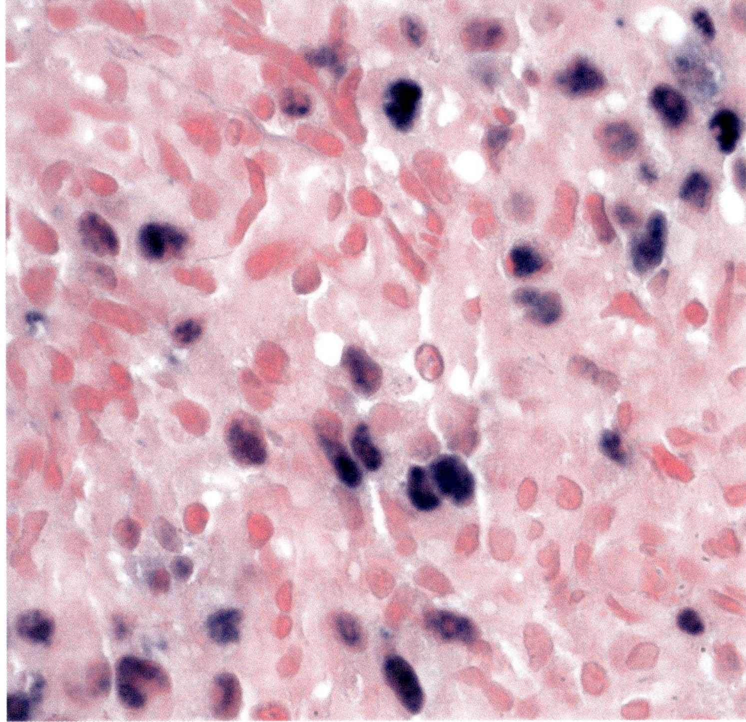

FIGURE 11-18

12

Histiocytic and Dendritic Cell Neoplasms

HISTIOCYTIC SARCOMA

LANGERHANS CELL HISTIOCYTOSIS (LCH)

LANGERHANS CELL SARCOMA

INTERDIGITATING DENDRITIC CELL SARCOMA

FOLLICULAR DENDRITIC CELL SARCOMA

Histiocytic Sarcoma

DEFINITION

This is a neoplasm of cells resembling mature histiocytes, morphologically and immunophenotypically.

CLINICAL FEATURES

- This is a rare tumor (0.15% of hematopoietic neoplasms) with a median age of 52 years (range: 0.5–89 years). There is no gender predilection.
- Gastrointestinal tract, skin, soft tissues and lymph nodes (LNs) are typically involved.
- Patients present with a solitary mass/skin lesion; some show intestinal obstruction or systemic symptoms.

HISTOLOGIC FINDINGS

- Lymph nodes display a diffuse proliferation of monomorphic or pleomorphic large cells with oval or irregular nuclei, vesicular chromatin, and abundant eosinophilic cytoplasm (Figures 12-1 and 12-2).
- Occasional cells are multinucleated.
- Phagocytic activity may be present, but this is a non-specific finding.
- Reactive lymphocytes, plasma cells, and eosinophils may be present in the background (Figure 12-3).
- The neoplastic cells are positive for CD4, CD45, CD68, CD163 (Figure 12-4), lysozyme; are sometimes positive for CD15, S100 (weak); and are negative for CD33, CD13, myeloperoxidase, CD1a, CD21, CD23, CD35, HMB45, EMA, cytokeratin, CD3, CD20, CD79a

DIFFERENTIAL DIAGNOSIS

- Follicular dendritic cell sarcoma
- Monocytic sarcoma
- Diffuse large B-cell lymphoma
- Anaplastic large cell lymphoma
- Hodgkin lymphoma
- Carcinoma

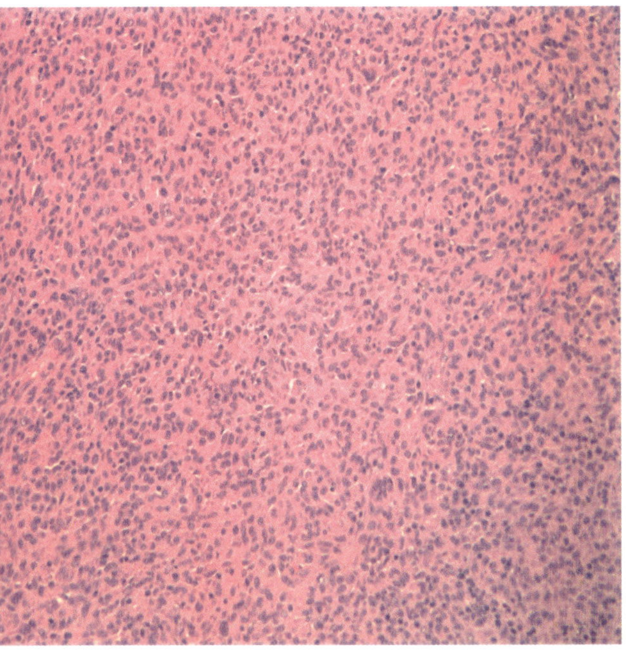

FIGURE 12-1

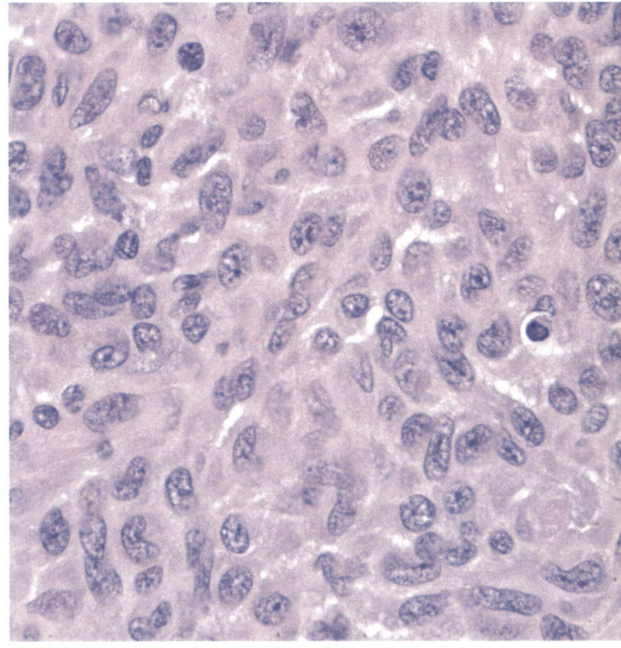

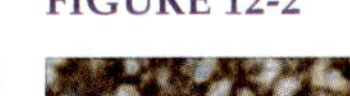

FIGURE 12-2

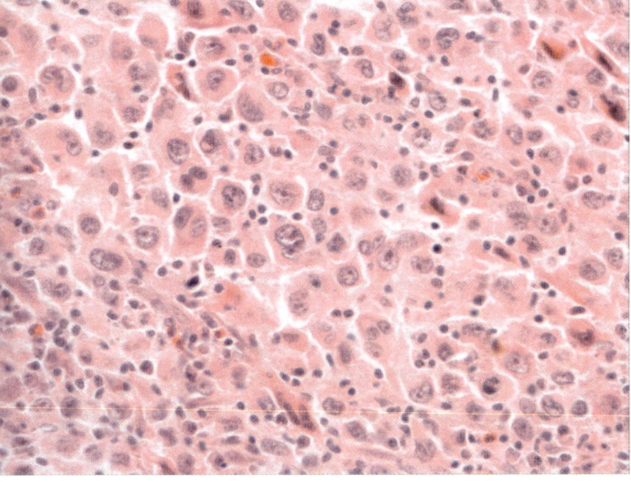

FIGURE 12-3

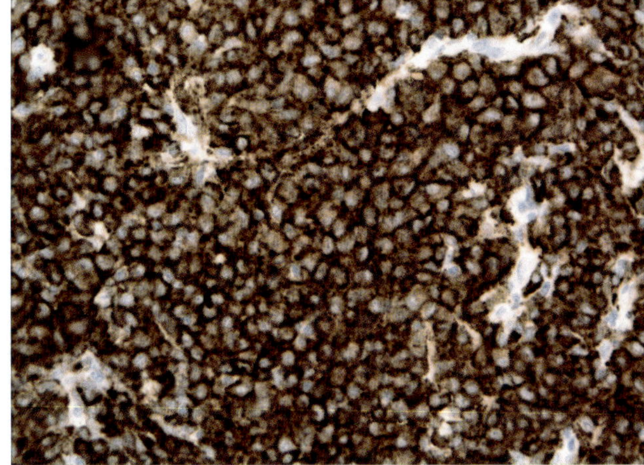

FIGURE 12-4

FIGURE 12-1 This lymph node has effaced architecture and a diffuse large cell infiltrate.

FIGURE 12-2 High-power shows neoplastic cells with large, oval nuclei, vesicular chromatin, and abundant eosinophilic, foamy cytoplasm.

FIGURE 12-3 This example manifests as a pleomorphic large cell malignancy with a broad differential diagnosis. There are background inflammatory cells, including lymphocytes, plasma cells, and eosinophils.

FIGURE 12-4 This is the same case as Figures 12-1 and 12-2; CD163, a specific marker of histiocytes, is strongly positive in all of the neoplastic cells.

Langerhans Cell Histiocytosis (LCH)

DEFINITION

LCH represents a neoplastic proliferation of Langerhans cells, characterized by specific immunophenotypic (CD1a, langerin, and S100 positive) and ultrastructural (Birbeck granules) features.

CLINICAL FEATURES

- LCH is common in children, and manifests a male to female ratio of 3.7:1.
- LCH can involve one site ("eosinophilic granuloma"); multiple sites within a single system ("Hand-Schuller-Christian disease"); or can be disseminated within multiple systems ("Letterer-Siwe disease"); lymph nodes can be involved occasionally in the solitary form of LCH.

HISTOLOGIC FINDINGS

- Involved lymph nodes demonstrate a sinusoidal and/or paracortical infiltrate of Langerhans cells, which are oval-shaped cells with folded, grooved nuclei, inconspicuous nucleoli, and abundant, pale cytoplasm (Figures 12-5 and 12-6); osteoclast-type giant cells and frequent eosinophils are present in the background (Figure 12-7).
- The typical immunophenotype is CD1a(+), langerin (+), S100(+), CD68(+), HLA-DR(+), CD45(+/−), lysozyme(+/−), CD21(−), CD35(−), CD163(−), CD4(+).

DIFFERENTIAL DIAGNOSIS

- Histiocytic sarcoma
- Langerhans cell sarcoma
- Follicular dendritic cell sarcoma
- Interdigitating dendritic cell sarcoma

FIGURE 12-5 This lymph node reveals paracortical infiltration and expansion.

FIGURE 12-6 High-power view shows bland Langerhans cells with grooved nuclei, delicate nuclear membranes, and abundant eosinophilic cytoplasm.

FIGURE 12-7 Langerhans cells are admixed with numerous eosinophils and an osteoclast-type multinucleated giant cell.

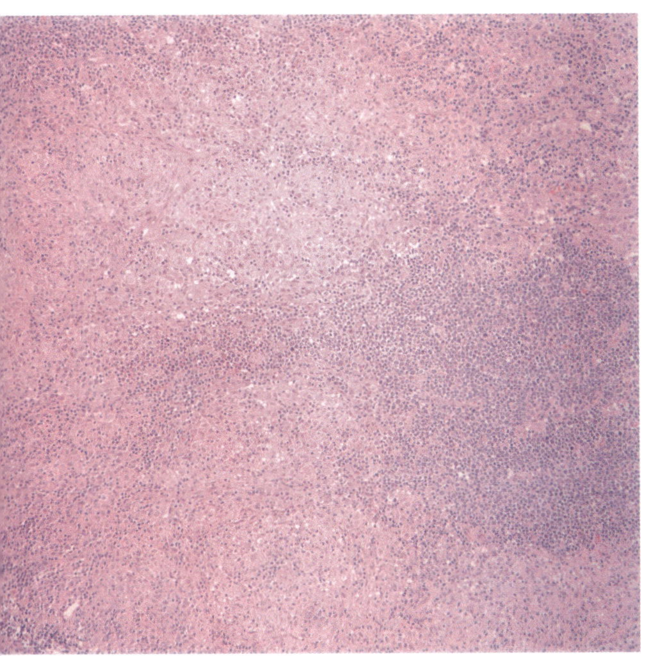
FIGURE 12-5

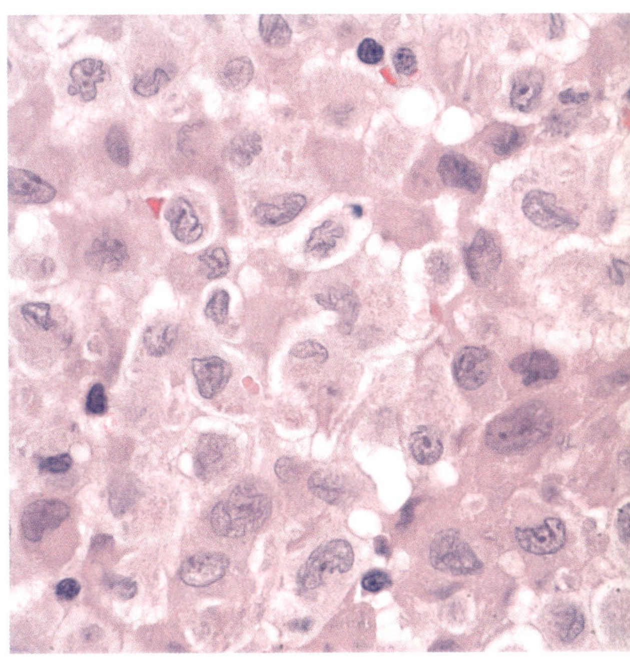
FIGURE 12-6

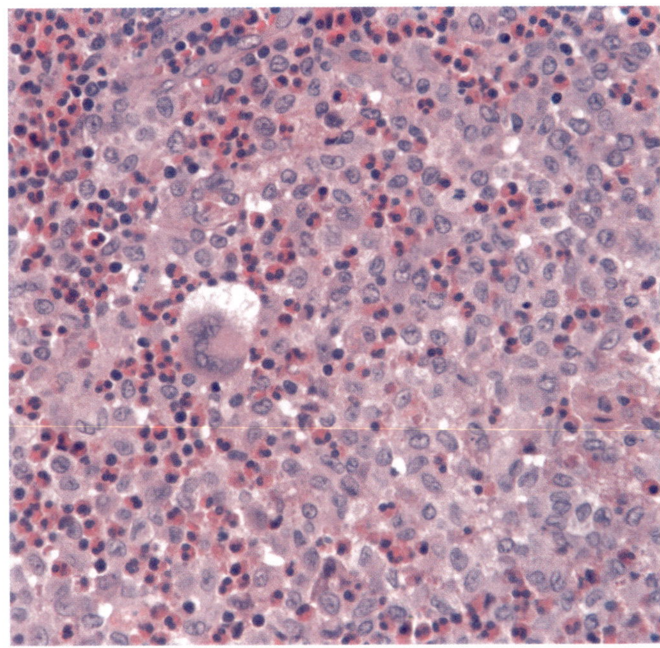
FIGURE 12-7

Langerhans Cell Sarcoma

DEFINITION

Langerhans cell carcoma is a high-grade malignancy composed of atypical cells with Langerhans cell immunophenotype.

CLINICAL FEATURES

- This is an extremely rare tumor with a median age of 39 years and a male to female ratio of 2:1.
- Langerhans cell sarcoma commonly presents in skin and/or soft tissue, with secondary lymph node and multiorgan involvement.

HISTOLOGIC FINDINGS

- These tumors consist of highly atypical cells, generally with distinct nucleoli, that may occasionally demonstrate the characteristic nuclear grooves of Langerhans cells (Figures 12-8 and 12-9).
- A high mitotic rate is characteristic.
- The immunophenotype is that of typical Langerhans cells: CD1a(+), langerin (+), S100(+), CD68(+), HLA-DR(+), CD45(+/−), lysozyme(+/−), CD21(−), CD35(−), CD163(−), CD4(+).

DIFFERENTIAL DIAGNOSIS

- Soft tissue sarcoma
- Langerhans cell histiocytosis

FIGURE 12-8 This lymph node has effaced architecture and an extensive spindle cell infiltrate.

FIGURE 12-9 The atypical neoplastic cells, have occasional nuclear grooves, similar to Langerhans cells. The nuclei contain distinct nucleoli, which is not a feature of Langerhans cell histiocytosis.

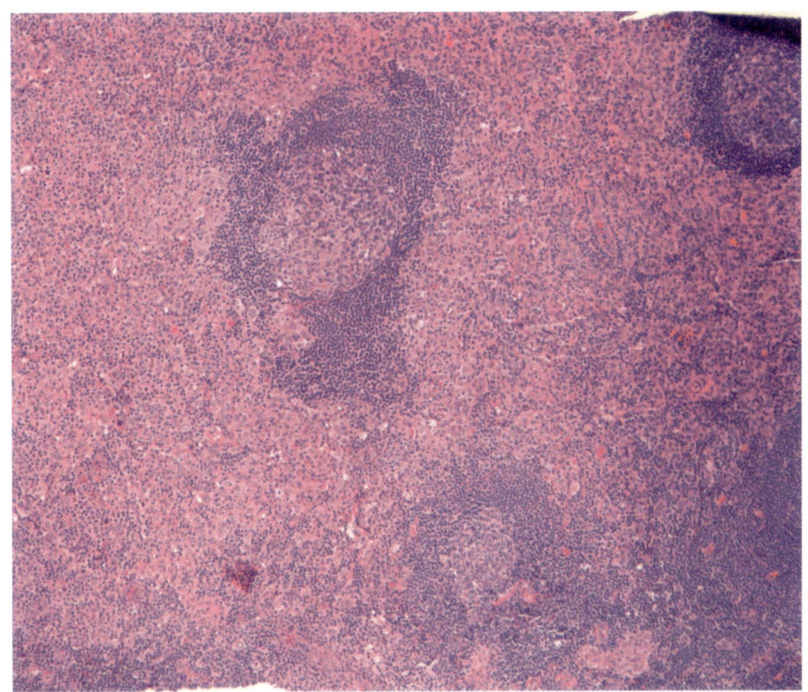

FIGURE 12-8

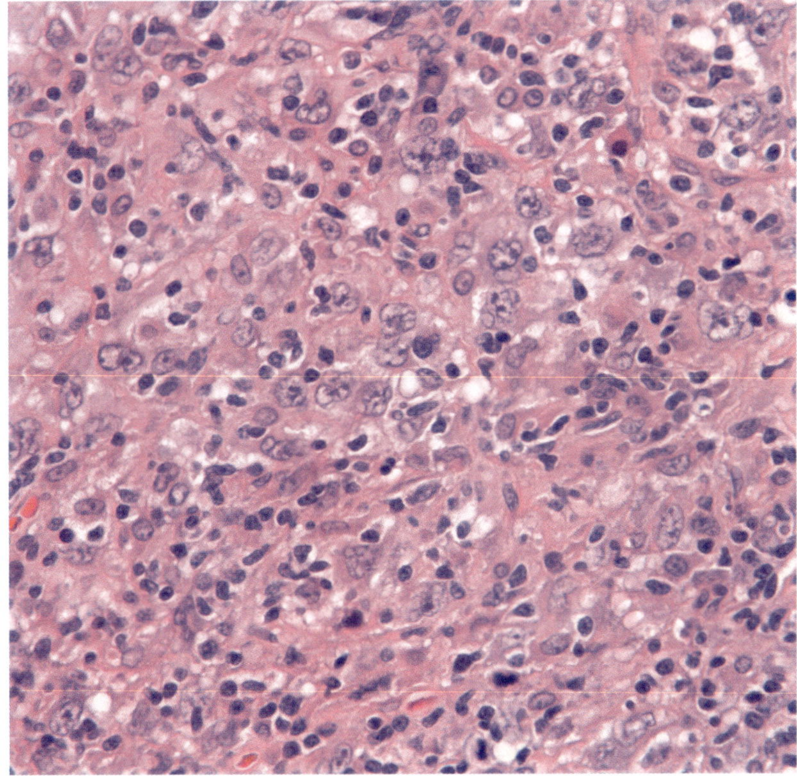

FIGURE 12-9

Interdigitating Dendritic Cell Sarcoma

DEFINITION

Interdigitating dendritic cell sarcoma is a high-grade neoplasm composed of spindle and oval-shaped cells with interdigitating dendritic cell immunophenotype.

CLINICAL FEATURES

- This extremely rare tumor occurs mostly in adults with a slight male predominance.
- Patients usually present with asymptomatic, solitary lymphadenopathy.

HISTOLOGIC FINDINGS

- Interdigitating dendritic cell sarcoma produces paracortical infiltrates composed of spindle to ovoid cells in a storiform or fascicle pattern (Figures 12-10 and 12-11).
- The neoplastic cells have regular, oval or spindle-shaped nuclei, vesicular chromatin, inconspicuous nucleoli, and abundant cytoplasm. Cytologic atypia varies from minimal to pronounced (Figures 12-12 and 12-13).
- The typical immunophenotype is S100(+), fascin (+), CD68(+/−), CD45(+/−), lysozyme (+/−), CD1a(−), langerin (−), CD21(−), CD23(−), CD35(−), MPO(−), CD34(−), CD30(−), CD123(−), CD163(−).

DIFFERENTIAL DIAGNOSIS

- Histiocytic sarcoma
- Langerhans cell sarcoma
- Follicular dendritic cell sarcoma
- Other sarcomas metastatic to lymph node

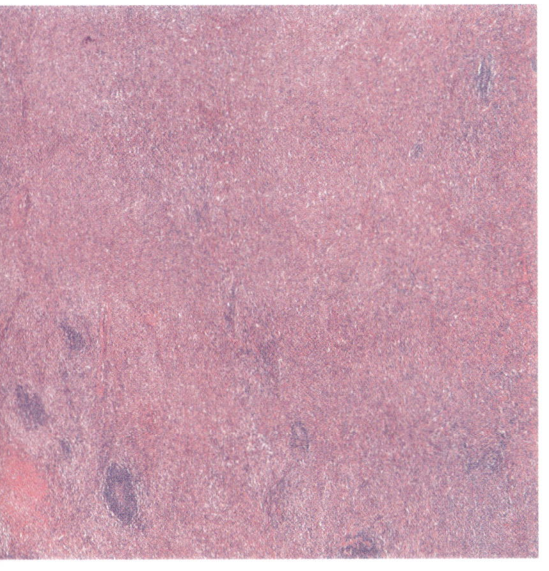

FIGURE 12-10

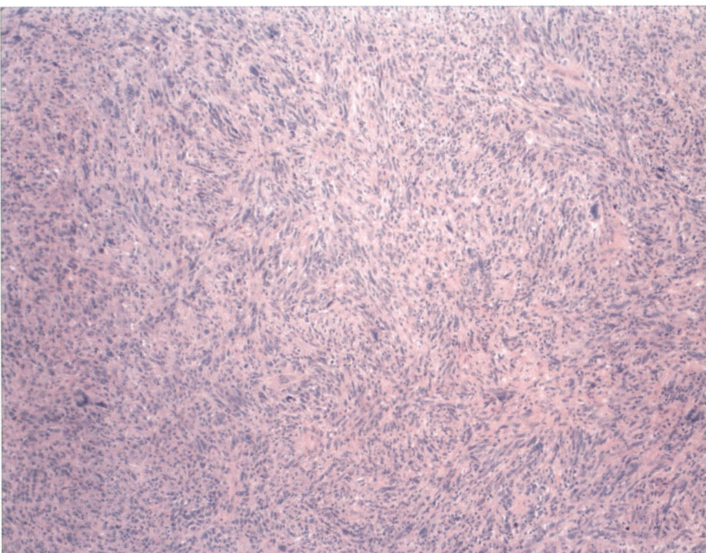

FIGURE 12-11

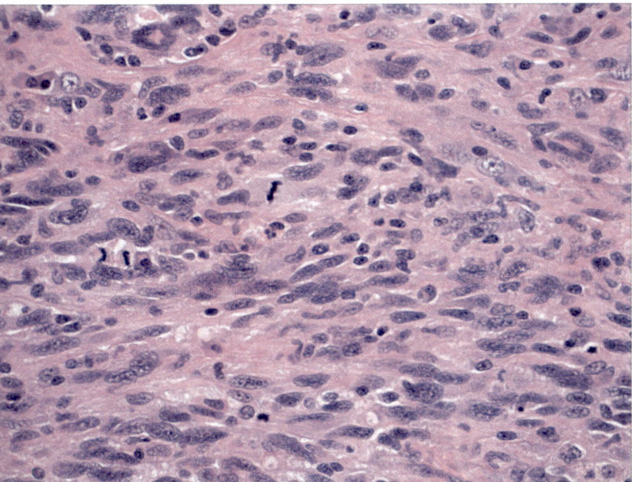

FIGURE 12-12

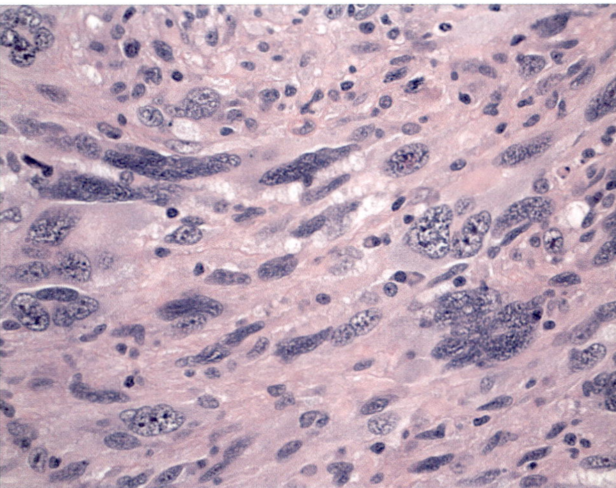

FIGURE 12-13

FIGURE 12-10 This lymph node contains a paracortical infiltrate producing sub-total effacement of the normal architecture.
FIGURE 12-11 This intermediate power image demonstrates a storiform architecture.
FIGURE 12-12 A high-power highlights atypical spindled cells and frequent mitotic figures.
FIGURE 12-13 Other areas of the tumor demonstrated dramatic cytologic atypia.

Follicular Dendritic Cell Sarcoma

DEFINITION

This is a neoplasm composed of spindle and oval-shaped cells with follicular dendritic cell morphology and immunophenotype.

CLINICAL FEATURES

- This is a rare tumor with a mean age of 44 years and no gender predilection.
- Patients present with asymptomatic lymphadenopathy in 50–66% of cases.

HISTOLOGIC FINDINGS

- Involved lymph nodes contain a neoplastic infiltrate with storiform, fascicular, or nodular distribution (Figure 12-14).
- The neoplastic cells have oval nuclei with vesicular chromatin, distinct eosinophilic nucleoli, eosinophilic cytoplasm, and frequent binucleation (Figure 12-15).
- Background small lymphocytes may be conspicuous.
- The typical immunophenotype is CD21(+), CD23(+), CD35(+), clusterin(+), fascin(+), HLA-DR(+), S100(+/−), CD68(+/−), CD1a(−), lysozyme(−), MPO(−), CD30(−), CD123(−), CD163(−) (Figure 12-16).

DIFFERENTIAL DIAGNOSIS

- Histiocytic sarcoma
- Langerhans cell sarcoma
- Interdigitating dendritic cell sarcoma
- Other sarcomas metastatic to lymph node

FIGURE 12-14 This lymph node is replaced by a spindle cell proliferation with focal storiform appearance.

FIGURE 12-15 High-power magnification of the infiltrate reveals cells with elongated nuclei, vesicular chromatin, small nucleoli, and eosinophilic cytoplasm with indistinct cells borders.

FIGURE 12-16 Immunohistochemistry demonstrates CD21 and CD35 expression in the neoplastic cells.

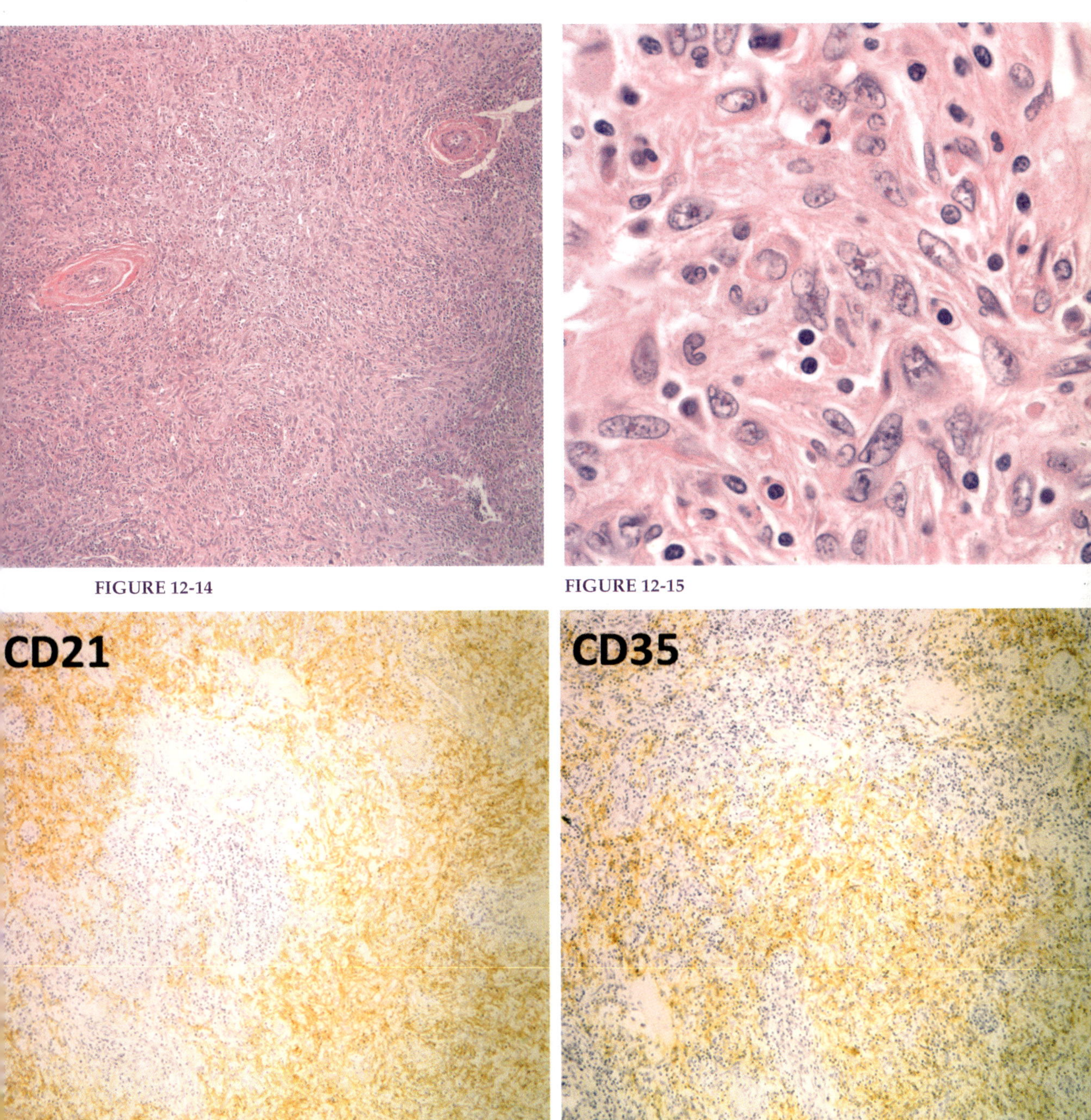

FIGURE 12-14

FIGURE 12-15

FIGURE 12-16

Precursor Lymphoid Neoplasms

13

LYMPHOBLASTIC LYMPHOMA

Lymphoblastic Lymphoma

DEFINITION

Lymphoblastic lymphoma (LBL) is defined as tissue involvement by malignant, immature T- or B-lineage cells, existing as either primary disease or secondary involvement by a leukemic process (>25% lymphoblasts in the bone marrow). The majority of primary LBLs are of T-lineage (85–90%), with B-lineage LBLs representing 10%, which contrasts with the leukemic phase wherein B-lymphoblastic leukemias account for 80–85% of cases. The 2008 WHO classifies both the leukemic and tissue phase under the same category: B- or T-lymphoblastic leukemia/lymphoma.

CLINICAL FEATURES

- T-LBLs present most commonly as bulky anterior mediastinal masses in young males during adolescence or early twenties and are frequently associated with pleural effusions. Supradiaphragmatic adenopathy is observed in approximately 50%.
- B-LBLs most commonly involve the skin, lymph nodes, and bone and soft tissue, with infrequent mediastinal involvement. Median age range of presentation is 10–20 years old.

HISTOLOGIC FINDINGS

- Lymph nodes show effaced architecture by a diffuse, monotonous proliferation of medium-sized cells with round to variably irregular nuclear contours, delicate, open chromatin, variably distinct, small nucleoli, and small amounts of cytoplasm (Figure 13-1). Rare cases may show atypical morphology, characterized by pleomorphic, immunoblastic or centroblastic histology.
- The tumor has a high proliferation index and is frequently associated with many mitotic figures. Low-power examination may reveal a "starry-sky" appearance with frequent tingible-body macrophages (Figures 13-2 and 13-3).
- CD34, TDT, and CD1a (for T-lineage) expression are used to define immaturity in LBLs.
- Histology cannot distinguish B- and T-lineage, so immunohistochemistry and/or flow cytometry are required. The majority of B-lineage LBLs express CD10, CD19, CD22, CD34, CD79a, PAX-5, and TDT; CD20 expression is observed in approximately one-third of cases. All cases of T-LBL are positive for CD3.

DIFFERENTIAL DIAGNOSIS

- Myeloid sarcoma
- Burkitt lymphoma
- Blastoid variant of mantle cell lymphoma
- Thymoma/Thymic tissue

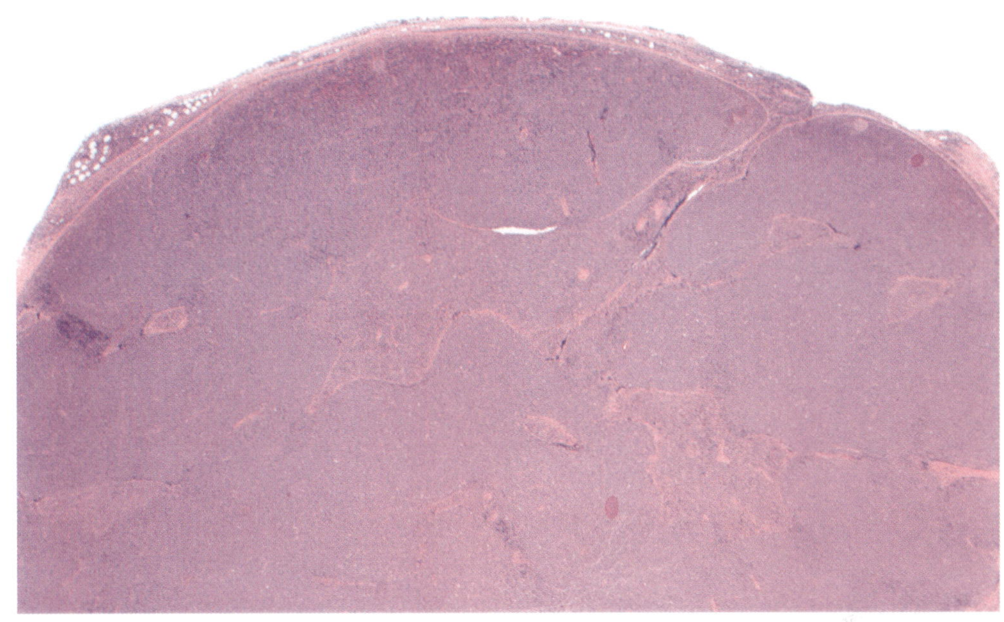

FIGURE 13-1

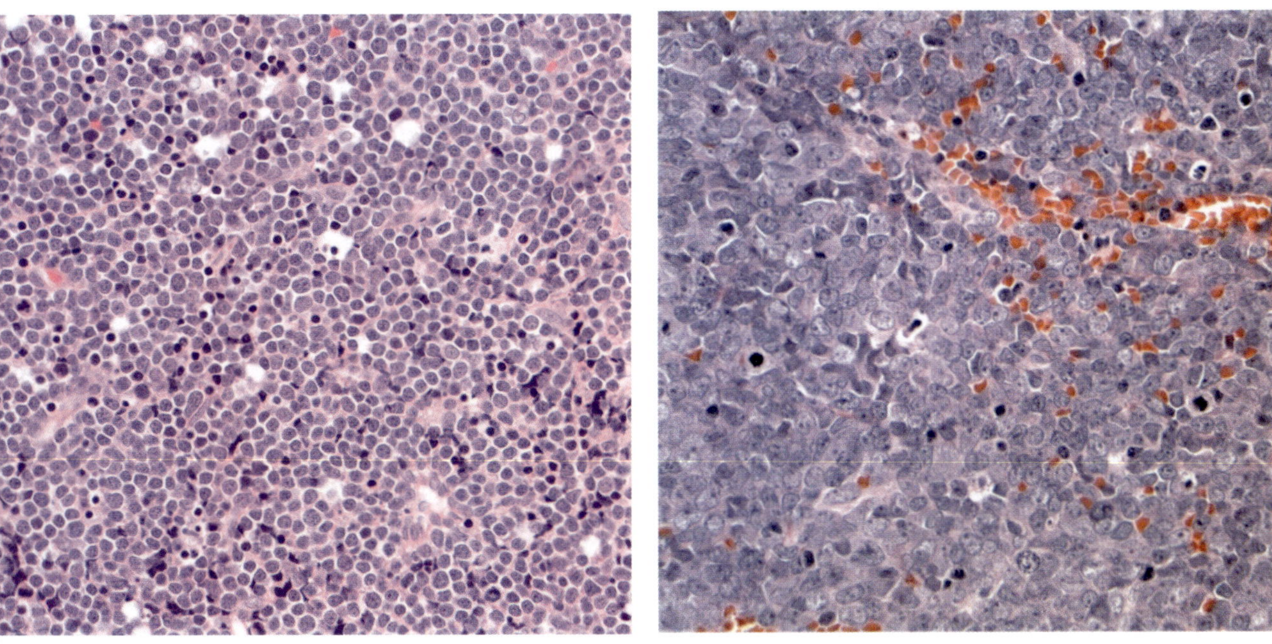

FIGURE 13-2

FIGURE 13-3

FIGURE 13-1 B-lymphoblastic lymphoma. The lymph node shows complete effacement by a densely cellular infiltrate with extension into the surrounding adipose tissue.

FIGURE 13-2 B-lymphoblastic lymphoma. High-power magnification reveals a monotonous population of medium-sized cells with round nuclear contours and delicate chromatin admixed with tingible-body macrophages, imparting a "starry sky" appearance.

FIGURE 13-3 B-lymphoblastic lymphoma. High-power magnification reveals monotonous cells with immature, delicate chromatin and numerous mitotic figures.

14

Acute Myeloid Leukemia and Related Precursor Neoplasms

MYELOID SARCOMA

BLASTIC PLASMACYTOID DENDRITIC CELL NEOPLASM (BPDCN)

Myeloid Sarcoma

DEFINITION

A myeloid sarcoma is a tumor mass consisting of immature cells (myeloblasts, monoblasts, or other myeloid blast equivalents) involving an extramedullary site.

CLINICAL FEATURES

- The median age of occurrence is 56 years with a male to female ratio of 1.2:1.
- De novo myeloid sarcoma is equivalent to a diagnosis of acute myeloid leukemia (AML); it can present prior to, or can coincide with blood/marrow presentation of AML, or can occur as a relapse manifestation of AML.
- It may represent acute transformation of a pre-existing myelodysplastic syndrome or myeloproliferative neoplasm.

HISTOLOGIC FINDINGS

- Lymph nodes show partial or total architectural effacement in a diffuse or interfollicular pattern by a neoplastic infiltrate composed of immature myeloid cells (Figures 14-1 and 14-2).
- Cytologic features vary, ranging from monotonous, medium to large cells with regular or mildly irregular nuclei, fine (blastic) chromatin, variably distinct nucleoli, and scanty cytoplasm (Figure 14-2) to cells with folded or irregular nuclei and more abundant cytoplasm, corresponding to monocytic differentiation (Figure 14-3). Admixed eosinophilic myelocytes may be present.
- Depending on the lineage of differentiation (granulocytic or monocytic), the neoplastic cells may express CD34, CD33 (>90%), CD117 (~80%), myeloperoxidase (~85%), CD68 (>95%), CD56 (~15%), or lysozyme (>90%).

DIFFERENTIAL DIAGNOSIS

- Diffuse large B-cell lymphoma
- Lymphoblastic lymphoma
- Anaplastic large cell lymphoma
- Carcinoma

FIGURE 14-1 This lymph node has effaced architecture and a diffuse neoplastic infiltrate with a vaguely storiform distribution.

FIGURE 14-2 High-power view demonstrates large atypical cells with irregular nuclei, finely dispersed chromatin, inconspicuous nucleoli, and pale cytoplasm. Frequent mitoses are present.

FIGURE 14-3 This high-power image of an acute monocytic leukemia in a lymph node demonstrates prominent nuclear folding and irregularity and abundant pale cytoplasm, corresponding to promonocytes.

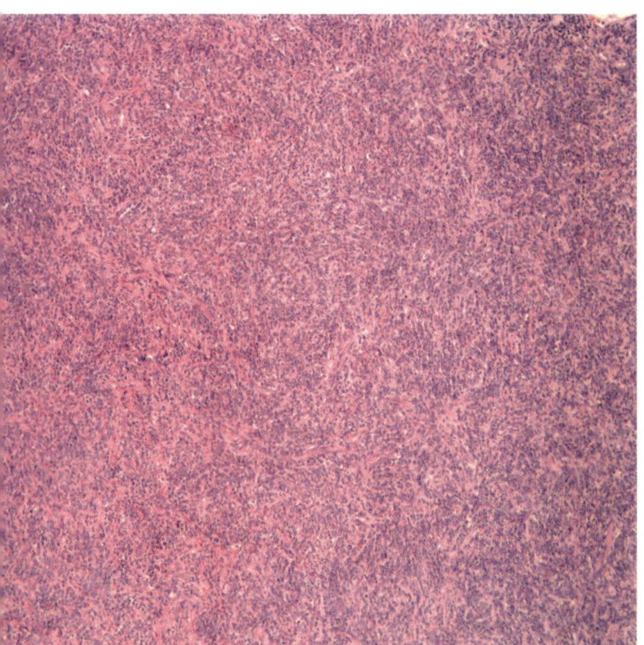

FIGURE 14-1

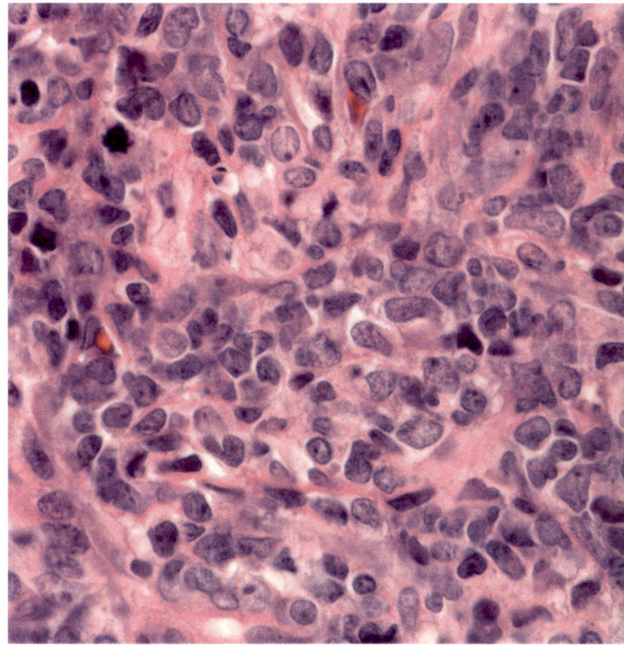

FIGURE 14-2

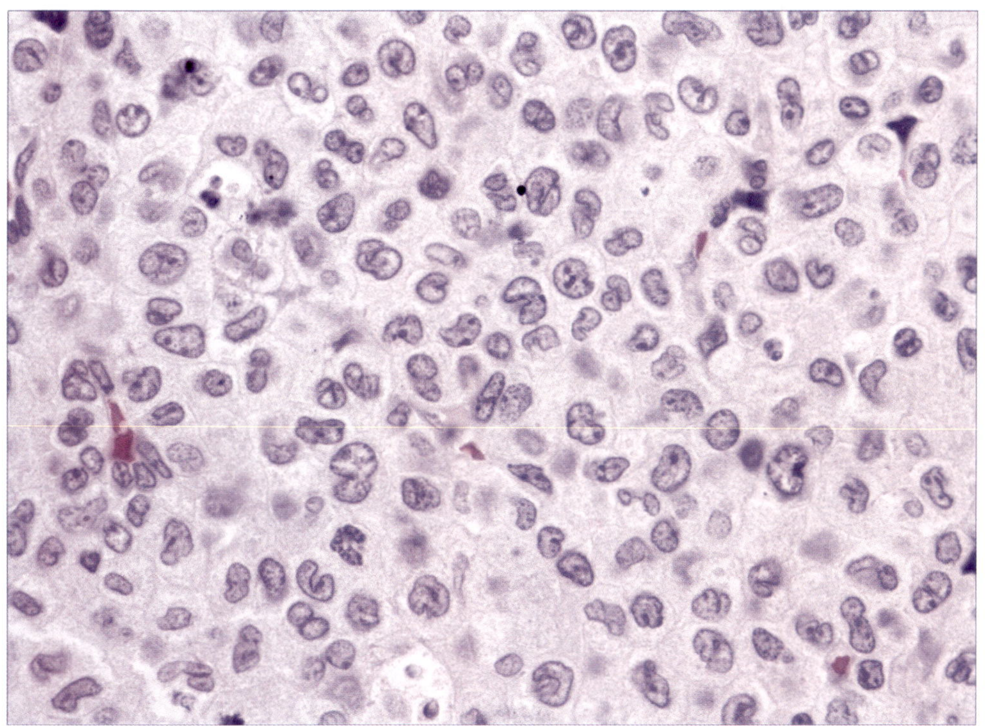

FIGURE 14-3

Blastic Plasmacytoid Dendritic Cell Neoplasm (BPDCN)

DEFINITION

This is an aggressive neoplasm of precursors of plasmacytoid dendritic cells.

CLINICAL FEATURES

- The median age of onset is 67 years, with a male predominance (male:female = 3.3:1).
- The typical presentation is with skin (100%), peripheral blood/bone marrow (60–90%), and lymph node involvement (40–50%).

HISTOLOGIC FINDINGS

- Involved lymph nodes show a leukemic pattern of infiltration in the interfollicular or medullary areas, with a diffuse infiltrate composed of medium-sized, monomorphic cells with irregular nuclear contours, finely dispersed chromatin, inconspicuous nucleoli, and scanty cytoplasm (Figures 14-4 and 14-5).
- The neoplastic cells are positive for: CD4, CD56, CD123, TCL1, CD45; sometimes positive for: CD68 (50%), CD7, CD33, CD2, CD36, CD38, TdT (33%); and negative for: CD34, CD117, CD13, myeloperoxidase, lysozyme, CD3, CD5, TIA-1, granzyme B, EBER, CD20, CD79a (Figures 14-6 and 14-7).

DIFFERENTIAL DIAGNOSIS

- Acute myeloid leukemia, NOS
- Lymphoblastic leukemia/lymphoma
- Mantle cell lymphoma, blastoid variant
- Extranodal NK/T cell lymphoma, nasal type
- Peripheral T-cell lymphoma, NOS

FIGURE 14-4 This lymph node contains a diffuse interfollicular neoplastic infiltrate. Frequent tingible body macrophages impart a "starry sky" appearance.

FIGURE 14-5 The malignant cells are monomorphous and medium-sized, with irregular nuclei, fine chromatin, and occasional nucleoli.

FIGURE 14-6 Immunohistochemistry demonstrates CD33, CD123, and TCL1 positivity in the neoplastic cells.

FIGURE 14-7 Immunohistochemistry demonstrates TdT and focal weak lysozyme (LYS) positivity in the neoplastic cells, which are also negative for CD34 and myeloperoxidase.

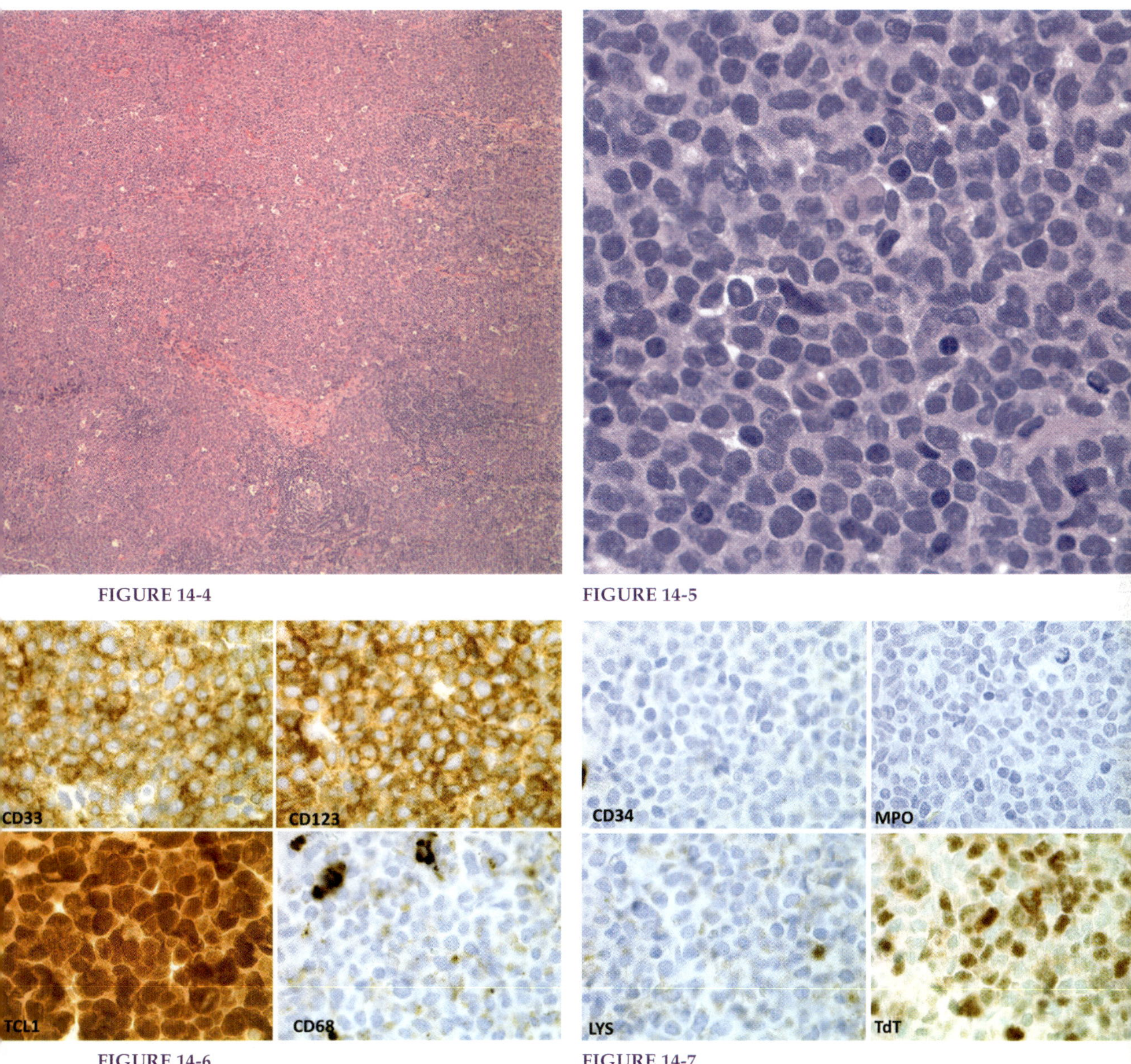

FIGURE 14-4

FIGURE 14-5

FIGURE 14-6

FIGURE 14-7

15

Metastatic Tumors in Lymph Nodes

Metastatic Tumors in Lymph Nodes

DEFINITION

This phenomenon represents involvement of lymph nodes by metastatic tumors.

CLINICAL FEATURES

- The location of involved lymph nodes may suggest the origin of the primary tumor (Table 15-1).
- Lymph node metastases may be the initial presentation of an unknown primary neoplasm.

HISTOLOGIC FINDINGS

- In early stages, metastases involve the lymph node sinuses; advanced cases may show subtotal replacement of normal architecture by metastatic neoplastic cells (Figure 15-1).
- The morphology is suggestive of the general type of primary tumor (e.g., adenocarcinoma vs. squamous cell carcinoma vs. melanoma).
- Immunohistochemistry is helpful in detecting occult metastases and in establishing the tumor of origin.

DIFFERENTIAL DIAGNOSIS

- Anaplastic large cell lymphoma
- Diffuse large B-cell lymphoma

TABLE 15-1 Likely primary tumor sites based on locations of lymph nodes with metastases

Anatomic site of metastasis	Anatomic site of primary tumor
Cervical lymph nodes	Head and neck, thoracic
Supraclavicular	Abdominal (gastric)
Axillary	Breast, upper extremity, trunk
Inguinal	Prostate, rectum, uterus, lower extremity
Pelvic	Prostate, testis, uterus, lower extremity

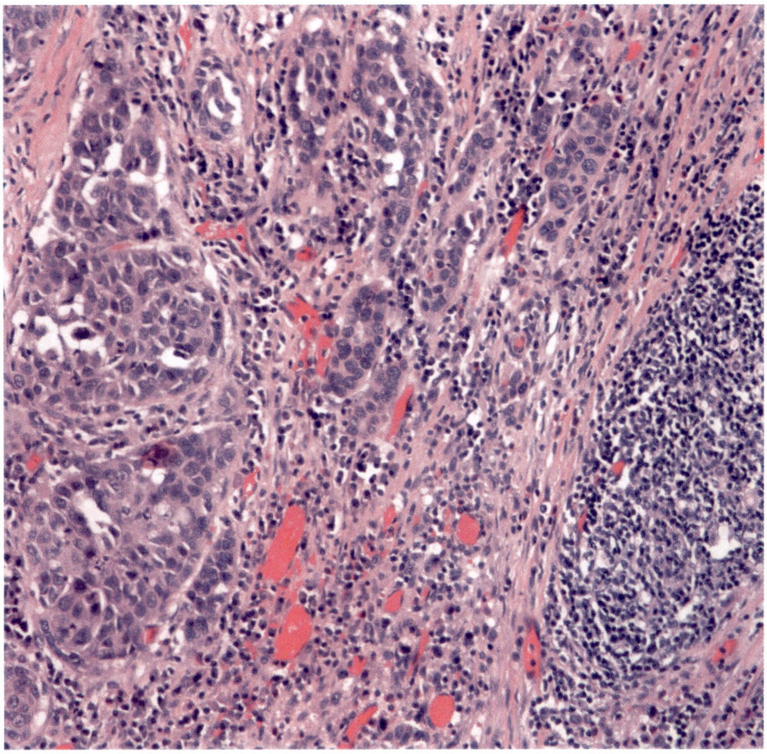

FIGURE 15-1

FIGURE 15-1 This cervical lymph node is almost entirely replaced by nested of poorly differentiated carcinoma cells.

References

1. INFECTIOUS LYMPHADENOPATHIES

INFECTIOUS MONONUCLEOSIS LYMPHADENITIS

Anagnostopoulos I, Hummel M, Falini B, Joehrens K, Stein H. Epstein-barr virus infection of monocytoid B-cell proliferates: an early feature of primary viral infection? *Am J Surg Pathol.* 2005;29(5) 595–601.

Niedobitek G, Herbst H, Young LS, et al. Patterns of Epstein-Barr virus infection in non-neoplastic lymphoid tissue. *Blood.* 1992;79(10):2520–2526.

CYTOMEGALOVIRUS LYMPHADENITIS

Kjeldsberg C. Reactive disorders of lymph nodes. In: Kjeldsberg C, ed. *Practical Diagnosis of Hematologic Disorders.* Vol. 1, 4th ed. Chicago: ASCP Press; 2006:277–298.

Younes M, Podesta A, Helie M, Buckley P. Infection of T but not B lymphocytes by cytomegalovirus in lymph node. An immunophenotypic study. *Am J Surg Pathol.* 1991;15(1):75–80.

HERPES SIMPLEX VIRUS LYMPHADENITIS

Gaffey MJ, Ben-Ezra JM, Weiss LM. Herpes simplex lymphadenitis. *Am J Clin Pathol.* 1991;95(5):709–714.

Oo K, Xiao W, Hameed A, Xiao P. Concurrent herpes simplex viral lymphadenitis and chronic lymphocytic leukemia/small lymphocytic lymphoma, mimicking large-cell (Richter) transformation. *Leuk Lymphoma.* 2009;50(9):1535–1537.

Tamaru J, Mikata A, Horie H, et al. Herpes simplex lymphadenitis. Report of two cases with review of the literature. *Am J Surg Pathol.* 1990;14(6):571–577.

HUMAN IMMUNODEFICIENCY VIRUS LYMPHADENITIS

Diebold J, Marche C, Audouin J, et al. Lymph node modification in patients with the acquired immunodeficiency syndrome (AIDS) or with AIDS related complex (ARC). A histological, immuno-histopathological and ultrastructural study of 45 cases. *Pathol Res Pract.* 1985;180(6):590–611.

Human immunodeficiency virus lymphadenitis. In: Ioachim HL, Medeiros LJ, eds. *Ioachim's Lymph Node Pathology.* 4th ed. Philadelphia: Lippincott Williams & Wilkins; 2009:99–105.

NONSPECIFIC BACTERIAL LYMPHADENITIS

Beiler HA, Eckstein TM, Roth H, Daum R. Specific and nonspecific lymphadenitis in childhood: etiology, diagnosis, and therapy. *Pediatr Surg Int.* 1997;12(2–3):108–112.

Ordinary bacterial lymphadenitis. In: Ioachim HL, Medeiros LJ, eds. *Ioachim's Lymph Node Pathology.* 4th ed. Philadelphia: Lippincott Williams & Wilkins; 2009:106–109.

CAT-SCRATCH LYMPHADENITIS

Cat-scratch disease in children–Texas, September 2000-August 2001. *MMWR Morb Mortal Wkly Rep.* 2002;51(10):212–214.

Qian X, Jin L, Hayden RT, Macon WR, Lloyd RV. Diagnosis of cat scratch disease with *Bartonella henselae* infection in formalin-fixed paraffin-embedded tissues by two different PCR assays. *Diagn Mol Pathol.* 2005;14(3):146–151.

Sander A, Posselt M, Bohm N, Ruess M, Altwegg M. Detection of *Bartonella henselae* DNA by two different PCR assays and determination of the genotypes of strains involved in histologically defined cat scratch disease. *J Clin Microbiol.* 1999;37(4):993–997.

BACILLARY ANGIOMATOSIS

Chan JK, Lewin KJ, Lombard CM, Teitelbaum S, Dorfman RF. Histopathology of bacillary angiomatosis of lymph node. *Am J Surg Pathol.* 1991;15(5):430–437.

Psarros G, Riddell J IV, Gandhi T, Kauffman CA, Cinti SK. *Bartonella henselae* infections in solid organ transplant recipients: report of 5 cases and review of the literature. *Medicine (Baltimore).* 2012;91(2):111–121.

SYPHILIS (LUETIC) LYMPHADENITIS

Facchetti F, Incardona P, Lonardi S, et al. Nodal inflammatory pseudotumor caused by luetic infection. *Am J Surg Pathol.* 2009;33(3):447–453.

Hartsock RJ, Halling LW, King FM. Luetic lymphadenitis: a clinical and histologic study of 20 cases. *Am J Clin Pathol.* 1970;53(3):304–314.

van Crevel R, Grefte JM, van Doorninck D, Sturm P. Syphilis presenting as isolated cervical lymphadenopathy: two related cases. *J Infect.* 2009;58(1):76–78.

MYCOBACTERIUM TUBERCULOSIS LYMPHADENITIS

Bayazit YA, Bayazit N, Namiduru M. Mycobacterial cervical lymphadenitis. *ORL J Otorhinolaryngol Relat Spec.* 2004;66(5):275–280.

MYCOBACTERIUM AVIUM-INTRACELLULARE LYMPHADENITIS

Klatt EC, Jensen DF, Meyer PR. Pathology of *Mycobacterium avium-intracellulare* infection in acquired immunodeficiency syndrome. *Hum Pathol.* 1987;18(7):709–714.

HISTOPLASMA CAPSULATUM LYMPHADENITIS

Case records of the Massachusetts General Hospital. Weekly clinicopathological exercises. Case 15-1991. A 48-year-old man with dysphagia, chest pain, fever, and a subcarinal mass. *N Engl J Med.* 1991;324(15):1049–1056.

Meijer JA, Sjogren EV, Kuijper E, Verbist BM, Visser LG. Necrotizing cervical lymphadenitis due to disseminated *Histoplasma capsulatum* infection. *Eur J Clin Microbiol Infect Dis.* 2005;24(8):574–576.

COCCIDIOIDES LYMPHADENITIS

D'Avino A, Di Giambenedetto S, Fabbiani M, Farina S. Coccidioidomycosis of cervical lymph nodes in an HIV-infected patient with immunologic reconstitution on potent HAART: a rare observation in a nonendemic area. *Diagn Microbiol Infect Dis.* 2012;72(2):185–187.

Kirkland TN, Fierer J. Coccidioidomycosis: a reemerging infectious disease. *Emerg Infect Dis.* 1996;2(3):192–199.

Robinson MJ, Fogel R. Granulomatous lymphadenitis caused by Coccidioides immitis. *J Am Osteopath Assoc.* 1994;94(7):578–582.

FILARIASIS

Filaria lymphadenitis. In: Ioachim HL, Medeiros LJ, eds. *Ioachim's Lymph Node Pathology*, 4th ed. Philadelphia: Lippincott Williams & Wilkins; 2009:168–171.

Filarial nematodes and filariasis. In: Winn WC, Koneman EW, Allen SD, Janda WM, Procop GW, Schreckenberger P, eds. *Koneman's Color Atlas and Textbook of Diagnostic Microbiology*, Baltimore: Lippincot Williams & Wilkins; 2006:1303–1305.

2. REACTIVE LYMPHADENOPATHIES

FOLLICULAR HYPERPLASIA

Osborne BM, Butler JJ, Variakojis D, Kott M. Reactive lymph node hyperplasia with giant follicles. *Am J Clin Pathol.* 1982;78(4):493–499.

Reactive lymphoid hyperplasia. In: Ioachim HL, Medeiros LJ, eds. *Ioachim's Lymph Node Pathology.* 4th ed. Philadelphia: Lippincott Williams & Wilkins; 2009:172–180.

PARACORTICAL HYPERPLASIA

Reactive lymphoid hyperplasia. In: Ioachim HL, Medeiros LJ, eds. *Ioachim's Lymph Node Pathology.* 4th ed. Philadelphia: Lippincott Williams & Wilkins; 2009:172–180.

SINUS HISTIOCYTOSIS

Reactive lymphoid hyperplasia. In: Ioachim HL, Medeiros LJ, eds. *Ioachim's Lymph Node Pathology.* 4th ed. Philadelphia: Lippincott Williams & Wilkins; 2009;172–180.

PROGRESSIVE TRANSFORMATION OF GERMINAL CENTERS (PTGC)

Chang CC, Osipov V, Wheaton S, Tripp S, Perkins SL. Follicular hyperplasia, follicular lysis, and progressive transformation of germinal centers. A sequential spectrum of morphologic evolution in lymphoid hyperplasia. *Am J Clin Pathol.* 2003;120(3):322–326.

Nguyen PL, Ferry JA, Harris NL. Progressive transformation of germinal centers and nodular lymphocyte predominance Hodgkin's disease: a comparative immunohistochemical study. *Am J Surg Pathol.* 1999;23(1):27–33.

Sweetenham JW, Polliack A. Progressive transformation of germinal centers and Hodgkin lymphoma: more insights but maybe more confusion? *Leuk Lymphoma.* 2011;52(11):2041–2042.

DERMATOPATHIC LYMPHADENOPATHY

Burke JS, Colby TV. Dermatopathic lymphadenopathy. Comparison of cases associated and unassociated with mycosis fungoides. *Am J Surg Pathol.* 1981;5(4):343–352.

Gould E, Porto R, Albores-Saavedra J, Ibe MJ. Dermatopathic lymphadenitis. The spectrum and significance of its morphologic features. *Arch Pathol Lab Med.* 1988;112(11):1145–1150.

3. LYMPHADENOPATHIES ASSOCIATED WITH SYSTEMIC DISORDERS

KIMURA LYMPHADENOPATHY

Chen H, Thompson LD, Aguilera NS, Abbondanzo SL. Kimura disease: a clinicopathologic study of 21 cases. *Am J Surg Pathol.* 2004;28(4):505–513.

Hui PK, Chan JK, Ng CS, Kung IT, Gwi E. Lymphadenopathy of Kimura's disease. *Am J Surg Pathol.* 1989;13(3):177–186.

SINUS HISTIOCYTOSIS WITH MASSIVE LYMPHADENOPATHY (ROSAI-DORFMAN DISEASE)

Eisen RN, Buckley PJ, Rosai J. Immunophenotypic characterization of sinus histiocytosis with massive lymphadenopathy (Rosai-Dorfman disease). *Semin Diagn Pathol.* 1990;7(1):74–82.

Foucar E, Rosai J, Dorfman R. Sinus histiocytosis with massive lymphadenopathy (Rosai-Dorfman disease): review of the entity. *Semin Diagn Pathol.* 1990;7(1):19–73.

Rosai J, Dorfman RF. Sinus histiocytosis with massive lymphadenopathy: a pseudolymphomatous benign disorder. Analysis of 34 cases. *Cancer.* 1972;30(5):1174–1188.

KIKUCHI-FUJIMOTO LYMPHADENOPATHY

Bosch X, Guilabert A, Miquel R, Campo E. Enigmatic Kikuchi-Fujimoto disease: a comprehensive review. *Am J Clin Pathol.* July 2004;122(1):141–152.

Dorfman RF, Berry GJ. Kikuchi's histiocytic necrotizing lymphadenitis: an analysis of 108 cases with emphasis on differential diagnosis. *Semin Diagn Pathol.* 1988;5(4):329–345.

Kuo TT. Kikuchi's disease (histiocytic necrotizing lymphadenitis). A clinicopathologic study of 79 cases with an analysis of histologic subtypes, immunohistology, and DNA ploidy. *Am J Surg Pathol.* 1995;19(7):798–809.

Tsang WY, Chan JK, Ng CS. Kikuchi's lymphadenitis. A morphologic analysis of 75 cases with special reference to unusual features. *Am J Surg Pathol.* 1994; 18(3):219–231.

SARCOIDOSIS

Costabel U, Ohshimo S, Guzman J. Diagnosis of sarcoidosis. *Curr Opin Pulm Med.* 2008;14(5):455–461.

Iannuzzi MC, Rybicki BA, Teirstein AS. Sarcoidosis. *N Engl J Med.* 2007;357(21):2153–2165.

Rosen Y. Pathology of sarcoidosis. *Semin Respir Crit Care Med.* 2007;28(1):36–52.

SYSTEMIC LUPUS ERYTHEMATOSUS LYMPHADENOPATHY

Fox RA, Rosahn PD. The lymph nodes in disseminated lupus erythematosus. *Am J Pathol.* 1943;19:74–99.

Klemperer P. Pathology of disseminated lupus erythematosus. *Arch Pathol Lab Med* 1941;32:569–631.

Shapira Y, Weinberger A, Wysenbeek AJ. Lymphadenopathy in systemic lupus erythematosus. Prevalence and relation to disease manifestations. *Clin Rheumatol.* 1996;15(4):335–338.

RHEUMATOID LYMPHADENOPATHY

McCluggage WG, Bharucha H. Lymph node hyalinisation in rheumatoid arthritis and systemic sclerosis. *J Clin Pathol.* 1994;47(2):138–142.

Nosanchuk JS, Schnitzer B. Follicular hyperplasia in lymph nodes from patients with rheumatoid arthritis. A clinicopathologic study. *Cancer.* 1969;24(2):243–254.

CASTLEMAN DISEASE

Casper C. The aetiology and management of Castleman disease at 50 years: translating pathophysiology to patient care. *Br J Haematol.* 2005;129(1):3–17.

Frizzera G. Castleman's disease and related disorders. *Semin Diagn Pathol.* 1988;5(4):346–364.

Peterson BA, Frizzera G. Multicentric Castleman's disease. *Semin Oncol.* 1993;20(6):636–647.

STILL'S DISEASE

Jeon YK, Paik JH, Park SS, et al. Spectrum of lymph node pathology in adult onset Still's disease: analysis of 12 patients with one follow up biopsy. *J Clin Pathol.* 2004;57(10):1052–1056.

Reichert LJ, Keuning JJ, van Beek M, van Rijthoven AW. Lymph node histology simulating T-cell lymphoma in adult-onset Still's disease. *Ann Hematol.* 1992;65(1):53–54.

Valente RM, Banks PM, Conn DL. Characterization of lymph node histology in adult onset Still's disease. *J Rheumatol.* 1989;16(3):349–354.

IGG4-RELATED SCLEROSING DISEASE

Cheuk W, Yuen HK, Chu SY, Chiu EK, Lam LK, Chan JK. Lymphadenopathy of IgG4-related sclerosing disease. *Am J Surg Pathol.* 2008;32(5):671–681.

Grimm KE, Barry TS, Chizhevsky V, et al. Histopathological findings in 29 lymph node biopsies with increased IgG4 plasma cells. *Mod Pathol.* 2012;25(3):480–491.

AUTOIMMUNE LYMPHOPROLIFERATIVE SYNDROME

Lim MS, Straus SE, Dale JK, et al. Pathological findings in human autoimmune lymphoproliferative syndrome. *Am J Pathol.* 1998;153(5):1541–1550.

Worth A, Thrasher AJ, Gaspar HB. Autoimmune lymphoproliferative syndrome: molecular basis of disease and clinical phenotype. *Br J Haematol.* 2006;133(2):124–140.

4. LYMPH NODE INCLUSIONS

EPITHELIAL CELL INCLUSIONS IN LYMPH NODES

Diaz NM, Cox CE, Ebert M, et al. Benign mechanical transport of breast epithelial cells to sentinel lymph nodes. *Am J Surg Pathol.* 2004;28(12):1641–1645.

Fellegara G, Carcangiu ML, Rosai J. Benign epithelial inclusions in axillary lymph nodes: report of 18 cases and review of the literature. *Am J Surg Pathol.* 2011;35(8):1123–1133.

NEVUS CELL INCLUSIONS IN LYMPH NODES

Biddle DA, Evans HL, Kemp BL, et al. Intraparenchymal nevus cell aggregates in lymph nodes: a possible diagnostic pitfall with malignant melanoma and carcinoma. *Am J Surg Pathol.* 2003;27(5):673–681.

Bautista NC, Cohen S, Anders KH. Benign melanocytic nevus cells in axillary lymph nodes. A prospective incidence and immunohistochemical study with literature review. *Am J Clin Pathol.* 1994;102(1):102–108.

5. SPINDLE CELL NEOPLASMS OF LYMPH NODES

PALISADED MYOFIBROBLASTOMA

Suster S, Rosai J. Intranodal hemorrhagic spindle-cell tumor with "amianthoid" fibers. Report of six cases of a distinctive mesenchymal neoplasm of the inguinal region that simulates Kaposi's sarcoma. *Am J Surg Pathol.* 1989;13(5):347–357.

Weiss SW, Gnepp DR, Bratthauer GL. Palisaded myofibroblastoma. A benign mesenchymal tumor of lymph node. *Am J Surg Pathol.* 1989;13(5):341–346.

INFLAMMATORY PSEUDOTUMOR OF LYMPH NODE

Davis RE, Warnke RA, Dorfman RF. Inflammatory pseudotumor of lymph nodes. Additional observations and evidence for an inflammatory etiology. *Am J Surg Pathol.* 1991;15(8):744–756.

Moran CA, Suster S, Abbondanzo SL. Inflammatory pseudotumor of lymph nodes: a study of 25 cases with emphasis on morphological heterogeneity. *Hum Pathol.* 1997;28(3):332–338.

6. VASCULAR LYMPHADENOPATHIES AND NEOPLASMS OF LYMPH NODES

VASCULAR TRANSFORMATION OF LYMPH NODE SINUSES

Chan JK, Warnke RA, Dorfman R. Vascular transformation of sinuses in lymph nodes. A study of its morphological spectrum and distinction from Kaposi's sarcoma. *Am J Surg Pathol.* 1991;15(8):732–743.

Cook PD, Czerniak B, Chan JK, et al. Nodular spindle-cell vascular transformation of lymph nodes. A benign process occurring predominantly in retroperitoneal lymph nodes draining carcinomas that can simulate Kaposi's sarcoma or metastatic tumor. *Am J Surg Pathol.* 1995;19(9):1010–1020.

ANGIOMYOMATOUS HAMARTOMA

Chan JK, Frizzera G, Fletcher CD, Rosai J. Primary vascular tumors of lymph nodes other than Kaposi's sarcoma. Analysis of 39 cases and delineation of two new entities. *Am J Surg Pathol.* 1992;16(4):335–350.

Mauro CS, McGough RL III, Rao UN. Angiomyomatous hamartoma of a popliteal lymph node: an unusual cause of posterior knee pain. *Ann Diagn Pathol.* 2008;12(5):372–374.

HEMANGIOMAS AND HEMANGIOENDOTHELIOMAS

Chan JK, Frizzera G, Fletcher CD, Rosai J. Primary vascular tumors of lymph nodes other than Kaposi's sarcoma. Analysis of 39 cases and delineation of two new entities. *Am J Surg Pathol.* 1992;16(4):335–350.

Tsang WY, Chan JK, Dorfman RF, Rosai J. Vasoproliferative lesions of the lymph node. *Pathol Annu.* 1994;29(Pt 1):63–133.

KAPOSI SARCOMA

Geraminejad P, Memar O, Aronson I, Rady PL, Hengge U, Tyring SK. Kaposi's sarcoma and other manifestations of human herpesvirus 8. *J Am Acad Dermatol.* 2002;47(5):641–655.

Sullivan RJ, Pantanowitz L, Casper C, Stebbing J, Dezube BJ. HIV/AIDS: epidemiology, pathophysiology, and treatment of Kaposi sarcoma-associated herpesvirus disease: kaposi sarcoma, primary effusion lymphoma, and multicentric Castleman disease. *Clin Infect Dis.* 2008;47(9):1209–1215.

7. FOREIGN BODY LYMPHADENOPATHIES

METAL DEBRIS-ASSOCIATED LYMPHADENOPATHY

Benz EB, Sherburne B, Hayek JE, Falchuk KH, Sledge CB, Spector M. Lymphadenopathy associated with total joint prostheses. A report of two cases and a review of the literature. *J Bone Joint Surg Am.* 1996;78(4):588–593.

Gray MH, Talbert ML, Talbert WM, Bansal M, Hsu A. Changes seen in lymph nodes draining the sites of large joint prostheses. *Am J Surg Pathol.* 1989;13(12):1050–1056.

LYMPHANGIOGRAPHY-ASSOCIATED LYMPHADENOPATHY

Lipid lymphadenopathy. In: Ioachim HL, Medeiros LJ, eds. *Ioachim's Lymph Node Pathology.* 4th ed. Philadelphia: Lippincott Williams & Wilkins; 2009:270–274.

Ravel R. Histopathology of lymph nodes after lymphangiography. *Am J Clin Pathol.* 1966;46(3):335–340.

8. MATURE B-CELL NEOPLASMS

CHRONIC LYMPHOCYTIC LEUKEMIA/SMALL LYMPHOCYTIC LYMPHOMA (CLL/SLL)

Ben-Ezra J, Burke JS, Swartz WG, et al. Small lymphocytic lymphoma: a clinicopathologic analysis of 268 cases. *Blood.* 1989;73(2):579–587.

Mature B-cell neoplasms. In: Swerdlow SH, Campo E, Harris NL, et al. eds. *WHO Classification of Tumours of Haematopoietic and Lymphoid Tissues*, Lyon: IARC Press; 2008:179.

Matutes E, Owusu-Ankomah K, Morilla R, et al. The immunological profile of B-cell disorders and proposal of a scoring system for the diagnosis of CLL. *Leukemia.* 1994;8(10):1640–1645.

SPLENIC B-CELL MARGINAL ZONE LYMPHOMA (SMZL)

Berger F, Felman P, Thieblemont C, et al. Non-MALT marginal zone B-cell lymphomas: a description of clinical presentation and outcome in 124 patients. *Blood.* 2000;95(6):1950–1956.

Piris MA, Arribas A, Mollejo M. Marginal zone lymphoma. *Semin Diagn Pathol.* 2011;28(2):135–145.

HAIRY CELL LEUKEMIA (HCL)

Sharpe RW, Bethel KJ. Hairy cell leukemia: diagnostic pathology. *Hematol Oncol Clin North Am.* 2006;20(5):1023–1049.

Summers TA, Jaffe ES. Hairy cell leukemia diagnostic criteria and differential diagnosis. *Leuk Lymphoma.* 2011;52(Suppl 2):6–10.

LYMPHOPLASMACYTIC LYMPHOMA (LPL)

Owens RC, Jr. Antimicrobial stewardship: concepts and strategies in the 21st century. *Diagn Microbiol Infect Dis.* 2008;61(1):110–128.

Sargent RL, Cook JR, Aguilera NI, et al. Fluorescence immunophenotypic and interphase cytogenetic characterization of nodal lymphoplasmacytic lymphoma. *Am J Surg Pathol.* 2008;32(11):1643–1653.

HEAVY CHAIN DISEASES (HCDS)

Bieliauskas S, Tubbs RR, Bacon CM, et al. Gamma heavy-chain disease: defining the spectrum of associated lymphoproliferative disorders through analysis of 13 cases. *Am J Surg Pathol.* 2012;36(4):534–543.

Wahner-Roedler DL, Witzig TE, Loehrer LL, Kyle RA. Gamma-heavy chain disease: review of 23 cases. *Medicine (Baltimore).* 2003;82(4):236–250.

EXTRAOSSEOUS PLASMACYTOMA

Lin BT, Weiss LM. Primary plasmacytoma of lymph nodes. *Hum Pathol.* 1997;28(9):1083–1090.

Menke DM, Horny HP, Griesser H, et al. Primary lymph node plasmacytomas (plasmacytic lymphomas). *Am J Clin Pathol.* 2001;115(1):119–126.

NODAL MARGINAL ZONE LYMPHOMA

Campo E, Miquel R, Krenacs L, Sorbara L, Raffeld M, Jaffe ES. Primary nodal marginal zone lymphomas of splenic and MALT type. *Am J Surg Pathol.* 1999;23(1):59–68.

Nathwani BN, Anderson JR, Armitage JO, et al. Marginal zone B-cell lymphoma: a clinical comparison of nodal and mucosa-associated lymphoid tissue types. Non-Hodgkin's Lymphoma Classification Project. *J Clin Oncol.* 1999;17(8):2486–2492.

Traverse-Glehen A, Felman P, Callet-Bauchu E, et al. A clinicopathological study of nodal marginal zone B-cell lymphoma. A report on 21 cases. *Histopathology.* 2006;48(2):162–173.

FOLLICULAR LYMPHOMA (FL)

Harris NL, Jaffe ES, Diebold J, et al. World Health Organization classification of neoplastic diseases of the hematopoietic and lymphoid tissues: report of the Clinical Advisory Committee meeting-Airlie House, Virginia, November 1997. *J Clin Oncol.* 1999;17(12):3835–3849.

Mann RB, Berard CW. Criteria for the cytologic subclassification of follicular lymphomas: a proposed alternative method. *Hematol Oncol.* 1983;1(2):187–192.

MANTLE CELL LYMPHOMA (MCL)

Sander B. Mantle cell lymphoma: recent insights into pathogenesis, clinical variability, and new diagnostic markers. *Semin Diagn Pathol.* 2011;28(3):245–255.

Williams ME, Connors JM, Dreyling MH, et al. Mantle cell lymphoma: report of the 2010 mantle cell lymphoma consortium workshop. *Leuk Lymphoma.* 2011;52(1):24–33.

DIFFUSE LARGE B-CELL LYMPHOMA, NOT OTHERWISE SPECIFIED (DLBCL, NOS)

Harris NL, Jaffe ES, Stein H, et al. A revised European-American classification of lymphoid neoplasms: a proposal from the International Lymphoma Study Group. *Blood.* 1994;84(5):1361–1392.

Lim MS, Beaty M, Sorbara L, et al. T-cell/histiocyte-rich large B-cell lymphoma: a heterogeneous entity with derivation from germinal center B cells. *Am J Surg Pathol.* 2002;26(11):1458–1466.

Shimoyama Y, Asano N, Kojima M, et al. Age-related EBV-associated B-cell lymphoproliferative disorders: diagnostic approach to a newly recognized clinicopathological entity. *Pathol Int.* 2009;59(12):835–843.

PRIMARY MEDIASTINAL LARGE B-CELL LYMPHOMA (PMLBCL)

Cazals-Hatem D, Lepage E, Brice P, et al. Primary mediastinal large B-cell lymphoma. A clinicopathologic study of 141 cases compared with 916 nonmediastinal large B-cell lymphomas, a GELA ("Groupe d'Etude des Lymphomes de l'Adulte") study. *Am J Surg Pathol.* 1996;20(7):877–888.

Pileri SA, Zinzani PL, Gaidano G, et al. Pathobiology of primary mediastinal B-cell lymphoma. *Leuk Lymphoma.* 2003;44(Suppl 3):S21–S26.

ALK POSITIVE LARGE B-CELL LYMPHOMA

Reichard KK, McKenna RW, Kroft SH. ALK-positive diffuse large B-cell lymphoma: report of four cases and review of the literature. *Mod Pathol.* 2007;20(3):310–319.

Laurent C, Do C, Gascoyne RD, et al. Anaplastic lymphoma kinase-positive diffuse large B-cell lymphoma: a rare clinicopathologic entity with poor prognosis. *J Clin Oncol.* 2009;27(25):4211–4216.

PLASMABLASTIC LYMPHOMA (PBL)

Castillo J, Pantanowitz L, Dezube BJ. HIV-associated plasmablastic lymphoma: lessons learned from 112 published cases. *Am J Hematol.* 2008;83(10):804–809.

Hsi ED, Lorsbach RB, Fend F, Dogan A. Plasmablastic lymphoma and related disorders. *Am J Clin Pathol.* 2011;136(2):183–194.

LARGE B-CELL LYMPHOMA ARISING IN HHV8-ASSOCIATED MULTICENTRIC CASTLEMAN DISEASE

Dupin N, Diss TL, Kellam P, et al. HHV-8 is associated with a plasmablastic variant of Castleman disease that is linked to HHV-8-positive plasmablastic lymphoma. *Blood.* 2000;95(4):1406–1412.

Oksenhendler E, Boulanger E, Galicier L, et al. High incidence of Kaposi sarcoma-associated herpesvirus-related non-Hodgkin lymphoma in patients with HIV infection and multicentric Castleman disease. *Blood.* 2002;99(7):2331–2336.

BURKITT LYMPHOMA (BL)

Bellan C, Stefano L, Giulia de F, Rogena EA, Lorenzo L. Burkitt lymphoma versus diffuse large B-cell lymphoma: a practical approach. *Hematol Oncol.* 2010;28(2):53–56.

Nakamura N, Nakamine H, Tamaru J, et al. The distinction between Burkitt lymphoma and diffuse large B-Cell lymphoma with c-myc rearrangement. *Mod Pathol.* 2002;15(7):771–776.

B-CELL LYMPHOMA, UNCLASSIFIABLE, WITH FEATURES INTERMEDIATE BETWEEN DIFFUSE LARGE B-CELL LYMPHOMA AND BURKITT LYMPHOMA

Harrington AM, Olteanu H, Kroft SH, Eshoa C. The unique immunophenotype of double-hit lymphomas. *Am J Clin Pathol.* 2011;135(4):649–650.

Snuderl M, Kolman OK, Chen YB, et al. B-cell lymphomas with concurrent IGH-BCL2 and MYC rearrangements are aggressive neoplasms with clinical and pathologic features distinct from Burkitt lymphoma and diffuse large B-cell lymphoma. *Am J Surg Pathol.* 2010;34(3):327–340.

B-CELL LYMPHOMA, UNCLASSIFIABLE, WITH FEATURES INTERMEDIATE BETWEEN DIFFUSE LARGE B-CELL LYMPHOMA AND CLASSICAL HODGKIN LYMPHOMA

Garcia JF, Mollejo M, Fraga M, et al. Large B-cell lymphoma with Hodgkin's features. *Histopathology.* 2005;47(1):101–110.

Traverse-Glehen A, Pittaluga S, Gaulard P, et al. Mediastinal gray zone lymphoma: the missing link between classic Hodgkin's lymphoma and mediastinal large B-cell lymphoma. *Am J Surg Pathol.* 2005;29(11):1411–1421.

9. MATURE T- AND NK-CELL NEOPLASMS

T-CELL PROLYMPHOCYTIC LEUKEMIA

Catovsky D, Muller-Hermelink HK, Ralfkiaer E. T-cell prolymphocytic leukemia. In: Swerdlow SH, Campo E, Harris NL, et al. eds. *WHO Classification of Tumours of Haematopoietic and Lymphoid Tissues*, Lyon: IARC Press; 2008:270–271.

Foucar K. Mature T-cell leukemias including T-prolymphocytic leukemia, adult T-cell leukemia/lymphoma, and Sezary syndrome. *Am J Clin Pathol.* 2007;127(4):496–510.

Valbuena JR, Herling M, Admirand JH, Padula A, Jones D, Medeiros LJ. T-cell prolymphocytic leukemia involving extramedullary sites. *Am J Clin Pathol.* 2005;123(3):456–464.

AGGRESSIVE NK-CELL LEUKEMIA/LYMPHOMA

Chan JK, Sin VC, Wong KF, et al. Nonnasal lymphoma expressing the natural killer cell marker CD56: a clinicopathologic study of 49 cases of an uncommon aggressive neoplasm. *Blood.* 1997;89(12):4501–4513.

Mori N, Yamashita Y, Tsuzuki T, et al. Lymphomatous features of aggressive NK cell leukaemia/lymphoma with massive necrosis, haemophagocytosis and EB virus infection. *Histopathology.* 2000;37(4):363–371.

ADULT T-CELL LEUKEMIA/LYMPHOMA

Ohshima K. Pathological features of diseases associated with human T-cell leukemia virus type I. *Cancer Sci.* 2007;98(6):772–778.

Ohshima K, Jaffe ES, Kikuchi M. Adult T-cell leukemia/lymphoma. In: Swerdlow SH, Campo E, Harris NL, et al. eds. *WHO Classification of Tumours of Haematopoietic and Lymphoid Tissues*, Lyon: IARC Press; 2008;281–284.

SEZARY SYNDROME/MYCOSIS FUNGOIDES

Olsen E, Vonderheid E, Pimpinelli N, et al. Revisions to the staging and classification of mycosis fungoides and Sezary syndrome: a proposal of the International Society for Cutaneous Lymphomas (ISCL) and the cutaneous lymphoma task force of the European Organization of Research and Treatment of Cancer (EORTC). *Blood.* 2007;110(6):1713–1722.

Ralfkiaer E, Cerroni L, Sander CA, Smoller BR, Willemze R. Mycosis fungoides. In: Swerdlow SH, Campo E, Harris NL, et al. eds. *WHO Classification of Tumours of Haematopoietic and Lymphoid Tissues*, Lyon: IARC Press; 2008:296–298.

PERIPHERAL T-CELL LYMPHOMA, NOT OTHERWISE SPECIFIED

Jamal S, Picker LJ, Aquino DB, McKenna RW, Dawson DB, Kroft SH. Immunophenotypic analysis of peripheral T-cell neoplasms. A multiparameter flow cytometric approach. *Am J Clin Pathol.* 2001;116(4):512–526.

Pileri SA, Weisenburger DD, Sing I, et al. Peripheral T-cell lymphoma, not otherwise specified. In: Swerdlow SH, Campo E, Harris NL, et al., eds. *WHO Classification of Tumours of Haematopoietic and Lymphoid Tissues*, Lyon: IARC Press; 2008;306–308.

Weisenburger DD, Savage KJ, Harris NL, et al. Peripheral T-cell lymphoma, not otherwise specified: a report of 340 cases from the International Peripheral T-cell Lymphoma Project. *Blood.* 2011;117(12):3402–3408.

ANGIOIMMUNOBLASTIC T-CELL LYMPHOMA

Attygalle A, Al-Jehani R, Diss TC, et al. Neoplastic T cells in angioimmunoblastic T-cell lymphoma express CD10. *Blood.* 2002;99(2):627–633.

Attygalle AD, Kyriakou C, Dupuis J, et al. Histologic evolution of angioimmunoblastic T-cell lymphoma in consecutive biopsies: clinical correlation and insights into natural history and disease progression. *Am J Surg Pathol.* 2007;31(7):1077–1088.

Chen W, Kesler MV, Karandikar NJ, McKenna RW, Kroft SH. Flow cytometric features of angioimmunoblastic T-cell lymphoma. *Cytometry B Clin Cytom.* 2006;70(3):142–148.

ANAPLASTIC LARGE CELL LYMPHOMA, ALK POSITIVE

Falini B. Anaplastic large cell lymphoma: pathological, molecular and clinical features. *Br J Haematol.* 2001;114(4):741–760.

Medeiros LJ, Elenitoba-Johnson KS. Anaplastic large cell lymphoma. *Am J Clin Pathol.* 2007;127(5):707–722.

Savage KJ, Harris NL, Vose JM, et al. ALK- anaplastic large-cell lymphoma is clinically and immunophenotypically different from both ALK+ ALCL and peripheral T-cell lymphoma, not otherwise specified: report from the International Peripheral T-Cell Lymphoma Project. *Blood.* 2008;111(12):5496–5504.

ANAPLASTIC LARGE CELL LYMPHOMA, ALK NEGATIVE

Medeiros LJ, Elenitoba-Johnson KS. Anaplastic large cell lymphoma. *Am J Clin Pathol.* 2007;127(5):707–722.

Savage KJ, Harris NL, Vose JM, et al. ALK- anaplastic large-cell lymphoma is clinically and immunophenotypically different from both ALK+ ALCL and peripheral T-cell lymphoma, not otherwise specified: report from the International Peripheral T-Cell Lymphoma Project. *Blood.* 2008;111(12):5496–5504.

10. HODGKIN LYMPHOMA

NODULAR LYMPHOCYTE PREDOMINANT HODGKIN LYMPHOMA

Ansell SM. Annual clinical updates in hematological malignancies: a continuing medical education series. Hodgkin lymphoma: 2011 update on diagnosis, risk-stratification, and management. *Am J Hematol.* 2011;86(10):851–858.

Eberle FC, Mani H, Jaffe ES. Histopathology of Hodgkin's lymphoma. *Cancer J.* 2009;15(2):129–137.

Poppema S, Delsol G, Pileri S, et al. Nodular lymphocyte predominant Hodgkin lymphoma. In: Swerdlow SH, Campo E, Harris NL, et al. eds. *WHO Classification of Tumours of Haematopoietic and Lymphoid Tissues*, Lyon: IARC Press; 2008;323–325.

NODULAR SCLEROSIS CLASSICAL HODGKIN LYMPHOMA

Eberle FC, Mani H, Jaffe ES. Histopathology of Hodgkin's lymphoma. *Cancer J.* 2009;15(2):129–137.

Shimabukuro-Vornhagen A, Haverkamp H, Engert A, et al. Lymphocyte-rich classical Hodgkin's lymphoma: clinical presentation and treatment outcome in 100 patients treated within German Hodgkin's Study Group trials. *J Clin Oncol.* 2005;23(24):5739–5745.

Stein H, von Wasielewski R, Poppema S, MacLennan KA, Guenova M. Nodular sclerosis classical Hodgkin lymphoma. In: Swerdlow SH, Campo E, Harris NL, et al. eds. *WHO Classification of Tumours of Haematopoietic and Lymphoid Tissues*, Lyon: IARC Press; 2008:330.

MIXED CELLULARITY CLASSICAL HODGKIN LYMPHOMA

Eberle FC, Mani H, Jaffe ES. Histopathology of Hodgkin's lymphoma. *Cancer J.* 2009;15(2):129–137.

Shimabukuro-Vornhagen A, Haverkamp H, Engert A, et al. Lymphocyte-rich classical Hodgkin's lymphoma: clinical presentation and treatment outcome in 100 patients treated within German Hodgkin's Study Group trials. *J Clin Oncol.* 2005;23(24):5739–5745.

Weiss LM, von Wasielewski R, Delsol G, Poppema S, Stein H. Mixed cellularity classical Hodgkin lymphoma. In: Swerdlow SH, Campo E, Harris NL, et al., eds. *WHO Classification of Tumours of Haematopoietic and Lymphoid Tissues*, Lyon: IARC Press; 2008;331.

LYMPHOCYTE-RICH CLASSICAL HODGKIN LYMPHO

Anagnostopoulos I, Isaacson PG, Stein H. Lymphocyte-rich classical Hodgkin lymphoma. In: Swerdlow SH, Campo E, Harris NL, et al., eds. *WHO Classification of Tumours of Haematopoietic and Lymphoid Tissues.* Lyon: IARC Press; 2008:332–333.

Eberle FC, Mani H, Jaffe ES. Histopathology of Hodgkin's lymphoma. *Cancer J.* 2009;15(2): 129–137.

Shimabukuro-Vornhagen A, Haverkamp H, Engert A, et al. Lymphocyte-rich classical Hodgkin's lymphoma: clinical presentation and treatment outcome in 100 patients treated within German Hodgkin's Study Group trials. *J Clin Oncol.* 2005;23(24):5739–5745.

LYMPHOCYTE-DEPLETED CLASSICAL HODGKIN LYMPHOMA

Benharroch D, Stein H, Peh SC. Lymphocyte-depleted classical Hodgkin lymphoma. In: Swerdlow SH, Campo E, Harris NL, et al. eds. *WHO Classification of Tumours of Haematopoietic and Lymphoid Tissues*, Lyon: IARC Press; 2008:334.

Klimm B, Franklin J, Stein H, et al. Lymphocyte-depleted classical Hodgkin's lymphoma: a comprehensive analysis from the German Hodgkin study group. *J Clin Oncol.* 2011;29(29): 3914–3920.

Shimabukuro-Vornhagen A, Haverkamp H, Engert A, et al. Lymphocyte-rich classical Hodgkin's lymphoma: clinical presentation and treatment outcome in 100 patients treated within German Hodgkin's Study Group trials. *J Clin Oncol.* 2005;23(24):5739–5745.

11. IMMUNODEFICIENCY-ASSOCIATED LYMPHOPROLIFERATIVE DISORDERS

LYMPHOMAS ASSOCIATED WITH HIV INFECTION

Carbone A, Cesarman E, Spina M, Gloghini A, Schulz TF. HIV-associated lymphomas and gamma-herpesviruses. *Blood.* 2009;113(6):1213–1224.

Carbone A, Gloghini A. AIDS-related lymphomas: from pathogenesis to pathology. *Br J Haematol.* 2005;130(5):662–670.

POST-TRANSPLANT LYMPHOPROLIFERATIVE DISORDERS (PTLD)

EARLY LESIONS: PLASMACYTIC HYPERPLASIA AND INFECTIOUS MONONUCLEOSIS (IM)—LIKE PTLD

Chadburn A, Chen JM, Hsu DT, et al. The morphologic and molecular genetic categories of posttransplantation lymphoproliferative disorders are clinically relevant. *Cancer.* 1998;82(10):1978–1987.

Lones MA, Mishalani S, Shintaku IP, Weiss LM, Nichols WS, Said JW. Changes in tonsils and adenoids in children with posttransplant lymphoproliferative disorder: report of three cases with early involvement of Waldeyer's ring. *Hum Pathol.* 1995;26(5):525–530.

POLYMORPHIC PTLD

Frizzera G, Hanto DW, Gajl-Peczalska KJ, et al. Polymorphic diffuse B-cell hyperplasias and lymphomas in renal transplant recipients. *Cancer Res.* 1981;41(11 Pt 1):4262–4279.

Hanto DW, Gajl-Peczalska KJ, Frizzera G, et al. Epstein-Barr virus (EBV) induced polyclonal and monoclonal B-cell lymphoproliferative diseases occurring after renal transplantation. Clinical, pathologic, and virologic findings and implications for therapy. *Ann Surg.* 1983;198(3):356–369.

MONOMORPHIC PTLD

Harris NL, Ferry JA, Swerdlow SH. Posttransplant lymphoproliferative disorders: summary of society for hematopathology workshop. *Semin Diagn Pathol.* 1997;14(1):8–14.

Swerdlow SH. T-cell and NK-cell posttransplantation lymphoproliferative disorders. *Am J Clin Pathol.* 2007;127(6):887–895.

CLASSICAL HODGKIN LYMPHOMA TYPE PTLD

Ranganathan S, Webber S, Ahuja S, Jaffe R. Hodgkin-like posttransplant lymphoproliferative disorder in children: does it differ from posttransplant Hodgkin lymphoma? *Pediatr Dev Pathol.* 2004;7(4):348–360.

Rowlings PA, Curtis RE, Passweg JR, et al. Increased incidence of Hodgkin's disease after allogeneic bone marrow transplantation. *J Clin Oncol.* 1999;17(10):3122–3127.

OTHER IATROGENIC IMMUNODEFICIENCY-ASSOCIATED LYMPHOPROLIFERATIVE DISORDERS

Salloum E, Cooper DL, Howe G, et al. Spontaneous regression of lymphoproliferative disorders in patients treated with methotrexate for rheumatoid arthritis and other rheumatic diseases. *J Clin Oncol.* 1996;14(6):1943–1949.

Wolfe F, Michaud K. The effect of methotrexate and anti-tumor necrosis factor therapy on the risk of lymphoma in rheumatoid arthritis in 19,562 patients during 89,710 person-years of observation. *Arthritis Rheum.* 2007;56(5):1433–1439.

12. HISTIOCYTIC AND DENDRITIC CELL NEOPLASMS

HISTIOCYTIC SARCOMA

Pileri SA, Grogan TM, Harris NL, et al. Tumours of histiocytes and accessory dendritic cells: an immunohistochemical approach to classification from the International Lymphoma Study Group based on 61 cases. *Histopathology.* 2002;41(1):1–29.

Vos JA, Abbondanzo SL, Barekman CL, Andriko JW, Miettinen M, Aguilera NS. Histiocytic sarcoma: a study of five cases including the histiocyte marker CD163. *Mod Pathol.* 2005;18(5):693–704.

LANGERHANS CELLS HISTIOCYTOSIS (LCH)

Edelweiss M, Medeiros LJ, Suster S, Moran CA. Lymph node involvement by Langerhans cell histiocytosis: a clinicopathologic and immunohistochemical study of 20 cases. *Hum Pathol.* 2007;38(10):1463–1469.

Pileri SA, Grogan TM, Harris NL, et al. Tumours of histiocytes and accessory dendritic cells: an immunohistochemical approach to classification from the International Lymphoma Study Group based on 61 cases. *Histopathology.* 2002;41(1):1–29.

LANGERHANS CELL SARCOMA

Ferringer T, Banks PM, Metcalf JS. Langerhans cell sarcoma. *Am J Dermatopathol.* 2006;28(1):36–39.

Pileri SA, Grogan TM, Harris NL, et al. Tumours of histiocytes and accessory dendritic cells: an immunohistochemical approach to classification from the International Lymphoma Study Group based on 61 cases. *Histopathology.* 2002;41(1):1–29.

INTERDIGITATING DENDRITIC CELL SARCOMA

Pillay K, Solomon R, Daubenton JD, Sinclair-Smith CC. Interdigitating dendritic cell sarcoma: a report of four paediatric cases and review of the literature. *Histopathology.* 2004;44(3):283–291.

Pileri SA, Grogan TM, Harris NL, et al. Tumours of histiocytes and accessory dendritic cells: an immunohistochemical approach to classification from the International Lymphoma Study Group based on 61 cases. *Histopathology.* 2002;41(1):1–29.

FOLLICULAR DENDRITIC CELL SARCOMA

Pileri SA, Grogan TM, Harris NL, et al. Tumours of histiocytes and accessory dendritic cells: an immunohistochemical approach to classification from the International Lymphoma Study Group based on 61 cases. *Histopathology.* 2002;41(1):1–29.

Soriano AO, Thompson MA, Admirand JH, et al. Follicular dendritic cell sarcoma: a report of 14 cases and a review of the literature. *Am J Hematol.* 2007;82(8):725–728.

13. PRECURSOR LYMPHOID NEOPLASMS

LYMPHOBLASTIC LYMPHOMA

Cortelazzo S, Ponzoni M, Ferreri AJ, Hoelzer D. Lymphoblastic lymphoma. *Crit Rev Oncol Hematol.* 2011;79(3):330–343.

Maitra A, McKenna RW, Weinberg AG, Schneider NR, Kroft SH. Precursor B-cell lymphoblastic lymphoma. A study of nine cases lacking blood and bone marrow involvement and review of the literature. *Am J Clin Pathol.* 2001;115(6):868–875.

Oschlies I, Burkhardt B, Chassagne-Clement C, et al. Diagnosis and immunophenotype of 188 pediatric lymphoblastic lymphomas treated within a randomized prospective trial: experiences and preliminary recommendations from the European childhood lymphoma pathology panel. *Am J Surg Pathol.* 2011;35(6):836–844.

14. ACUTE MYELOID LEUKEMIA AND RELATED PRECURSOR NEOPLASMS

MYELOID SARCOMA

Campidelli C, Agostinelli C, Stitson R, Pileri SA. Myeloid sarcoma: extramedullary manifestation of myeloid disorders. *Am J Clin Pathol.* 2009;132(3):426–437.

Hoyer JD, Grogg KL, Hanson CA, Gamez JD, Dogan A. CD33 detection by immunohistochemistry in paraffin-embedded tissues: a new antibody shows excellent specificity and sensitivity for cells of myelomonocytic lineage. *Am J Clin Pathol.* 2008;129(2):316–323.

Pileri SA, Ascani S, Cox MC, et al. Myeloid sarcoma: Clinico-pathologic, phenotypic and cytogenetic analysis of 92 adult patients. *Leukemia.* 2007;21(2):340–350.

BLASTIC PLASMACYTOID DENDRITIC CELL NEOPLASM (BPDCN)

Benet C, Gomez A, Aguilar C, et al. Histologic and immunohistologic characterization of skin localization of myeloid disorders: a study of 173 cases. *Am J Clin Pathol.* 2011;135(2):278–290.

Jegalian AG, Buxbaum NP, Facchetti F, et al. Blastic plasmacytoid dendritic cell neoplasm in children: diagnostic features and clinical implications. *Haematologica.* 2010;95(11):1873–1879.

Index

NOTE: *Page numbers followed by 'f' indicate figures and 't' indicate tables*

Abdominal lymph node, 139f
Abnormal lymph nodes, 150
Acute myeloid leukemia (AML), diagnosis of, 218
Adenopathy, 12
Adjacent nodal parenchyma, 84
Adult onset Still's disease (AOSD), 64
Adult T-cell leukemia/lymphoma (ATLL), 148
Aggressive B-cell lymphoma, 136
Aggressive NK-cell leukemia/lymphoma, 146
AITL. *See* Angioimmunoblastic T-cell lymphoma
ALK+ ALCL. *See* Anaplastic large cell lymphoma (ALCL), ALK positive
ALK- ALCL. *See* Anaplastic large cell lymphoma (ALCL), ALK negative
ALK positive large B-cell lymphoma, 130
Alpha heavy chain diseases (Alpha HCD), 114
ALPS. *See* Autoimmune lymphoproliferative syndrome
Amianthoid bodies, 78
AML. *See* Acute myeloid leukemia
Anaplastic large cell lymphoma (ALCL), ALK negative, 166
Anaplastic large cell lymphoma (ALCL), ALK positive, 160, 162, 164
  lymphohistiocytic variant of, 163f
  neoplastic cells, 165f
  small cell variant of, 163f
Angioimmunoblastic T-cell lymphoma (AITL), 148, 156, 158
  "angioimmunoblastic-like," 8
  histologic patterns, 156
  Reed-Sternberg-like cells in, 159f
Angiomatosis, bacillary. *See* Bacillary angiomatosis
Angiomyomatous hamartoma, 86
  hilar lesion, 87f
AOSD. *See* Adult onset Still's disease
Apoptosis, cellular, 68
Autoimmune lymphoproliferative syndrome (ALPS), 68

Bacillary angiomatosis, 14, 16
Bacterial lymphadenitis, 10
Bartonella henselae, 12, 14
B-cell lymphoma, 138
B-cells
  clonal, 106, 124
  in histiocytes, 126
  neoplasm, 102, 108, 118
  non-Hodgkin lymphoma, 124
Benign disorder, 48
BL. *See* Burkitt lymphoma
Blastic plasmacytoid dendritic cell neoplasm (BPDCN), 220
B-lineage cells, 214
Blue nevus cell clusters, 74
B-lymphoblastic lymphoma, 215f
BPDCN. *See* Blastic plasmacytoid dendritic cell neoplasm
Breast carcinoma, 74
Bulky disease, 172
Burkitt lymphoma (BL), 136, 138, 184, 185f

Capillary hemangiomas, 88, 89f
Capsular connective tissue, 74
Carcinoma, breast, 74
Cardinal immunophenotypic feature, ALPS, 68
Castleman disease, 58, 60, 62
Cat scratch lymphadenitis, 12
Cavernous hemangiomas, 88, 89f
CD20 immunohistochemistry, 127f
CD57(+) T cells, 170
Cellular apoptosis, 68
Cervical lymph nodes, 170
cHL. *See* Classical Hodgkin lymphoma
Chronic inflammatory disease, 46, 64
Chronic lymphocytic leukemia/small lymphocytic lymphoma (CLL/SLL), 102, 104
Classical Hodgkin lymphoma (cHL), 142, 180
Classical Hodgkin lymphoma type PTLD, 196

CLL/SLL. *See* Chronic lymphocytic leukemia/small lymphocytic lymphoma
Clonal B cells, 106, 124
Coccidioides lymphadenitis, 28
Congenital disorder, ALPS, 68
Cytomegalovirus lymphadenitis, 4

Dendritic cells, 36, 36f, 42
Dermatopathic lymphadenopathy (DL), 42, 150
Diffuse large B-cell lymphoma (DLBCL), 124, 128, 138, 140, 155f, 184, 193f
  in AITL, 156
  subtypes, 126, 127f
Diffuse large B-cell lymphoma, not otherwise specified (NOS), 124
Diffuse pattern of FL, 118, 119f
DL. *See* Dermatopathic lymphadenopathy
DLBCL. *See* Diffuse large B-cell lymphoma
DLBCL, NOS. *See* Diffuse large B-cell lymphoma, not otherwise specified

EBER. *See* Epstein-Barr virus small encoded RNA
EBV. *See* Epstein-Barr virus
Emperipolesis, 48
Endemic BL, 136
Eosinophilic infiltrates, 46
Eosinophilic lymphogranuloma. *See* Kimura lymphadenopathy
Eosinophils, 202, 203f, 204, 205f
Epithelial cell inclusions in lymph nodes, 72
Epithelioid hemangioendothelioma, 89f
Epstein-Barr virus (EBV), 2
Epstein-Barr virus positive diffuse large B-cell lymphoma, 124, 126
  B-cell lymphoma, 127f
Epstein-Barr virus small encoded RNA (EBER), 2
European Organization of Research and Treatment of Cancer (EORTC), 150
Extraosseous plasmacytoma, 114

Felty syndrome, 56
Filariasis, 30
FL. *See* Follicular lymphoma
Florid follicular hyperplasia. *See* Follicular hyperplasia
Follicular dendritic cell (FDC), 156
Follicular dendritic cell sarcoma, 210
Follicular hyperplasia, 8, 9f, 18f, 34
Follicular lymphoma (FL), 48, 118, 121f
Follicular pattern of FL, 118, 121f

Gamma heavy chain disease (Gamma HCD), 112
Gene
  mutations, 68
  translocation, 136
Germinal center, 34, 40
Giant cells
  multinucleated, 53f
  osteoclast-type, 204
Granular eosinophilic material, 5f
Granulomas, non-necrotizing, 52

Hairy cell leukemia (HCL), 108
Hamartomatous lesion, 86
HCDs. *See* Heavy chain diseases
HCL. *See* Hairy cell leukemia
Heavy chain diseases (HCDs), definition, 112
Hemangioendotheliomas, 88
Hemangiomas, 88
  capillary, 88, 89f
  cavernous, 88, 89f
Hematolymphoid neoplasms, WHO classification of, 124, 186
Herpes simplex virus (HSV), 6
Herpes simplex virus lymphadenitis, 6
Heterogeneous group of disorders, 186
HHV8 immunohistochemistry, 137f
High-grade B-cell lymphoma, 138
Highly active antiretroviral therapy (HAART), 184
Histiocytic necrotizing lymphadenitis. *See* Kikuchi-Fujimoto lymphadenopathy
Histiocytic sarcoma, 202
Histiocytosis, sinus. *See* Sinus histiocytosis
Histoplasma lymphadenitis, 26
HIV. *See* Human immunodeficiency virus
Hodgkin lymphoma (HL), 184, 185f
  LDCHL, 180–181
  LRCHL, 178–179
  MCCHL, 176–177
  NLPHL, 170–171
  NSCHL, 172–175
HSV. *See* Herpes simplex virus
Human immunodeficiency virus (HIV) infection, 8
  lymphomas associated with. *See* Lymphomas associated with HIV infection
Human immunodeficiency virus lymphadenitis, 8

Human T-cell leukemia virus (HTLV-1), 148
Hyaline vascular Castleman disease, 58
Hyperplastic follicles, AITL with, 156

Iatrogenic immunodeficiency-associated lymphoproliferative disorders, 198
IgG antibodies, 12
IgG4-related sclerosing disease, 66
IgM antibodies, 12
IM. *See* Infectious mononucleosis
Immature myeloid cells, 218, 219f
Immunoblasts, 51f, 64, 65f, 69f
Immunodeficiency-associated BL, 136
Immunohistochemistry, 50, 112, 113f, 114, 131f, 139f, 224
Infectious mononucleosis (IM), 2
Infectious mononucleosis-like PTLD, 188
Infectious mononucleosis-like syndrome, 4
Infectious mononucleosis lymphadenitis, 2
Inflammatory pseudotumor of lymph node, 80
Inguinal lymph node, neoplastic infiltration in, 147f
In situ hybridization, 112, 113f
Interdigitating dendritic cells, 42, 43f
Interdigitating dendritic cell sarcoma, 208
Interfollicular mature plasmacytosis, 62
International Society for Cutaneous Lymphomas (ISCL), 150

Juvenile rheumatoid arthritis, 64

Kaposi sarcoma, 90
Karyorrhectic debris, 50
Kikuchi-Fujimoto lymphadenopathy, 50
Kimura lymphadenopathy, 46

Langerhans cell histiocytosis (LCH), 204
Langerhans cells, 42, 43f
Langerhans cell sarcoma, 206
Large B-cell lymphoma in HHV8-associated multicentric Castleman disease, 134
Large cell transformation, 150, 151f
LBL. *See* Lymphoblastic lymphoma
LCH. *See* Langerhans cell histiocytosis
Lofgren's syndrome, 52
LP cells, 40, 170
LPL. *See* Lymphoplasmacytic lymphoma
LRCHL. *See* Lymphocyte rich classical Hodgkin lymphoma
Luetic lymphadenitis, 18, 20
Lymphadenopathy, 34, 36, 40
  lymphangiography-associated, 96–97
  metal debris-associated, 94–95
  T-cell prolymphocytic leukemia, 144
Lymphangiography-associated lymphadenopathy, 96
Lymphatic filariasis. *See* Filariasis
Lymphoblastic lymphoma (LBL), 214, 215f
Lymphocyte-depleted classical Hodgkin lymphoma (LDCHL), 180
Lymphocyte rich classical Hodgkin lymphoma (LRCHL), 178
Lymphocytes, 156, 157f, 202, 203f
  neoplastic, 144, 145f
Lymphoid proliferations, 186
Lymphoma, 118. *See also* Aggressive NK-cell leukemia/lymphoma
  ALCL, ALK$^+$, 160
  non-Hodgkin, 68, 184
Lymphomas associated with HIV infection, 184
Lymphomatous variants, 148
Lymphoplasmacytic infiltrates, 66
Lymphoplasmacytic lymphoma (LPL), 110
Lymphoproliferative disorders, 58
  iatrogenic immunodeficiency-associated. *See* Iatrogenic immunodeficiency-associated lymphoproliferative disorders

Macroglobulinemia, Waldenstrom, 110
Mantle cell lymphoma (MCL), 122
Mantle layer cells, 40, 41
Mantle zone, 8
Marginal zone lymphoma (MZL), 116
Mature B-cell neoplasms, nomenclature and classification, 100, 101t
MCCHL. *See* Mixed cellularity classical Hodgkin lymphoma
MCL. *See* Mantle cell lymphoma
Metal debris-associated lymphadenopathy, 94
Metastasis, anatomic site of, 224t
Metastatic neoplastic cells, 224, 225f
Metastatic tumors in lymph nodes, 224
Microfilariae, filariasis, 30
Microlymphoma, 135f
Mixed cellularity classical Hodgkin lymphoma (MCCHL), 176
Monocytes, plasmacytoid, 50
Monocytoid B-cells, 4, 5f
Monomorphic B-cell PTLD, 192
Monomorphic medium-sized cells, 137f
Monomorphic PTLD, 186, 192
Monomorphic T/NK-cell PTLD, 194
Multicentric Castleman disease, 62, 134

Multinucleated giant cell, 53f
Mutations, gene, 68
Mycobacterium avium-intracellulare (MAI) lymphadenitis, 24
Mycobacterium tuberculosis (Mtb) lymphadenitis, 22
Mycosis fungoides (MF). *See* Sezary syndrome (SS)/mycosis fungoides
Myeloid sarcoma, 218
MZL. *See* Marginal zone lymphoma

Necrosis, 6, 7f, 23f, 172f, 181f
Neoplasms, hematolymphoid, 124, 186
Neoplastic cells, 107f, 109f, 116, 117f, 131f, 146, 170
  ALK+ ALCL, 165f
  anaplastic variant consists of, 148
  in follicular dendritic cell sarcoma, 210, 211f
  histiocytic sarcoma, 202, 203f
  PTCL, NOS, 153f
Neoplastic follicles, 118, 119f
Neoplastic infiltration, 145f
  in inguinal lymph node, 147f
Neoplastic lymphocytes, 144, 145f
Neoplastic proliferation of Langerhans cells, 204
Neoplastic spindle cells, 90
Nevus cell inclusions in lymph nodes, 74
NLPHL. *See* Nodular lymphocyte predominant Hodgkin lymphoma
Nodal marginal zone lymphoma (Nodal MZL), 116
Nodular lymphocyte predominant Hodgkin lymphoma (NLPHL), 40, 170
Nodular sclerosis classical Hodgkin lymphoma (NSCHL), 172, 174
Noncaseating granulomas, 20, 21f
Non-Hodgkin lymphomas (NHLs), 68, 184
Non-necrotizing granulomas, 52
Non-treponemal antibody tests, 18
NSCHL. *See* Nodular sclerosis classical Hodgkin lymphoma

Osteoclast-type giant cells, 204, 205f
Ovoid cells in storiform/fascicle pattern, 208, 209f

Pale cytoplasm, 218, 219f
Palisaded myofibroblastoma, 78
Paracortex, 36, 36f, 42, 156
  cytomegalovirus. *See* Cytomegalovirus lymphadenitis
  HIV lymphadenitis, 8
  infectious mononucleosis (IM), 2
Paracortical hyperplasia, 34, 56, 64, 68
Parenchyma, adjacent nodal, 84
PCR. *See* Polymerase chain reaction
Perilymphadenitis, 56
Peripheral T-cell lymphoma, not otherwise specified (PTCL, NOS), 152, 154
  lymphoepithelioid variant in, 155f
  morphological spectrum, 153f
Plasmablastic lymphoma (PBL), 132
Plasmablasts, 134
  diffuse infiltrate of, 135f
Plasma cells, 20, 110, 202, 203f
  infiltrate, 48
Plasma cell variant, 60
Plasmacytic hyperplasia, 188
Plasmacytic proliferations, 186
Plasmacytoid monocytes, 50
Plasmacytoma. *See* Extraosseous plasmacytoma
Plasmacytosis, interfollicular mature, 62
PMLBCL. *See* Primary mediastinal large B-cell lymphoma
Polykaryocytes, Warthin-Finkeldey, 46
Polylobate nuclei, 125f
Polymerase chain reaction (PCR), 12
Polymorphic PTLD, 190
Post-transplant lymphoproliferative disorders (PTLD), 186
  cHL. *See* Classical Hodgkin lymphoma type PTLD
  classification, 186
  monomorphic. *See* Monomorphic PTLD
  polymorphic. *See* Polymorphic PTLD
Primary mediastinal large B-cell lymphoma (PMLBCL), 126, 128
Primary tumor, anatomic site of, 224t
Progressive transformation of germinal centers (PTGC), 40, 170
Proliferation centers, 102
Prolymphocytes, 102
Pseudofollicles, 102
PTCL, NOS. *See* Peripheral T-cell lymphoma, not otherwise specified
PTGC. *See* Progressive transformation of germinal centers
PTLD. *See* Post-transplant lymphoproliferative disorders

RA. *See* Rheumatoid arthritis
Rare Reed-Stenberg cells, 185f
Reactive follicles, 56
Red cells, extravasat, 90
Reed-Sternberg (RS) cells, 148
in AITL, 161f
classic immunophenotype of, 180
LRCHL, 178, 179f
MCCHL, 176, 177f
morphology, 128, 140
NSCHL, 172, 173f, 174, 175f
Rheumatoid arthritis (RA), 56
juvenile, 64
Rheumatoid lymphadenopathy, 56
Rosai-Dorfman disease. *See* Sinus histiocytosis with massive lymphadenopathy
Rosai-Dorfman histiocytes, 48, 49f
RS cells. *See* Reed-Sternberg cells

Sarcoidosis, 52
Secondary follicle, 57f
Sezary syndrome (SS)/mycosis fungoides, 150
dermatopathic lymphadenopathy, 151f
Sinus histiocytosis, 38
Sinus histiocytosis with massive lymphadenopathy, 48
SLE lymphadenopathy. *See* Systemic lupus erythematosus lymphadenopathy
SMZL. *See* Splenic B-cell marginal zone lymphoma
Spindle cells, 80, 81f
fascicles of, 78
Spirochetes, 20
Splenic B-cell marginal zone lymphoma (SMZL), 106
Sporadic BL, 136
Still's disease, 64
Superficial lymph node, 74
Syphilis lymphadenitis. *See* Luetic lymphadenitis
Systemic lupus erythematosus (SLE) lymphadenopathy, 54

T cell/histiocyte-rich large B-cell lymphoma (TCHRLBCL), 126
T-cell lymphoma, angioimmunoblastic. *See* Angioimmunoblastic T-cell lymphoma
T-cell prolymphocytic leukemia (T-PLL), 144
TCHRLBCL. *See* T cell/histiocyte-rich large B-cell lymphoma
T-lineage cells, 214
T-PLL. *See* T-cell prolymphocytic leukemia
Tuberculous lymphadenitis, 22
Tumor, anatomic site of primary, 224t
Tumor cells, 130
immunophenotype, 144
PTCL, NOS, 153f

Unicentric Castleman disease, 60

Vacuoles, 96, 97f
Vascular proliferation, 84
Vascular spaces, 84
Vascular structures, bacillary angiomatosis, 14, 15f
Vascular transformation of lymph node sinuses (VTS), 84

Waldenstrom macroglobulinemia, 110
Warthin-Finkeldey polykaryocytes, 46
Warthin-Starry stain, 12, 13f, 20

Yeast organisms, 26, 28